A Clinician's Guide to Breast Cancer

A Clinician's Guide to Breast Cancer

Edited by Eliza Harrison

STATES
ACADEMIC PRESS
www.statesacademicpress.com

States Academic Press,
109 South 5th Street,
Brooklyn, NY 11249, USA

Visit us on the World Wide Web at:
www.statesacademicpress.com

ISBN: 978-1-63989-000-2

Cataloging-in-Publication Data

A clinician's guide to breast cancer / edited by Eliza Harrison.
p. cm.
Includes bibliographical references and index.
ISBN 978-1-63989-000-2
1. Breast--Cancer. 2. Breast--Cancer--Treatment. I. Harrison, Eliza.
RC280.B8 C55 2022
616.994 49--dc23

Table of Contents

Preface

The world is advancing at a fast pace like never before. Therefore, the need is to keep up with the latest developments. This book was an idea that came to fruition when the specialists in the area realized the need to coordinate together and document essential themes in the subject. That's when I was requested to be the editor. Editing this book has been an honour as it brings together diverse authors researching on different streams of the field. The book collates essential materials contributed by veterans in the area which can be utilized by students and researchers alike.

The cancer which begins in the breast is termed as breast cancer. The cells start developing uncontrollably and do not die off at their usual age. Breast cancer can begin in the milk ducts, and are known as ductal cancers, or the glands which make breast milk, also known as lobular cancers. There are various types of imaging tests which can be used to detect and diagnose breast cancer such as MRI, mammogram and ultrasound. A biopsy can also be used for the diagnosis of breast cancer, as well as finding out the type and stage of cancer. Some of the different ways in which it can be treated are surgery, hormone therapy and chemotherapy. This book includes some of the vital pieces of work being conducted across the world, on various topics related to breast cancer. It strives to provide a fair idea about this discipline and to help develop a better understanding of the latest advances within this field. Scientists and students actively engaged in this field will find this book full of crucial and unexplored concepts.

Each chapter is a sole-standing publication that reflects each author´s interpretation. Thus, the book displays a multi-facetted picture of our current understanding of application, resources and aspects of the field. I would like to thank the contributors of this book and my family for their endless support.

Editor

1

The Biological and Clinical Significance of Glutaminase in Luminal Breast Cancer

Brendah K. Masisi [1], Rokaya El Ansari [1], Lutfi Alfarsi [1], Madeleine L. Craze [1], Natasha Jewa [1], Andrew Oldfield [1], Hayley Cheung [1], Michael Toss [1], Emad A. Rakha [1,2] and Andrew R. Green [1,*]

1 Nottingham Breast Cancer Research Centre, Academic Unit for Translational Medical Sciences, School of Medicine, University of Nottingham Biodiscovery Institute, University Park, Nottingham NG7 2RD, UK; msxbkma@nottingham.ac.uk (B.K.M.); rokayaelansari@gmail.com (R.E.A.); alfarsil@yahoo.com (L.A.); mszmc@nottingham.ac.uk (M.L.C.); mzytnj@nottingham.ac.uk (N.J.); andrewoldfield1998@gmail.com (A.O.); mzyhcc@nottingham.ac.uk (H.C.); michael.toss@nottingham.ac.uk (M.T.); emad.rakha@nottingham.ac.uk (E.A.R.)

2 Cellular Pathology, Nottingham University Hospitals NHS Trust, Hucknall Road, Nottingham NG5 1PB, UK

* Correspondence: andrew.green@nottingham.ac.uk;

Simple Summary: Certain nutrients are needed by cancers to grow. Some breast cancers need the nutrient glutamine to grow and without it they don't grow as quickly. In this study, we wanted to know the role of an enzyme, glutaminase, which is a substance produced by the body that breaks down glutamine so it can be used by cancers to grow. This enzyme occurs as two different types but we don't know what their roles are in breast cancer. We therefore looked at the two types of enzyme in over 7000 breast cancers. We found that patients with high amounts of enzyme in early forms of breast cancer died earlier. Therefore, this enzyme has an important role in breast cancer and could be used to identify cancers which will get worse. We also think that using a drug to stop this enzyme will stop cancers growing. More studies are needed to confirm this.

Abstract: The glutamine metabolism has a key role in the regulation of uncontrolled tumour growth. This study aimed to evaluate the expression and prognostic significance of glutaminase in luminal breast cancer (BC). The glutaminase isoforms (GLS/GLS2) were assessed at genomic/transcriptomic levels, using METABRIC (n = 1398) and GeneMiner datasets (n = 4712), and protein using immunohistochemistry in well-characterised cohorts of Oestrogen receptor-positive/HER2-negative BC patients: ductal carcinoma in situ (DCIS; n = 206) and invasive breast cancer (IBC; n = 717). Glutaminase expression was associated with clinicopathological features, patient outcome and glutamine-metabolism-related genes. In DCIS, GLS alone and GLS+/GLS2- expression were risk factors for shorter local recurrence-free interval ($p < 0.0001$ and $p = 0.001$, respectively) and remained prognostic factors independent of tumour size, grade and comedo necrosis ($p = 0.0008$ and $p = 0.003$, respectively). In IBC, *GLS* gene copy number gain with high mRNA expression was associated with poor patient outcome ($p = 0.011$), whereas high GLS2 protein was predictive of a longer disease-free survival ($p = 0.006$). Glutaminase plays a role in the biological function of luminal BC, particularly GLS in the early non-invasive stage, which could be used as a potential biomarker to predict disease progression and a target for inhibition. Further validation is required to confirm these observations, and functional assessments are needed to explore their specific roles.

Keywords: glutaminase; DCIS; IBC; prognosis

---

1. Introduction

Metabolic reprogramming has been recognised as a hallmark of cancer [1]. Malignant transformation and progression require alteration of signalling pathways related to cellular metabolism to meet the demand for both energy and biomass for proliferating malignant cells. Glutamine is the second most utilised source of energy after glucose used by cancer cells to support tumour cell proliferation and survival, and some breast cancers are known to exhibit glutamine addiction [2]. Glutamine plays a role in the replenishment of biosynthetic intermediates to maintain a functioning tricarboxylic-acid (TCA) cycle, and it allows for the synthesis of macromolecules and antioxidants for rapidly proliferating cells [3,4]. Glutamine is catabolised to glutamate by the mitochondrial enzyme glutaminase, which presents as two isoforms; kidney-type (GLS/KGA) and liver-type (GLS2/LGA) [5].

Both the prognostic and the therapeutic significance of these two glutaminase isoforms remain an active area of research. GLS is the main isoform expressed in cancer cells, and there is increasing evidence suggesting it plays an important role in carcinogenesis and tumour progression in various solid cancers. Previous studies have established that high GLS correlates with higher rates of tumour growth and is associated with advanced tumour stage and poor patient outcomes [6–8]. In contrast, although studies are limited on GLS2, it tends to have opposing functions, as it is markedly increased in tumours that are more differentiated and less aggressive [9,10]. High GLS2 expression is associated with a significantly longer survival time in hepatocellular carcinoma [11].

In breast cancer (BC), GLS is expressed at different levels in molecular subtypes and appears to play an important role in the aggressive subclass of luminal BC in addition to triple-negative BC (TNBC) [12]. It has also been observed that patients with high *GLS* but not *GLS2* mRNA expression in highly proliferative luminal BC have the worst patient outcome compared with those classified as low proliferative [13]. BC is a heterogeneous group of diseases with histological types and metabolic pathways together sustaining the initiation and progression [14,15]. The progression from ductal carcinoma in situ (DCIS) to invasive disease is a complex multifactorial process that involves different mechanisms, including metabolic pathways. Whilst glutamine dependency has been confirmed in TNBC, there remains a need to explore the role of GLS isoforms in luminal Oestrogen receptor-positive (ER +) and human epidermal growth factor receptor 2-negative (HER2-) breast tumours which show higher glutamine metabolic activity in in vitro studies [16]. The prognostic significance of GLS isoforms in luminal DCIS and invasive disease also remain to be validated. Therefore, we hypothesised that both GLS and GLS2 play a role in the tumour progression and prognosis in luminal BC. This study aimed to assess the expression levels and prognostic significance of GLS and GLS2 in ER+/HER2- patients in well-characterised DCIS and BC cohorts.

2. Materials and Methods

2.1. Study Cohorts

Protein expression was conducted on two cohorts of ER+/HER2− BC comprising DCIS and IBC. Supplementary Tables S1 and S2 summarises the clinicopathological parameters of the two study cohorts. Patients were presented and managed at Nottingham City Hospital, Nottingham, UK. Clinicopathological, treatment and outcome data were collected and were prospectively maintained.

The DCIS cohort included primary DCIS (n = 206), without synchronous IBC as previously described [17,18]. Clinicopathological data included age at diagnosis, method of diagnosis, either screening or symptomatic presentation, tumour grade, size and comedo-type necrosis. Expression of ER, progesterone receptor (PR), HER2 and Ki67 were previously determined for this cohort [18]. Local recurrence-free interval (LRFI) was defined as any event of ipsilateral local recurrence (either DCIS or IBC) occurring after 6 months from the primary treatment.

The IBC cohort includes a well-characterised series of tumours from patients (n = 717) with long-term follow-up [19]. Outcome data included recurrence-free interval (RFI) and BC specific survival (BCSS), which was defined as the time (in months) from the date of primary surgical treatment to the time of recurrence or death from BC, respectively.

2.2. *Transcriptomic Data*

GLS and *GLS2* gene copy number (CN) aberrations and gene expression were evaluated in a cohort of 1398 ER +/HER2- BC cases in the Molecular Taxonomy of Breast Cancer International Consortium (METABRIC) cohort. Data were pre-processed and normalised as described previously [20]. Dichotomisation of *GLS*/*GLS2* mRNA expression was determined using the mean value. In addition, Breast Cancer Gene-Expression Miner v4.5 (bc-GenExMiner v4.5) incorporating TCGA and SCAN-B RNA sequencing data ($n = 4712$) was used. Correlation between *GLS* and *GLS2* mRNA expression with glutamine-associated genes was also investigated. The selection of these genes was based on previous publications, as either regulatory genes or supporting the biological function of GLS or GLS2 in the glutamine metabolism [13,21–23].

2.3. *Glutaminase Protein Expression*

Prior to immunohistochemistry (IHC) staining, the specificity for rabbit monoclonal GLS (Clone EP7212, Abcam, UK) and GLS2 (Ab169954, Abcam Plc, Cambridge, UK) primary antibodies was validated by western blotting (WB) using IBC (MCF7, ZR751, BT474, MDA-MB-231, T47D, UACC-812, MDA-MB-175, BT549, HCC1500 and SKBR3) and DCIS (MCF10DCIS) lysates obtained from cells from the American Type Culture Collection (Rockville, MD, USA), as previously described [13]. GLS was used at a dilution of 1:1000 overnight at 4 °C, while GLS2 was diluted at 1:1500 and incubated for 1hr at room temperature. Mouse monoclonal anti-β-actin antibody (Sigma, Life Sciences) (1:5000) was included as a positive control. Donkey anti-rabbit and Donkey anti-mouse fluorescent secondary peroxidase-conjugated antibodies (1:15,000 IRDye 680RD and IRDye 800CW, LI-COR Biosciences) were applied for 1hr at room temperature. Images were detected using the LI-COR Odyssey Fc machine with Image Studio 4.0 (LI-COR Biosciences) at wavelengths 700 nm and 800 nm. Specific bands were observed at the predicted size of 73 kDa and 65 kDa corresponding to KGA and GAC isoforms of GLS and 65 kDa and 31 kDa corresponding to LGA and GAB isoforms of GLS2 (Supplementary Figure S1). In addition, peptide blocking using IHC was performed to validate the specificity of GLS and GLS2 antibodies (Supplementary Figure S2). GLS and GLS2 antibodies were incubated with GLS (Ab206976) and GLS2 (Ab169954) peptides, respectively (Abcam Plc, Cambridge UK). There were no visible bands in Western blotting and an absence of staining in IHC compared to the antibody alone, which displayed bands and positive staining. GLS2 antibody was additionally incubated with GLS peptide (1:2 ratio), which showed positive staining, further confirming that GLS and GLS2 antibodies do not cross-react.

Tissue microarray (TMA) was constructed from both cohorts as previously described [17,24]. IHC was performed on 4μm TMA sections from both cohorts using the Novocastra Novolink TM Polymer Detection Systems Kit (Code: RE7280-K, Leica, Biosystems, UK) according to manufacturer instructions and as previously described [13]. Each antibody was used in a separate set of slides (non-dual staining). Heat-induced antigen epitope retrieval was performed in citrate buffer (pH 6.0) for 20min using a microwave oven (Whirlpool JT359 Jet Chef 1000 W) for both antibodies. Tissues were incubated with either GLS antibody 1:50 (Clone EP7212, Abcam, UK) or GLS2 antibody 1:400 (Ab169954, Abcam Plc, Cambridge, UK) diluted in Leica antibody diluent (RE AR9352, Leica Biosystems, Newcastle upon Tyne, UK) at 4 °C overnight and at room temperature for 1hr respectively. Negative (omission of the primary antibody) and positive control (liver tissue) were included according to the manufacturer's datasheet.

2.4. *Scoring of GLS and GLS2 Expression*

Stained TMA slides were scanned using a high-resolution digital scanner (NanoZoomer; Hamamatsu Photonics, Welwyn Garden City, UK) at x20 magnification and viewed using Xplore viewing software (Philips Healthcare, Belfast, UK). Assessment of staining for GLS and GLS2 in DCIS and invasive BC was based on a semi-quantitative assessment using a modified histochemical score (H-score), which included an assessment of both the intensity of staining and the percentage of stained tumour cells. For the intensity, a score index of 0, 1, 2 and 3 which corresponded to negative, weak, moderate and strong staining, was used, and the percentage of positively stained tumour cells for each intensity was estimated subjectively. The final H-score was calculated by multiplying the percentage of positively stained cells (0–100) by the intensity (0–3), producing a total range of 0–300 [25]. A pathologist blind scored 10% of the cases for inter-observer concordance. GLS and GLS2 protein expression were dichotomised into a low and high expression using the median H-score as per previous publications [26,27]. Breast cancer luminal subtypes were defined based on the IHC profile as: luminal A: ER +/HER2- low proliferation (Ki67 < 10%) and luminal B: ER +/HER2- high proliferation (Ki67 > 10%). For GLS expression, an H-score of 20 for DCIS and 100 for IBC were used. The median H-score for GLS2 expression was 103 and 90 in DCIS and IBC, respectively.

2.5. Statistical Analysis

SPSS version 25 (Chicago, IL, USA) was used to carry out statistical analyses. Continuous levels of *GLS* and *GLS2* mRNA and protein expressions were correlated with other parameters using Pearson's correlation coefficient. Differences in the mean between three or more groups were assessed using one-way analysis of variance (ANOVA) with the post-hoc Tukey multiple comparison test (for normalised data), while Mann–Whitney and Kruskal–Wallis tests were applied for non-parametric data. Kaplan–Meier survival curves and a log-rank test were used to investigate the association of glutaminase mRNA/protein expression with the clinical outcome. The Cox regression model was applied for the multivariate analysis against LRFI. A two-tailed *p*-value < 0.05 for all the tests was considered significant.

3. Results

3.1. Patterns of GLS and GLS2 Protein Expression

When present, GLS and GLS2 were located predominantly in the cytoplasm of tumour cells of both DCIS and IBC, with intensity levels varying from low to high (Figure 1). GLS showed negative or faint staining in the adjacent apparently normal terminal duct lobular units (TDLUs), while GLS2 showed moderate expression. Occasional stained inflammatory cells and surrounding stromal fibroblasts were sometimes evident (Figure 1). GLS expression was significantly higher in IBC than DCIS ($F = 332.4$, $p < 0.0001$) and GLS2 was higher in DCIS than IBC ($F = 9.8$, $p = 0.002$).

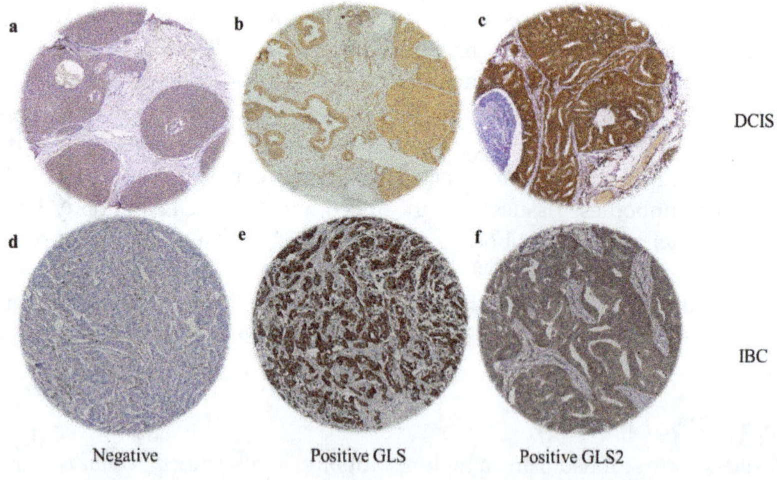

Figure 1. GLS and GLS2 protein expression in ER +/HER2- DCIS and invasive breast cancer. Representative TMA images (×20 magnification) depicting (**a**) negative immunostaining, positive GLS (**b**) and GLS2 (**c**) immunostaining in DCIS cases. (**d**) Negative immunostaining, positive GLS (**e**) and GLS2 (**f**) expression in invasive breast tumours.

3.2. *Glutaminase Expression in ER +/HER2- DCIS*

There was a weak positive linear correlation between GLS and GLS2 protein expression (Figure 2a; $r = 0.202$, $p = 0.009$). However, there were no associations between GLS or GLS2 with other clinical parameters, including tumour size or DCIS grade (Figure 2b–g). There was no difference in GLS expression between luminal subtypes (Figure 2h), but GLS2 expression was significantly higher in luminal B compared with luminal A tumours (Figure 2i, $p = 0.004$).

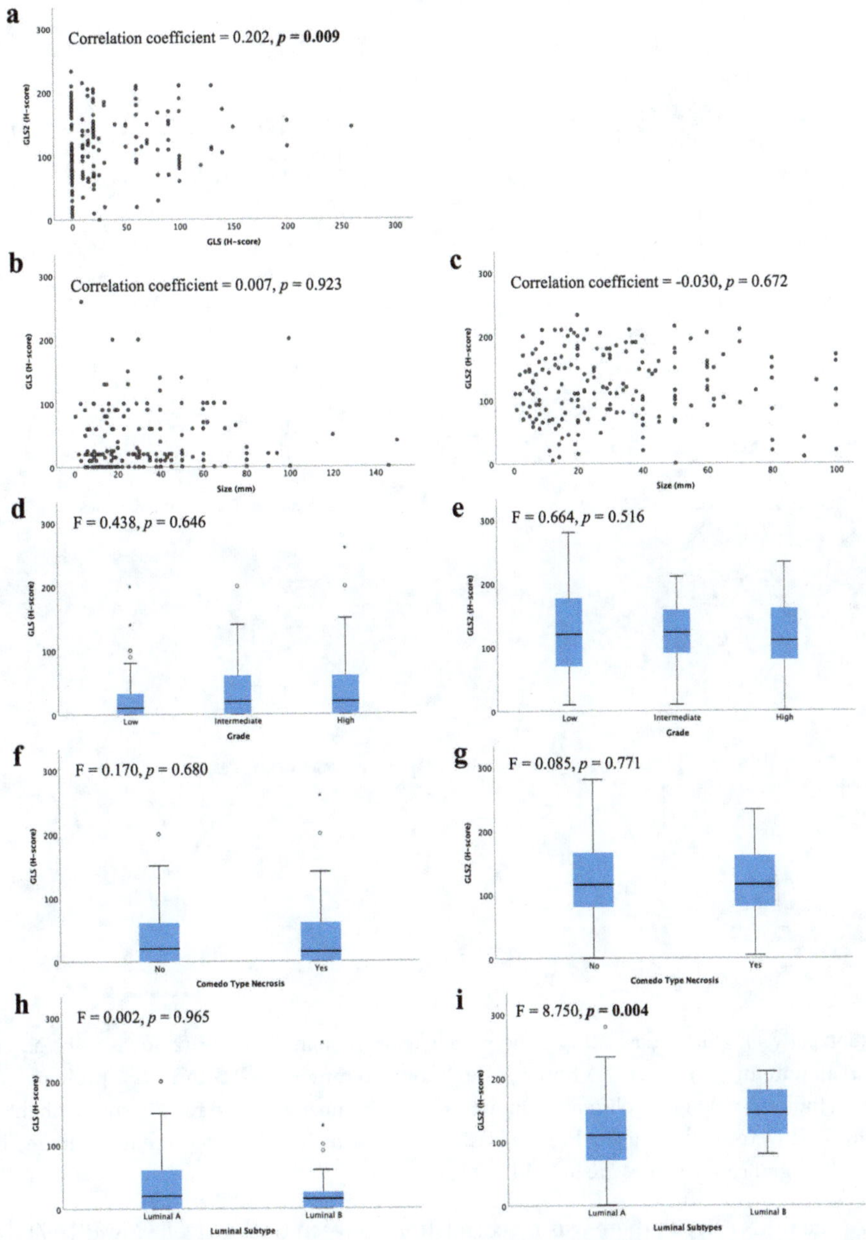

Figure 2. Glutaminase protein expression and its association with clinicopathological parameters and molecular subtypes in ER +/HER2- DCIS: (**a**) GLS and GLS2, GLS and (**b**) tumour size, (**d**) tumour grade, (**f**) comedo type necrosis, (**h**) luminal subtypes; GLS2 and (**c**) tumour size, (**e**) tumour grade, (**g**) comedo type necrosis, (**i**) luminal subtypes using Kruskal–Wallis test. Statistically significant p values are in **bold**.

3.3. Glutaminase Expression in ER +/HER2- Invasive BC

In the METABRIC cohort, a total of 19/1398 IBC (1.4%) showed *GLS* CN gain, whereas 16 cases (1.1%) showed CN loss. Regarding *GLS2*, CN gain was observed in 50 cases (3.6%) and loss observed in only 7 cases (0.5%). There was an association between *GLS* and *GLS2* CN variations and their corresponding mRNA expression (Figure 3g, $p = 0.006$ and Figure 3h, $p = 0.032$, respectively).

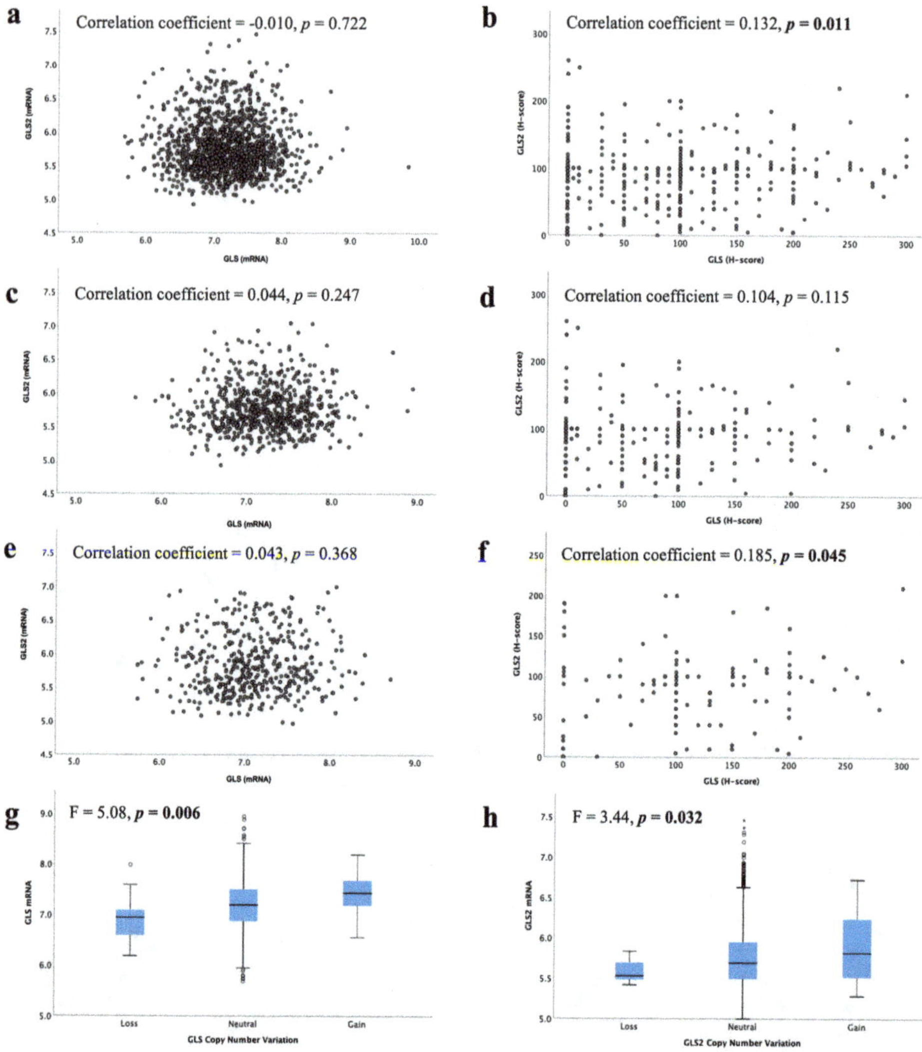

Figure 3. Correlation between glutaminase mRNA and protein expression in ER +/HER2- invasive breast cancer: *GLS* and *GLS2* mRNA in (**a**) all tumours, (**c**) luminal A tumours, (**e**) luminal B tumours; GLS and GLS2 protein in (**b**) all tumours, (**d**) low proliferation tumours, (**f**) high proliferation tumours. Copy number gain and relationship with mRNA expression for (**g**) *GLS* and (**h**) *GLS2* were analysed using Pearson's correlation coefficient. Data represented with median ± standard deviation. Statistically significant *p* values are in **bold**.

At the mRNA level, there was no correlation between *GLS* and *GLS2* in ER +/HER2- BC, luminal A or luminal B tumours (Figure 3a,c,e, all $p > 0.05$). However, in the Gene-Miner dataset, there was a very weak negative correlation between *GLS* and *GLS2* in all ER+ ($p < 0.00001$) and luminal A ($p = 0.003$) BC classes, but not the luminal B tumours (Supplementary Figure S3, $p = 0.202$). At the protein level, there was a weak positive linear correlation between GLS and the GLS2 protein in ER +/HER2- BC cases (Figure 3b, $p = 0.011$). When biological subtypes were considered, GLS and GLS2 proteins remained positively correlated, albeit weakly, in the high proliferation/luminal B tumours (Figure 3f, $p = 0.045$), but not the low proliferation/luminal A tumours (Figure 3d, $p = 0.115$).

3.4. Association of Glutaminase with Clinicopathological Parameters in Invasive BC

High *GLS* and *GLS2* mRNA were associated with lower tumour grade (Figure 4c, $p = 0.017$, Figure 4d, $p = 0.026$, respectively). There was no association between *GLS* or *GLS2* mRNA expression with tumour size (Figure 4a,b) or nodal stage (Figure 4e,f).

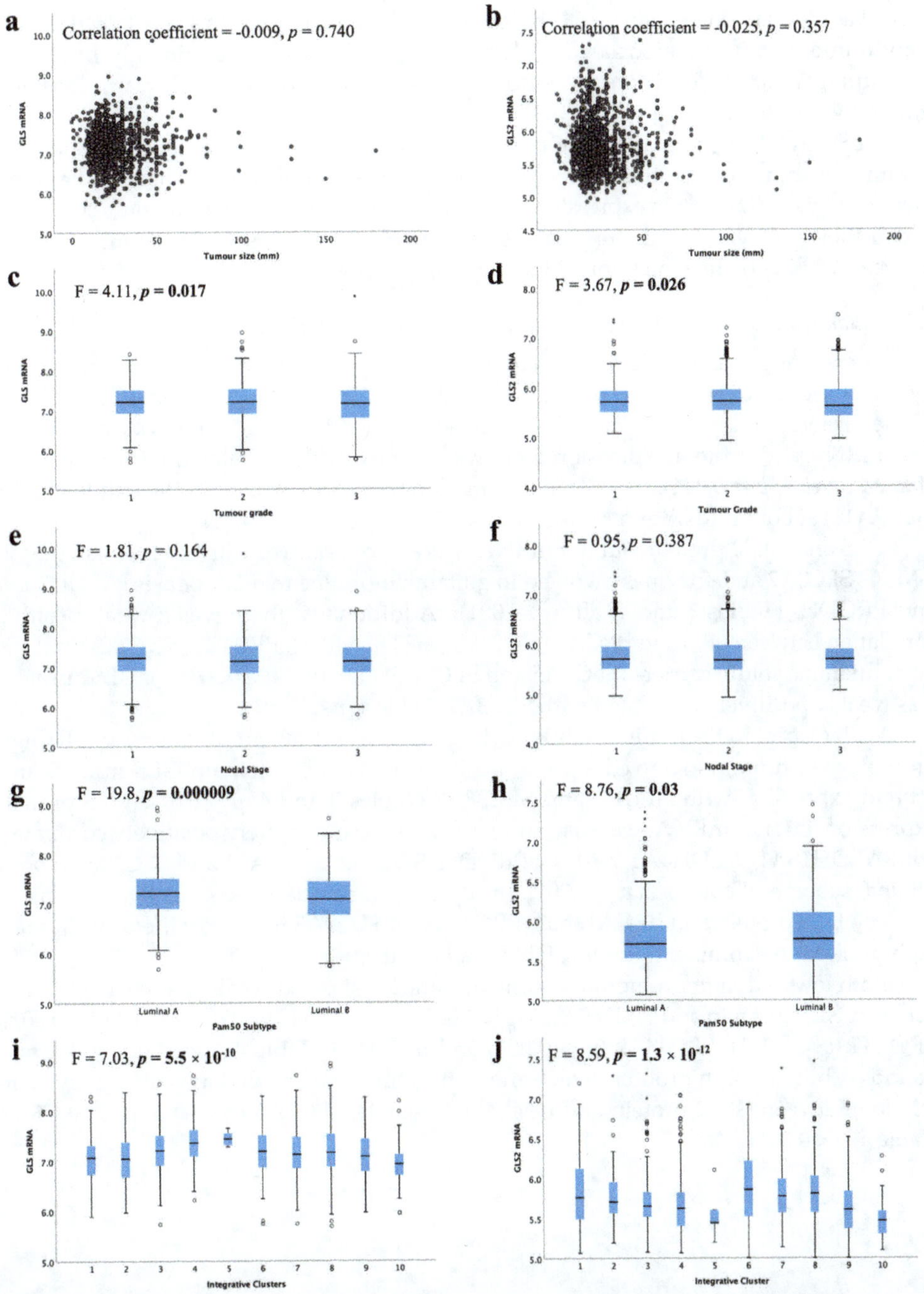

Figure 4. Glutaminase mRNA expression and its association with clinicopathological parameters: *GLS* and (**a**) tumour size, (**c**) tumour grade, (**e**) lymph node stage, (**g**) luminal subtypes, (**i**) METABRIC Integrative clusters; *GLS2* and (**b**) tumour size, (**d**) tumour grade, (**f**) lymph node stage, (**h**) luminal subtypes, (**j**) METABRIC Integrative clusters were analysed using Pearson's correlation coefficient. Data represented with median ± standard deviation. Statistically significant *p* values are in **bold**.

When comparing the levels of glutaminase mRNA expression in biological subtypes, there was a significantly lower level of *GLS* in luminal B compared with luminal A tumours (Figure 4g, $p < 0.001$). In contrast, luminal B tumours showed higher *GLS2* expression than luminal A tumours (Figure 4h, $p = 0.03$). Luminal B tumours were more likely to have *GLS* CNV, either gain or loss, compared with luminal A tumours ($p = 0.019$). Similarly, *GLS2* CN gains were primarily observed in luminal B tumours ($p = 0.00004$).

Within the METABRIC Integrative clusters, high *GLS* mRNA expression was associated with cluster 4 (predominately luminal A) (Figure 4i, $p < 0.0001$). In contrast, high *GLS2* was associated with cluster 6 (predominately luminal B) (Figure 4j, $p < 0.0001$). *GLS2* copy number gain was associated with cluster 1, which are predominantly luminal B tumours ($p = 0.000006$). There were no other associations between CN variations and Integrative clusters.

GLS and GLS2 protein were not associated with any of the key clinicopathological parameters: tumour size, tumour grade or nodal stage (Figure 5a–f). There was a trend towards higher GLS protein expression in the high proliferative luminal tumours compared with the low proliferative tumours (Figure 5g, $p = 0.051$). There was no significant difference between GLS2 protein expression in the luminal subtypes (Figure 5b).

3.5. Glutaminase and Glutamine Metabolism-Related Genes and Proteins

There was a weak positive correlation between GLS and GLS2 with Glutamate Dehydrogenase (GLUD1) and the solute carriers (SLC38A2 and SLC7A8) at both the mRNA (Tables 1 and 2, all $p < 0.05$) and protein levels ($p < 0.01$; Tables 3 and 4). In addition, GLS mRNA and protein expression were weakly positively correlated with ALDH4A1 (Tables 1 and 3, $p < 0.001$) and GLS2 was moderately correlated with the solute carrier (SLC7A11) at both mRNA and protein levels (Tables 2 and 4, $p < 0.01$).

GLS and GLS2 protein, but not mRNA, were also weakly positively correlated with c-MYC, SLC3A2 and enzymes involved in glutamine-proline regulatory axis (ALDH18A1 and PRODH) (Tables 3 and 4, all $p < 0.001$). Additionally, there was a weak positive correlation between GLS and BRCA1 ($p < 0.001$), p53 ($p < 0.01$), PIK3CA ($p < 0.001$) and the key glutamine solute carriers (SLC1A5 and SLC7A5) (Table 3, all $p < 0.001$). GLS2 protein was weakly positively correlated with SLC3A2 (Table 4, $p < 0.001$).

With respect to the luminal subtypes, both luminal A (low proliferative) and B (high proliferative) tumours showed a weak positive correlation between GLS mRNA and protein expression with GLUD1 and SLC38A2 (Tables 3 and 4, $p < 0.01$). GLS protein expression, but not mRNA, was also similarly weak to moderately positively correlated with ALDH18A1, ALDH4A1, c-MYC, PRODH, SLC3A2, SLC7A11 and SLC7A5 in both luminal subtypes (Table 3, all $p \leq 0.001$). In addition, there was a weak positive correlation between GLS protein and BRCA1, p53, PIK3CA and SLC1A5 in low proliferative but not high proliferative luminal tumours (Table 3, all $p \leq 0.001$).

Both low and high proliferative luminal tumours showed weak positive correlation between GLS2 protein and ALDH18A1 ($p < 0.001$), ALDH4A1 ($p < 0.01$), ATF4 ($p = 0.001$), PRODH ($p < 0.001$), SLC38A2 ($p \leq 0.001$) and SLC7A11 (Table 4, $p < 0.001$). Low proliferative, but not high proliferative, luminal tumours also showed a weak positive correlation between GLS2 protein and c-MYC ($p < 0.001$), SLC1A5 ($p < 0.05$) and SLC3A2 (Table 4, $p < 0.001$).

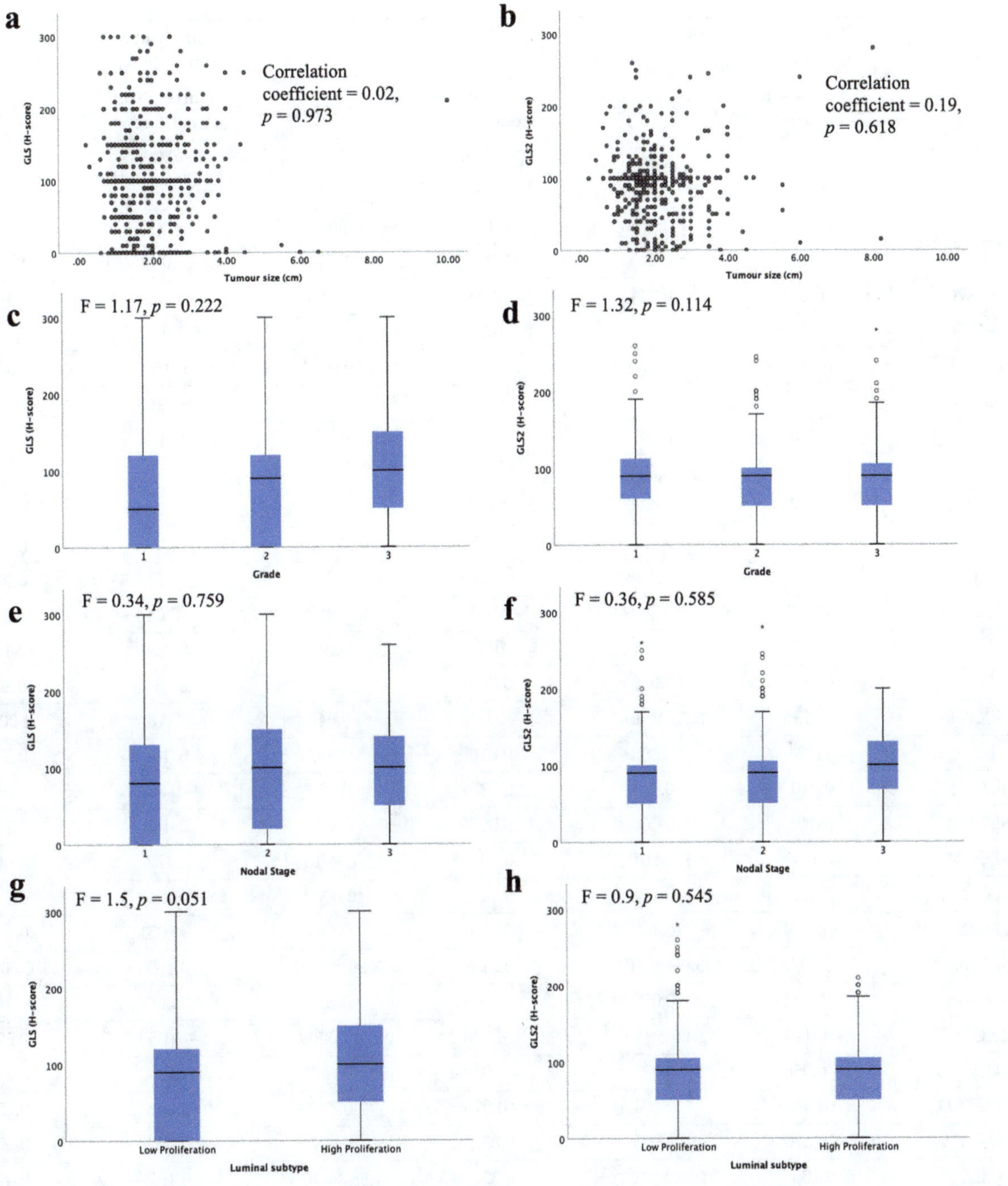

Figure 5. Glutaminase protein expression and its association with clinicopathological parameters and molecular subtypes in ER +/HER2- invasive breast cancer: GLS and (**a**) tumour size, (**c**), tumour grade, (**e**) lymph node stage, (**g**) luminal subtypes; GLS2 and (**b**) tumour size, (**d**) tumour grade, (**f**) lymph node stage, (**h**) luminal subtypes using one-way analysis of variance with the post-hoc Tukey test. Data represented with median ± standard deviation. Statistically significant p values are in **bold**.

Table 1. Correlation of *GLS* mRNA expression with glutamine-metabolism-related mRNA in invasive luminal breast cancer.

GLS vs	ER+/HER2- (n = 1398)		Luminal A (n = 693)		Luminal B (n = 443)	
	Correlation Coefficient	p Value	Correlation Coefficient	p Value	Correlation Coefficient	p Value
AKT1	−0.012	0.675	−0.034	0.376	−0.005	0.923
ALDH18A1	0.040	0.139	0.066	0.081	0.026	0.591
ALDH4A1	0.101	**0.000148**	0.136	**0.000331**	0.006	0.908
ATF4	0.031	0.245	0.042	0.272	0.095	**0.046**
BRCA1	−0.054	0.044	0.064	0.092	0.022	0.642
c-MYC	0.018	0.497	−0.005	0.903	0.070	0.141
GLUD1	0.141	**1.24×10^{-7}**	0.147	**0.0001**	0.168	**0.0004**
GLUL	−0.138	**2.25×10^{-7}**	−0.194	**2.84×10^{-7}**	−0.109	0.022
MTOR	0.028	0.292	0.044	0.244	−0.047	0.324
p53	−0.169	**<0.0001**				
PIK3CA	0.047	0.078	0.117	**0.002**	0.058	0.220
PRODH	−0.210	0.425	−0.052	0.175	−0.092	0.054
PYCR1	−0.097	**0.000282**	−0.010	0.799	−0.124	**0.009**
SLC1A1	−0.025	0.349	−0.007	0.857	−0.048	0.316
SLC1A2	0.022	0.421	0.071	0.063	0.064	0.179
SLC1A3	0.066	**0.014**	0.094	**0.013**	0.060	0.209
SLC1A5	−0.135	**3.78×10^{-7}**	−0.078	**0.040**	−0.183	**0.0001**
SLC1A6	−0.24	0.363	0.010	0.803	0.043	0.370
SLC1A7	0.010	0.713	0.038	0.319	−0.092	0.054
SLC38A1	0.049	0.066	0.057	0.131	0.052	0.272
SLC38A2	0.191	**6.33×10^{-13}**	0.250	**2.24×10^{-11}**	0.127	**0.007**
SLC38A3	0.041	0.124	0.141	**0.0002**	−0.047	0.326
SLC38A5	−0.004	0.893	0.056	0.140	−0.031	0.511
SLC38A7	0.157	**3.95×10^{-9}**	0.219	**5.69×10^{-9}**	0.169	**0.0004**
SLC38A8	−0.052	0.053	−0.049	0.201	0.009	0.849
SLC3A2	−0.144	**6.06×10^{-8}**	−0.148	**0.00009**	−0.052	0.276
SLC6A19	−0.056	0.035	−0.018	0.641	−0.050	0.296
SLC7A11	0.014	0.604	−0.013	0.735	0.068	0.151
SLC7A5	−0.230	0.383	0.032	0.407	0.052	0.278
SLC7A6	0.180	**1.32×10^{-11}**	0.220	**4.55×10^{-9}**	0.107	0.024
SLC7A7	−0.99	**0.000218**	−0.109	**0.004**	−0.075	0.113
SLC7A8	0.065	**0.016**	0.063	0.096	0.075	0.113
SLC7A9	−0.005	0.862	−0.021	0.588	−0.007	0.888

Statistically significant p values are in **bold**.

Table 2. Correlation of *GLS2* mRNA expression with glutamine-metabolism-related mRNA in invasive luminal breast cancer.

GLS2 vs	ER +/HER2- (n = 1398)		Luminal A (n = 693)		Luminal B (n = 443)	
	Correlation Coefficient	p Value	Correlation Coefficient	p Value	Correlation Coefficient	p Value
AKT1	0.038	0.157	0.066	0.083	0.021	0.656
ALDH18A1	−0.001	0.958	0.030	0.427	−0.035	0.463
ALDH4A1	−0.055	**0.042**	−0.037	0.325	−0.037	0.435
ATF4	0.042	0.120	0.072	0.058	−0.001	0.987
BRCA1	0.203	**1.72×10^{-14}**	0.120	**0.002**	0.169	**0.0003**
c-MYC	−0.104	**0.0001**	−0.150	**0.00007**	−0.040	0.399
GLUD1	0.224	**2.55×10^{-17}**	0.242	**1.02×10^{-10}**	0.151	**0.001**
GLUL	−0.017	0.519	−0.047	0.219	−0.055	0.246
MTOR	0.000	1.000	0.053	0.167	−0.052	0.279
p53	0.034	0.200				
PIK3CA	−0.12	0.649	0.016	0.674	−0.090	0.059
PRODH	-0.148	**2.69×10^{-8}**	-0.114	**0.003**	-0.114	**0.016**
PYCR1	0.009	0.731	−0.016	0.672	−0.031	0.516
SLC1A1	0.070	**0.009**	0.046	0.224	0.035	0.468
SLC1A2	0.191	**6.14×10^{-13}**	0.205	**5.28×10^{-8}**	0.146	**0.002**
SLC1A3	−0.190	**8.55×10^{-13}**	−0.163	**0.00002**	−0.249	**1.11×10^{-7}**
SLC1A5	0.211	**1.42×10^{-15}**	0.249	**2.87×10^{-11}**	0.157	**0.001**
SLC1A6	−0.012	0.655	0.005	0.898	−0.007	0.889
SLC1A7	−0.041	0.127	−0.060	0.112	−0.035	0.461
SLC38A1	−0.075	**0.005**	−0.110	**0.004**	−0.132	**0.005**
SLC38A2	−0.021	0.425	−0.017	0.654	−0.014	0.766
SLC38A3	0.095	**0.0004**	0.125	**0.001**	0.077	0.104
SLC38A5	−0.102	**0.0001**	−0.105	**0.006**	−0.098	**0.038**
SLC38A7	0.029	0.281	0.079	0.037	0.058	0.226
SLC38A8	0.051	0.055	0.036	0.348	0.024	0.615
SLC3A2	0.018	0.495	−0.039	0.308	0.014	0.769
SLC6A19	0.002	0.930	−0.032	0.406	−0.007	0.880
SLC7A11	0.089	0.001	0.091	0.017	0.085	0.075
SLC7A5	−0.038	0.158	−0.008	0.826	−0.062	0.190
SLC7A6	−0.103	0.158	−0.054	0.158	−0.031	0.522
SLC7A7	−0.200	**4.14×10^{-14}**	−0.211	**1.97×10^{-8}**	−0.257	**4.29×10^{-8}**
SLC7A8	0.061	**0.022**	0.074	0.500	0.020	0.681
SLC7A9	0.008	0.761	0.032	0.406	−0.095	0.045

Statistically significant p values are in **bold**.

Table 3. Correlation of GLS protein expression with glutamine-metabolism-related proteins in invasive luminal breast cancer.

GLS vs	ER +/HER2- (n = 668)		Low Proliferation (n = 275)		High Proliferation (n = 124)	
	Correlation Coefficient	p Value	Correlation Coefficient	p Value	Correlation Coefficient	p Value
pAKTs473	−0.003	0.958	0.006	0.913	0.017	0.842
ALDH18A1	0.347	$\mathbf{9.77 \times 10^{-17}}$	0.303	$\mathbf{1.02 \times 10^{-8}}$	0.348	**0.000002**
ALDH4A1	0.235	$\mathbf{4.53 \times 10^{-8}}$	0.249	**0.000004**	0.232	**0.002**
ATF4	0.224	$\mathbf{1.34 \times 10^{-7}}$	0.205	**0.0001**	0.244	**0.001**
BRCA1	0.151	**0.0005**	0.186	**0.001**	0.115	0.129
c-MYC	0.256	$\mathbf{1.42 \times 10^{-9}}$	0.240	**0.000005**	0.288	**0.0001**
GLUD1	0.170	**0.00002**	0.142	**0.004**	0.230	**0.001**
MTORC1	−0.032	0.463	0.009	0.864	−0.038	0.622
p53	0.137	**0.007**	0.227	**0.0004**	0	1
PIK3CA	0.231	**0.000002**	0.239	**0.00009**	0.121	0.152
PRODH	0.312	$\mathbf{2.60 \times 10^{-12}}$	0.308	$\mathbf{4.04 \times 10^{-8}}$	0.323	**0.00003**
PYCR1	0.023	0.652	0.076	0.222	−0.086	0.340
SLC1A5	0.244	$\mathbf{1.57 \times 10^{-9}}$	0.250	$\mathbf{6.96 \times 10^{-7}}$	0.141	0.050
SLC38A2	0.293	$\mathbf{1.08 \times 10^{-8}}$	0.188	**0.004**	0.333	**0.0003**
SLC3A2	0.355	$\mathbf{2.56 \times 10^{-16}}$	0.387	$\mathbf{5.96 \times 10^{-13}}$	0.269	**0.001**
SLC7A11	0.395	$\mathbf{1.34 \times 10^{-16}}$	0.402	$\mathbf{8.22 \times 10^{-12}}$	0.503	$\mathbf{1.78 \times 10^{-10}}$
SLC7A5	0.236	$\mathbf{3.87 \times 10^{-7}}$	0.188	**0.001**	0.256	**0.002**
SLC7A8	0.201	**0.001**	0.153	0.051	0.119	0.302

Statistically significant p values are in **bold**.

Table 4. Correlation of GLS2 protein expression with glutamine-metabolism-related proteins in invasive luminal breast cancer.

GLS2 vs	ER +/HER2- (n = 415)		Low Proliferation (n = 275)		High Proliferation (n = 124)	
	Correlation Coefficient	p Value	Correlation Coefficient	p Value	Correlation Coefficient	p Value
pAKTs473	−0.061	0.295	−0.149	**0.038**	0.084	0.441
ALDH18A1	0.342	$\mathbf{6.16 \times 10^{-12}}$	0.263	**0.00002**	0.050	$\mathbf{8.35 \times 10^{-9}}$
ALDH4A1	0.229	**0.000007**	0.210	**0.001**	0.292	**0.002**
ATF4	0.261	$\mathbf{8.71 \times 10^{-7}}$	0.227	**0.001**	0.323	**0.001**
BRCA1	0.049	0.372	0.040	0.551	0.055	0.584
c-MYC	0.205	**0.0001**	0.230	**0.0004**	0.184	0.060
GLUD1	0.176	**0.0005**	0.106	0.089	0.311	**0.001**
MTORC1	0.069	0.204	0.029	0.655	0.142	0.171
p53	−0.042	0.508	0.023	0.766	0.039	0.742
PIK3CA	0.071	0.234	0.0125	0.091	0.059	0.586
PRODH	0.358	$\mathbf{4.18 \times 10^{-11}}$	0.353	$\mathbf{1.76 \times 10^{-7}}$	0.378	**0.0001**
PYCR1	0.082	0.196	0.067	0.383	0.117	0.317
SLC1A5	0.061	0.232	0.128	**0.041**	−0.024	0.799
SLC38A2	0.284	$\mathbf{1.04 \times 10^{-7}}$	0.234	**0.001**	0.376	**0.00007**
SLC3A2	0.178	**0.0004**	0.273	**0.000009**	0.106	0.253
SLC7A11	0.285	$\mathbf{7.19 \times 10^{-8}}$	0.266	**0.00005**	0.339	**0.0004**
SLC7A5	0.029	0.579	0.021	0.747	0.075	0.433
SLC7A8	0.175	**0.006**	0.156	0.051	0.229	0.048

Statistically significant p values are in **bold**.

3.6. Glutaminase and Outcome in ER +/HER2- DCIS

High GLS expression in DCIS was associated with shorter LRFI for all recurrences (Figure 6a, $p < 0.0001$), whereas there was no association between GLS2 and DCIS outcome

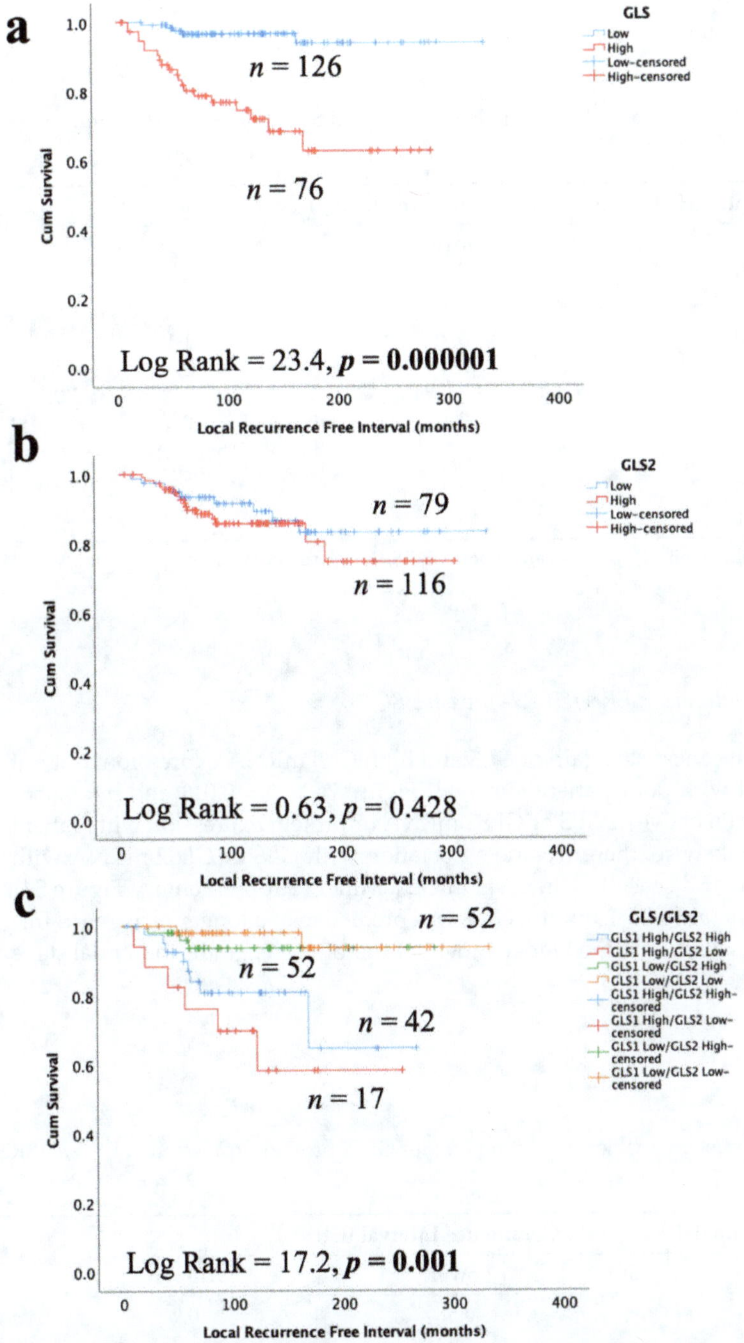

Figure 6. Kaplan–Meier of GLS and GLS2 protein expression with tumour recurrence in ER +/HER2- DCIS patients: (**a**) GLS, (**b**) GLS2, and (**c**) combined expression of GLS and GLS2. Statistically significant *p* values are in **bold**.

(Figure 6b, $p = 0.428$). When stratifying patients, taking into account both GLS and GLS2 co-expression, DCIS with GLS high/GLS2 low expression was associated with the shortest LRFI with GLShigh/GLS2 high showing moderate outcome and those tumors without GLS expression, irrespective of GLS2 expression, having the best outcome (Figure 6c, $p = 0.0001$). In multivariate Cox regression, GLS and GLS/GLS2 co-expression remained predictors of shorter LRFI independent of tumour size, grade and comedo necrosis (Table 5, $p = 0.0008$ and $p = 0.003$, respectively).

Table 5. Multivariate survival analysis of variables predicting LRFI for GLS and GLS/GLS2 protein co-expression in ER +/HER2- DCIS.

Parameters	Hazard Ratio (HR)	95% Confidence Interval (CI)		*p* Value
		Lower	Upper	
GLS	7.4	2.7	20.0	**0.0008**
Comedo type necrosis	0.7	0.3	1.6	0.397
Tumour size	0.5	0.2	1.1	0.080
Tumour grade	1.3	0.6	2.4	0.445
GLS/GLS2 co-expression	0.5	0.4	0.8	**0.003**
Comedo type necrosis	0.9	0.3	2.7	0.884
Tumour size	0.5	0.2	1.2	0.111
Tumour grade	1.1	0.5	2.4	0.745

Statistically significant *p* values are in **bold**. DCIS, ductal carcinoma in situ.

3.7. *Glutaminase and Outcome in ER +/HER2- Invasive BC*

In invasive breast cancer, CN gain of *GLS* and high *GLS* mRNA expression, but not *GLS2*, was associated with poor patient survival (Figure 7a,b, $p = 0.011$ and $p = 0.056$). There was no association between GLS or GLS2 mRNA or protein expression with patient BCSS (Figure 7c–f). Likewise, there was no association with *GLS* or *GLS2* mRNA with either patient survival or disease-free interval in GeneMiner (Supplementary Figure S4). However, GLS2 protein ($p = 0.006$), but not GLS, was predictive of a longer recurrence-free interval (Figure 7g,h), which remained independent of tumour size, grade and nodal stage ($p = 0.003$, Table 6).

Table 6. Multivariate survival analysis of variables predicting DFI for GLS2 protein expression in ER +/HER2- invasive breast cancer.

Parameters	Hazard Ratio (HR)	95% Confidence Interval (CI)		*p* Value
		Lower	Upper	
GLS2	0.6	0.5	0.9	**0.003**
Tumour size	1.3	0.9	1.7	0.141
Tumour grade	1.3	1.0	1.6	**0.033**
Nodal stage	1.5	1,2	1.9	**0.0003**

Statistically significant *p* values are in **bold**.

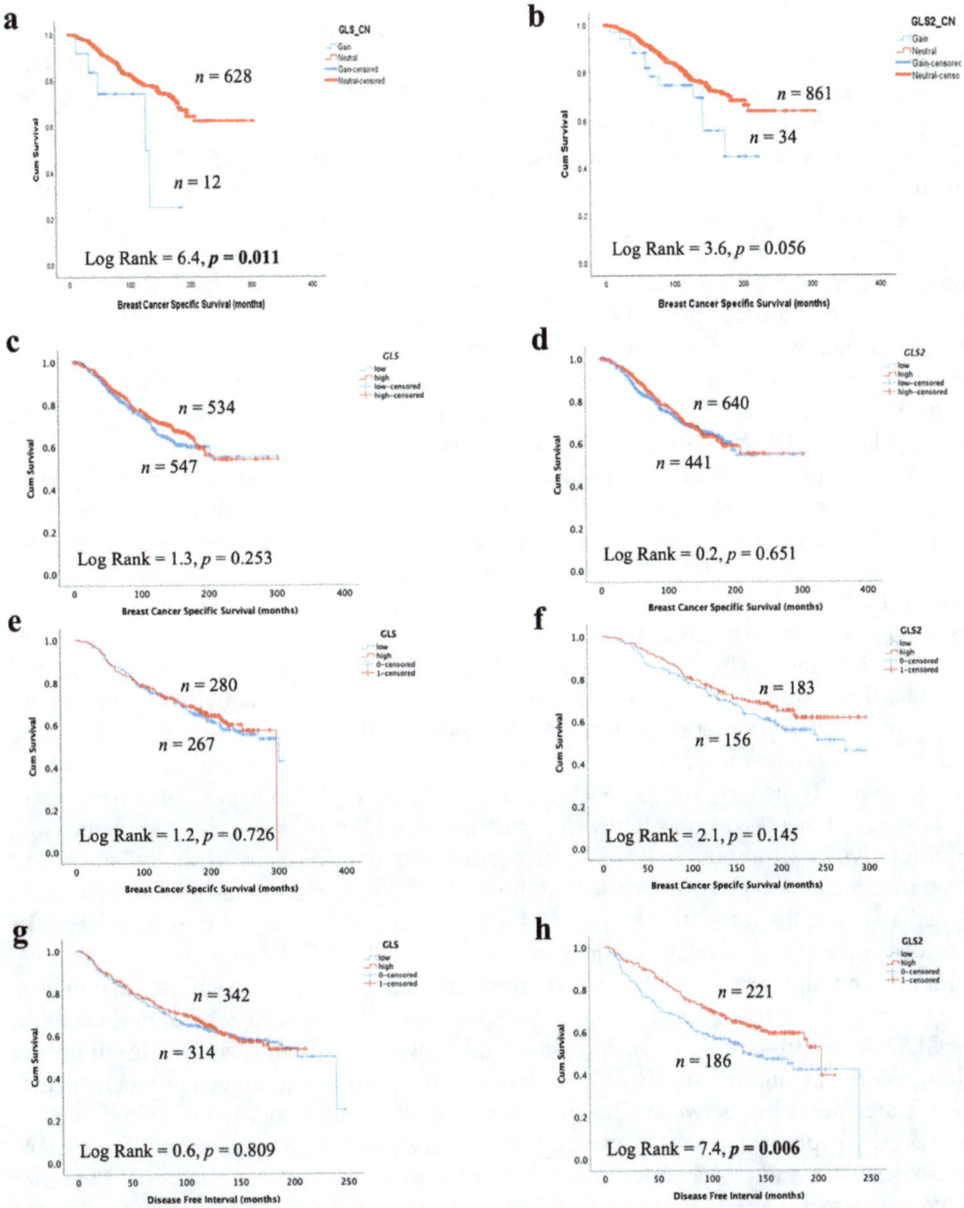

Figure 7. Association of glutaminase expression with patient outcome in ER +/HER2- invasive breast cancer in the METABRIC and Nottingham series: breast cancer-specific survival of (**a**) *GLS* copy number gain, (**b**) *GLS2* copy number gain, (**c**) *GLS* mRNA, (**d**) *GLS2* mRNA, (**e**) GLS protein and (**f**) GLS2 protein, a disease-free interval of (**g**) GLS protein and (**h**) GLS2 protein. Statistically significant p values are in **bold**.

4. Discussion

The glutamine metabolism is important in cancer cell proliferation and in promoting invasiveness [28]. It has been well established that glutamine synthesis is upregulated in most cancers, including BC, and consequently, glutaminase catalytic activity and levels are upregulated [5]. Several studies demonstrate that glutaminase contributes to cancer tumour growth in various human cancers such as prostate, lung and colorectal [7,8]. Despite these findings, the role of glutaminase in the progression of DCIS into the invasive disease stage remains poorly understood. In addition, studies on GLS2 expression in BC are limited. The current study evaluated the transcriptomic and proteomic expression of GLS and GLS2 and their association with various clinicopathological parameters and linked each biomarker to the patient outcome to provide an understanding of the prognostic significance of GLS and GLS2 in BC. To our knowledge, this is the first study to evaluate the role of both GLS and GLS2 in pre-invasive and invasive ER+/HER2- tumours. The ER +/luminal tumours are the most common type of BC, accounting for about 55–80% of all BC types and have varied tumour biology, disease prognosis and recurrence [29].

This study has revealed for the first time that that high GLS and GLShigh/GL2low expression are associated with shorter LRFI in DCIS independent from other clinicopathological variables. Our preliminary results, therefore, suggest that glutaminase Ftrcould be used as prognostic markers in early-stage disease to predict patient outcome, and this warrants further validation in external DCIS cohorts. The findings highlighted the importance of GLS in breast tumour proliferation and invasiveness and could potentially be used as a target for inhibition via the potent and non-competitive allosteric GLS inhibitor CB−839 (telaglenastat). CB-839 has anti-proliferative activity in triple-negative BC [7], and several clinical trials for solid cancers are ongoing [30]. In vitro and in vivo investigations using appropriate models are necessary to confirm this.

With respect to invasive tumours, increased expression of GLS2 protein predicted longer recurrence-free intervals. This finding concurs with previous results that GLS2 has been linked to a role in suppressing tumour growth. It has been demonstrated that overexpression of GLS2 decreases HCC cell invasiveness by counteracting the small GTPase Rac1 [31]. Nevertheless, consistent with a previous study, copy number gain of GLS was associated with poor outcomes in IBC [13].

Previous reports [5,7] have shown that high proliferative tumours such as TNBC and luminal B have higher glutamine metabolism and show increased activity of glutaminase compared to low proliferating tumours. It is noteworthy that although GLS and GLS2 catalyse the conversion of glutamine to glutamate, the expression and regulation of the two isozymes is distinct. The former is the frequently upregulated isoform in most cancers. This study showed a strong trend towards higher GLS protein expression in the high proliferative ER+ tumours in invasive breast cancer and in DCIS. In addition, High GLS2 protein expression was associated with luminal B compared to luminal A tumours in DCIS. When assessing the correlation between GLS and GLS2 and the two cohorts, we observed a positive correlation between the high expression of GLS and GLS2 protein in pre-invasive tumours and high proliferative invasive tumours. This finding could suggest that in both the pre-invasive stage and the invasive stage, tumour cells might be overcoming the effect of GLS2 overexpression by overexpressing GLS. However, further mechanistic studies for this scenario are highly warranted to understand the underlying molecular mechanisms.

The relationship between GLS and GLS2 and other regulatory genes at both mRNA and protein expression was also investigated. A weak positive correlation between glutaminase isozymes and c-Myc in luminal types at the protein level was observed. Evidence from various studies suggests that GLS is directly activated by c-Myc enabling sustained uncontrolled tumour cell proliferation. c-Myc is known as an important driver in maintaining a glutaminolysis phenotype, particularly in ER- tumours, and enhances GLS activity indirectly via suppressing the expression of miR-23a/b [21,32]. Our data suggest that this regulation might also occur in the ER +/luminal subtype. We observed a weak positive correlation between GLS with PI3KCa within the low proliferation subgroup. PI3KCa, a known oncogene, has a role in regulating cell proliferation and survival as well as an important role in regulating glucose and glutamine uptake and metabolism in different cancers. In BC, PIK3Ca mutations tend to be associated with hormone receptor-positive tumours, and a study carried out by Lau et al. has provided further evidence of the importance of PIK3Ca mutations in metabolic reprogramming, specifically increasing glutamine uptake and glutamate production by modulating pyruvate dehydrogenase activity [33]. *TP53* has been linked to regulating the glutamine metabolism by mediating the *GLS2* gene and having a tumour suppression effect on tumour cells [22]. Interestingly, in the current study, a weak positive association between wild type *TP53* and GLS expression in the low proliferating tumour was observed.

The association of both GLS and GLS2 with glutamine transporters and other enzymes involved in the glutamine metabolism is not surprising. Our analysis demonstrated weak to moderate associations between glutaminase with most of the glutamine metabolism-related enzymes and solute carriers. Among these is GLUD1, which was weakly associated with GLS and GLS2 at both mRNA and protein levels in the low and high proliferative tumours. Craze and colleagues [34] have shown that there is a relationship between GLUD1 and luminal tumours compared to HER2+ tumours. Furthermore, a weak positive correlation with both ALDH18A1 and PRODH was observed. Previously Craze et al. demonstrated that these enzymes were highly expressed in a subset of ER+ tumours that have high proliferation and were related to poor patient outcomes [13]. We also show that high expression of GLS and GLS2 were weakly associated with high expression of SLC7A5, SLC3A2 and SLC1A5. In their findings, El Ansari et al. demonstrated that the combination of SLC1A5, SLC7A5 and SLC3A2, defined as high SLCs cluster, was associated with poor prognostic markers in highly proliferative ER-positive tumours [23]. Our observation in this subset of BC is consistent with the previous studies. Although our findings did not show correlation with key clinicopathological features in invasive BC, mostly association with glutamine-metabolism-related genes, the findings may suggest that glutaminase isozymes expression in this subset of breast cancer is important in tumour biology rather than a clinical outcome in invasive BC. Further investigation studies are needed to understand the underlying molecular mechanisms.

5. Conclusions

This study provides strong evidence for the use of GLS as a prognostic biomarker for invasive progression of luminal DCIS and a potential target for inhibition. Further validation in external cohorts is warranted along with functional studies to decipher the role of GLS and its mechanism of action as a driver of disease progression.

Author Contributions: B.K.M.: Writing, methodology, data analysis and interpretation of the results, R.E.A.: data analysis, review and editing, L.A. and M.L.C. review, N.J., A.O., H.C.: methodology, M.T.: data analysis, review and editing, E.A.R.: review and editing. A.R.G.: conceived and designed the study, data analysis, and review and editing. All authors have read and agreed to the published version of the manuscript.

References

1. Hanahan, D.; Weinberg, R.A. Hallmarks of Cancer: The Next Generation. *Cell* **2011**, *144*, 646–674. [CrossRef]
2. Wise, D.R.; Thompson, C.B. Glutamine addiction: A new therapeutic target in cancer. *Trends Biochem. Sci.* **2010**, *35*, 427–433. [CrossRef]
3. Daye, D.; Wellen, K.E. Metabolic reprogramming in cancer: Unraveling the role of glutamine in tumorigenesis. *Semin. Cell Dev. Biol.* **2012**, *23*, 362–369. [CrossRef]
4. DeBerardinis, R.J.; Lum, J.J.; Hatzivassiliou, G.; Thompson, C.B. The Biology of Cancer: Metabolic Reprogramming Fuels Cell Growth and Proliferation. *Cell Metab.* **2008**, *7*, 11–20. [CrossRef]
5. Masisi, B.K.; El Ansari, R.; Alfarsi, L.; Rakha, E.A.; Green, A.R.; Craze, M.L. The role of glutaminase in cancer. *Histopathology* **2020**, *76*, 498–508. [CrossRef] [PubMed]
6. Kim, J.Y.; Heo, S.-H.; Choi, S.K.; Song, I.H.; Park, I.A.; Kim, Y.-A.; Park, H.S.; Park, S.Y.; Bang, W.S.; Gong, G.; et al. Glutaminase expression is a poor prognostic factor in node-positive triple-negative breast cancer patients with a high level of tumor-infiltrating lymphocytes. *Virchows Archiv* **2017** *470*, 381–389. [CrossRef] [PubMed]
7. Gross, M.I.; Demo, S.D.; Dennison, J.B.; Chen, L.; Chernov-Rogan, T.; Goyal, B.; Janes, J.R.; Laidig, G.J.; Lewis, E.R.; Li, J.; et al. Antitumor Activity of the Glutaminase Inhibitor CB-839 in Triple-Negative Breast Cancer. *Mol. Cancer Ther.* **2014**, *13*, 890–901. [CrossRef] [PubMed]

8. Huang, F.; Zhang, Q.; Ma, H.; Lv, Q.; Zhang, T. Expression of glutaminase is upregulated in colorectal cancer and of clinical significance. *Int. J. Clin. Exp. Pathol.* **2014**, *7*, 1093–1100. [PubMed]
9. Szeliga, M.; Bogacińska-Karaś, M.; Różycka, A.; Hilgier, W.; Marquez, J.; Albrecht, J. Silencing of GLS and overexpression of GLS2 genes cooperate in decreasing the proliferation and viability of glioblastoma cells. *Tumor Biol.* **2014**, *35*, 1855–1862. [CrossRef]
10. Martín-Rufián, M.; Nascimento-Gomes, R.; Higuero, A.; Crisma, A.R.; Campos-Sandoval, J.A.; Gomez, F.J.M.; Cardona, C.; Cheng, T.; Lobo, C.; Segura, J.A.; et al. Both GLS silencing and GLS2 overexpression synergize with oxidative stress against proliferation of glioma cells. *J. Mol. Med.* **2014**, *92*, 277–290. [CrossRef] [PubMed]
11. Yu, D.; Shi, X.; Meng, G.; Chen, J.; Yan, C.; Jiang, Y.; Wei, J.; Ding, Y. Kidney-type glutaminase (GLS1) is a biomarker for pathologic diagnosis and prognosis of hepatocellular carcinoma. *Oncotarget* **2015**, *6*, 7619–7631. [CrossRef] [PubMed]
12. Saha, S.K.; Islam, S.R.; Abdullah-Al-Wadud, M.; Ali, F.; Park, K.S. Multiomics Analysis Reveals that GLS and GLS2 Differentially Modulate the Clinical Outcomes of Cancer. *J. Clin. Med.* **2019**, *8*, 355. [CrossRef] [PubMed]
13. Craze, M.L.; Cheung, H.; Jewa, N.; Coimbra, N.; Soria, D.; El-Ansari, R.; Aleskandarany, M.; Cheng, K.W.; Diez-Rodriguez, M.; Nolan, C.C.; et al. MYC regulation of glutamine–proline regulatory axis is key in luminal B breast cancer. *Br. J. Cancer* **2018**, *118*, 258–265. [CrossRef] [PubMed]
14. Polyak, K. Heterogeneity in breast cancer. *J. Clin. Investig.* **2011**, *121*, 3786–3788. [CrossRef]
15. Haukaas, T.H.; Euceda, L.R.; Giskeødegård, G.F.; Lamichhane, S.; Krohn, M.; Jernström, S.; Aure, M.R.; Lingjærde, O.C.; Schlichting, E.; Garred, Ø. Metabolic clusters of breast cancer in relation to gene-and protein expression subtypes. *Cancer Metab.* **2016**, *4*, 12. [CrossRef]
16. Kung, H.-N.; Marks, J.R.; Chi, J.-T. Glutamine Synthetase Is a Genetic Determinant of Cell Type–Specific Glutamine Independence in Breast Epithelia. *PLoS Genet.* **2011**, *7*, e1002229. [CrossRef] [PubMed]
17. Miligy, I.M.; Gorringe, K.L.; Toss, M.S.; Al-Kawaz, A.A.; Simpson, P.; Diez-Rodriguez, M.; Nolan, C.C.; Ellis, I.; Green, A.; Rakha, E.A. Thioredoxin-interacting protein is an independent risk stratifier for breast ductal carcinoma in situ. *Mod. Pathol.* **2018**, *31*, 1807–1815. [CrossRef]
18. Hammond, M.E.H.; Hayes, D.F.; Dowsett, M.; Allred, D.C.; Hagerty, K.L.; Badve, S.; Fitzgibbons, P.L.; Francis, G.; Goldstein, N.S.; Hayes, M.; et al. American Society of Clinical Oncology/College of American Pathologists guideline recommendations for immunohistochemical testing of estrogen and progesterone receptors in breast cancer (unabridged version). *Arch. Pathol. Lab. Med.* **2010**, *134*, e48–e72. [CrossRef] [PubMed]
19. Alfarsi, L.H.; El Ansari, R.; Craze, M.L.; Masisi, B.K.; Ellis, I.O.; Rakha, E.A.; Green, A.R. PPFIA1 expression associates with poor response to endocrine treatment in luminal breast cancer. *BMC Cancer* **2020**, *20*, 1–8. [CrossRef]
20. Curtis, C.; Shah, S.P.; Chin, S.-F.; Turashvili, G.; Rueda, O.M.; Dunning, M.J.; Speed, D.; Lynch, A.G.; Samarajiwa, S.A.; Yuan, Y.; et al. The genomic and transcriptomic architecture of 2000 breast tumours reveals novel subgroups. *Nature* **2012**, *486*, 346–352. [CrossRef]
21. Gao, P.; Tchernyshyov, I.; Chang, T.-C.; Lee, Y.-S.; Kita, K.; Ochi, T.; Zeller, K.I.; De Marzo, A.M.; Van Eyk, J.E.; Mendell, J.T.; et al. c-Myc suppression of miR-23a/b enhances mitochondrial glutaminase expression and glutamine metabolism. *Nat. Cell Biol.* **2009**, *458*, 762–765. [CrossRef] [PubMed]
22. Suzuki, S.; Tanaka, T.; Poyurovsky, M.V.; Nagano, H.; Mayama, T.; Ohkubo, S.; Lokshin, M.; Hosokawa, H.; Nakayama, T.; Suzuki, Y.; et al. Phosphate-activated glutaminase (GLS2), a p53-inducible regulator of glutamine metabolism and reactive oxygen species. *Proc. Natl. Acad. Sci. USA* **2010**, *107*, 7461–7466. [CrossRef]
23. El-Ansari, R.; Craze, M.L.; Alfarsi, L.; Soria, D.; Diez-Rodriguez, M.; Nolan, C.C.; Ellis, I.O.; Rakha, E.A.; Green, A.R. The combined expression of solute carriers is associated with a poor prognosis in highly proliferative ER+ breast cancer. *Breast Cancer Res. Treat.* **2019**, *175*, 27–38. [CrossRef]
24. El-Rehim, D.M.A.; Ball, G.; Pinder, S.E.; Rakha, E.; Paish, C.; Robertson, J.F.; Macmillan, D.; Blamey, R.W.; Ellis, I.O. High- throughput protein expression analysis using tissue microarray technology of a large well-characterised series identifies bi- ologically distinct classes of breast cancer confirming recent cDNA expression analyses. *Int. J. Cancer* **2005**, *116*, 340–350. [CrossRef]
25. Dang, C.V. MYC on the Path to Cancer. *Cell* **2012**, *149*, 22–35. [CrossRef] [PubMed]
26. Aleskandarany, M.; Rakha, E.A.; Macmillan, R.D.; Powe, D.G.; Ellis, I.; Green, A.R. MIB1/Ki-67 labelling index can classify grade 2 breast cancer into two clinically distinct subgroups. *Breast Cancer Res. Treat.* **2010**, *127*, 591–599. [CrossRef]

27. Green, A.R.; Aleskandarany, M.; Agarwal, D.; Elsheikh, S.; Nolan, C.C.; Diez-Rodriguez, M.; Macmillan, R.D.; Ball, G.R.; Caldas, C.; Madhusudan, S.; et al. MYC functions are specific in biological subtypes of breast cancer and confers resistance to endocrine therapy in luminal tumours. *Br. J. Cancer* **2016**, *114*, 917–928. [CrossRef]
28. Dornier, E.; Rabas, N.; Mitchell, L.; Novo, D.; Dhayade, S.; Marco, S.; Mackay, G.; Sumpton, D.; Pallares, M.; Nixon, C.; et al. Glutaminolysis drives membrane trafficking to promote invasiveness of breast cancer cells. *Nat. Commun.* **2017**, *8*, 2255. [CrossRef]
29. Dawson, S.-J.; Rueda, O.M.; Aparicio, S.; Caldas, C. A new genome-driven integrated classification of breast cancer and its implications. *EMBO J.* **2013**, *32*, 617–628. [CrossRef]
30. Song, M.; Kim, S.-H.; Im, C.Y.; Hwang, H.-J. Recent Development of Small Molecule Glutaminase Inhibitors. *Curr. Top. Med. Chem.* **2018**, *18*, 432–443. [CrossRef] [PubMed]
31. Zhang, C.; Liu, J.; Zhao, Y.; Yue, X.; Zhu, Y.; Wang, X.; Wu, H.; Blanco, F.; Li, S.; Bhanot, G.; et al. Glutaminase 2 is a novel negative regulator of small GTPase Rac1 and mediates p53 function in suppressing metastasis. *eLife* **2016**, *5*, e10727. [CrossRef] [PubMed]
32. Wise, D.R.; DeBerardinis, R.J.; Mancuso, A.; Sayed, N.; Zhang, X.-Y.; Pfeiffer, H.K.; Nissim, I.; Daikhin, E.; Yudkoff, M.; McMahon, S.B.; et al. Myc regulates a transcriptional program that stimulates mitochondrial glutaminolysis and leads to glutamine addiction. *Proc. Natl. Acad. Sci. USA* **2008**, *105*, 18782–18787. [CrossRef]
33. Lau, C.-H.E.; Tredwell, G.; Ellis, J.K.; Lam, E.; Keun, H.C. Metabolomic characterisation of the effects of oncogenic PIK3CA transformation in a breast epithelial cell line. *Sci. Rep.* **2017**, *7*, 46079. [CrossRef] [PubMed]
34. Craze, M.L.; El-Ansari, R.; Aleskandarany, M.; Cheng, K.W.; Alfarsi, L.; Masisi, B.; Diez-Rodriguez, M.; Nolan, C.C.; Ellis, I.O.; Rakha, E.A.; et al. Glutamate dehydrogenase (GLUD1) expression in breast cancer. *Breast Cancer Res. Treat.* **2018**, *174*, 79–91. [CrossRef] [PubMed]

2

Application of the 21-Gene Recurrence Score in Patients with Early HR-Positive/HER2-Negative Breast Cancer: Chemotherapy and Survival Rate According to Clinical Risk

Soong June Bae [1,2,†], Sung Gwe Ahn [1,2,†], Jung Hwan Ji [1,2], Chihhao Chu [1,2], Dooreh Kim [3], Janghee Lee [4], Yoon Jin Cha [2,5] and Joon Jeong [1,2,*]

1 Department of Surgery, Gangnam Severance Hospital, Yonsei University College of Medicine, 211 Eonju-ro, Gangnam-gu, Seoul 06273, Korea; mission815815@yuhs.ac (S.J.B.); ASG2004@yuhs.ac (S.G.A.); SHEVCHENCKO@yuhs.ac (J.H.J.); WONYHAPPY@yuhs.ac (C.C.)
2 Institute for Breast Cancer Precision Medicine, Yonsei University College of Medicine, 237 Dogok-ro, Gangnam-gu, Seoul 06230, Korea; YOONCHA@yuhs.ac
3 Department of Surgery, Seoul St. Mary's Hospital, College of Medicine, The Catholic University of Seoul, Seoul 06591, Korea; rlaenfpd@naver.com
4 Department of Surgery, Sacred Heart Hospital, Hallym University, Hwaseong 18450, Korea; Doctorlee85@outlook.kr
5 Department of Pathology, Gangnam Severance Hospital, Yonsei University College of Medicine, 211 Eonju-ro, Gangnam-gu, Seoul 06273, Korea
* Correspondence: gsjjoon@yuhs.ac;
† Soong June Bae and Sung Gwe Ahn have contributed equally to this work.

Simple Summary: It is important to address the influence of 21-gene Recurrence Score (RS) on chemotherapy decision-making stratified by clinical risk in patients with hormone receptor (HR)-positive/human epidermal growth factor receptor 2 (HER2)-negative early breast cancer. Our study presented that the application of the 21-gene RS assay significantly reduced the chemotherapy rate in patients with high clinical risk. Meanwhile, there was no significant difference in the chemotherapy rate according to the implementation of the 21-gene RS assay in those with low clinical risk. Furthermore, we observed no difference in prognosis according to the application of 21-gene RS for either clinical risk. These results suggest that the 21-gene RS could be considered more positively in HR+/HER2- patients with high clinical risk to reduce chemotherapy rates without increasing the occurrence of relapse.

Abstract: We assessed the impact of 21-gene Recurrence Score (RS) assay on chemotherapy decision-making according to binary clinical risk stratification in patients with hormone receptor (HR)-positive/human epidermal growth factor receptor 2 (HER2)-negative early breast cancer. We included patients with tumors measuring 1–5 cm, N0-1, and HR+/HER2- breast cancer who underwent surgery followed by adjuvant treatment. The clinical risk was determined by a modified version of Adjuvant! Online. We performed propensity score matching (PSM) according to the application of 21-gene RS separately in the low and high clinical risk groups. Before PSM, 342 (39.0%) of 878 patients were classified as having high clinical risk. In the high clinical risk group, 21-gene RS showed a significantly reduced chemotherapy rate of 39.3%, without increasing the recurrence. After PSM, the 21-gene RS application significantly reduced chemotherapy rate by 34.0% in 200 patients with high clinical risk (21-gene RS application, 32.0% vs. no 21-gene RS application, 66.0%, $p < 0.001$). There was also no significant difference in RFS according to 21-gene RS status in the high clinical risk group (log-rank test, $p = 0.467$). These results support the usefulness of the 21-gene RS to reduce the chemotherapy rate without adversely affecting prognosis in a high clinical risk group.

Keywords: breast neoplasms; adjuvant treatment; 21-gene recurrence score; chemotherapy; clinical risk

1. Introduction

The 21-gene recurrence score (RS) assay (Oncotype DX, Genomic Heal, Redwood City, CA, USA) is one of the most frequently used commercially available gene-expression assays in breast cancer [1,2]. The 21-gene RS based on Oncotype DX assay was initially developed to quantify the likelihood of distant recurrence in women with hormone receptor (HR)-positive/human epidermal growth factor receptor 2 (HER2)-negative, node-negative breast cancer, with a high RS on a scale of 0 to 100 indicating a higher risk of distant recurrence [3,4]. Although the adjuvant chemotherapy reduced the risk of distant recurrence [5–7], there is a concern that the chemotherapy is unnecessary in the majority of patients with HR-positive, HER2-negative breast cancer. The predictive value of the 21-gene RS for chemotherapy benefit in women with ER-positive, HER2-negative breast cancer has been validated in several prospective clinical trials, including the National Surgical Adjuvant Breast and Bowel Project B-20 trial, Southwest Oncology Group (SWOG)-8814 trial, and Trial Assigning Individualized Options for Treatment (TAILORx) [8–11]. The chemotherapy benefit was observed when the 21-gene RS was high, whether a high 21-gene RS was defined as 31 or higher, or 26 or higher. Based on these results, the National Comprehensive Cancer Network guidelines recommend strong consideration of the 21-gene RS assay to determine the adjuvant chemotherapy in patients with tumor size > 0.5 cm, N0, and HR-positive/HER2-negative breast cancer [12]. Consequently, the use of the 21-gene RS has led to a decline in the chemotherapy rate sparing serious toxicities for HR-positive, HER-negative breast cancer in clinical practice [13–16].

The TAILORx trial was designed to address whether the adjuvant chemotherapy is beneficial for patients with HR+/HER2-, node-negative breast cancer with a midrange RS of 11 to 25, and revealed that adjuvant endocrine therapy alone was not inferior compared to adjuvant chemotherapy plus endocrine therapy [6]. Moreover, the results of a secondary analysis of the TAILORx suggested that the integration of the 21-gene RS and clinical risk provided more accurate information on the prognosis and the chemotherapy benefit of individual patients [17]. However, whether the application of 21-gene RS has an advantage in terms of reduction for adjuvant chemotherapy without adverse survival outcomes stratified by clinical risk has not yet been reported.

This study investigated the chemotherapy rates in the patient groups stratified by clinical risk according to 21-gene RS use. We also analyzed the impact of 21-gene RS on survival outcomes according to clinical risk.

2. Materials and Methods

2.1. Study Population

Following the Good Clinical Practice guidelines and the principles of the Declaration of Helsinki, our study was approved by the Institutional Review Board at Gangnam Severance Hospital, Yonsei University, Seoul, Republic of Korea (IRB no. 3-2021-0042), which waived the requirement for informed consent due to the retrospective study design.

The medical records of patients with breast cancer who underwent breast surgery followed by adjuvant treatment at Gangnam Severance Hospital between January 2014 and December 2018 were reviewed. We identified 878 patients with tumor size of 1–5 cm, pathologic node stage 0–1, HR-positive, HER2-negative breast cancer (Figure 1). The available clinicopathologic data included age, type of surgery, adjuvant treatment including chemotherapy and endocrine therapy, survival, ER status, progesterone receptor (PR) status, HER2 status, Ki-67 levels, histologic type, histologic grade (HG), lymphovascular invasion (LVI) status, pathologic stage, and 21-gene RS. The clinical risk was assessed using the Adjuvant! Algorithm as described in the MINDACT trial [18,19]. We classified the clinical risk as low or high based on the tumor size, nodal metastasis, and HG. Briefly, in N0 patients, the clinical risk was defined as low if the tumor was $\leq$3 cm in diameter and had a low HG, $\leq$2 cm in diameter and had an intermediate HG, or $\leq$1 cm in diameter and had a high HG. In N1 patients, the clinical risk was defined as low if the tumor was $\leq$2 cm in diameter and had a low HG. The clinical risk was defined as high if the low-risk criteria were not met.

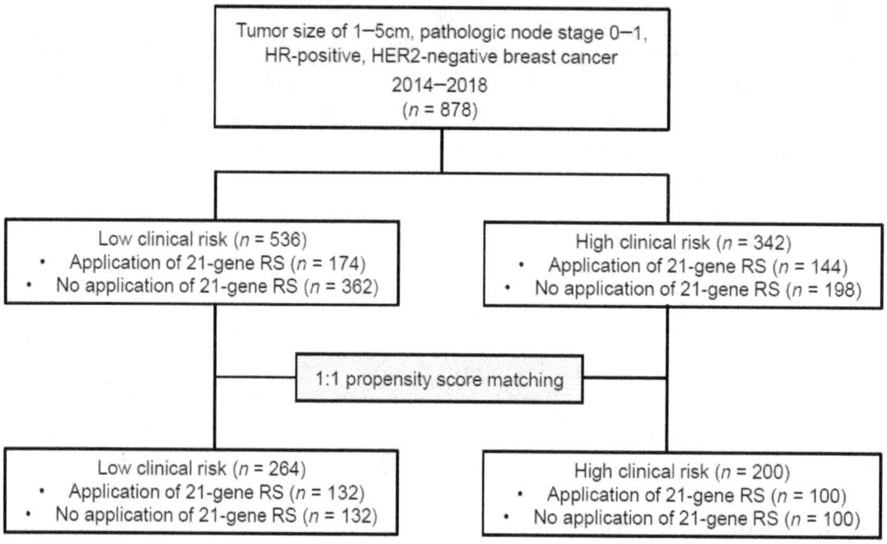

Figure 1. Study flowchart.

Oncotype DX 21-gene RS assays were not routinely performed in our institution because they are not covered by insurance. The clinicians discussed the use of the 21-gene RS with the patient based on the patient's clinicopathologic risk factors as well as their personal preferences. Previous studies, which predicted 21-gene RS results with clinicopathologic data, reported that the age, tumor size, HG, PR, LVI, and Ki-67 were related to the RS [20–22]. Based on these, the Oncotype DX assay was frequently omitted in patients whose clinicopathologic features were either mostly favorable or poor because their 21-gene RS was strongly expected to be low or high. In contrast, the clinicians generally recommended the application of the 21-gene RS assay to patients with intermediate or mixed clinicopathologic data. Consequently, 318 (36.2%) patients underwent 21-gene RS testing.

2.2. Immunohistochemistry

In our immunohistochemistry study, formalin-fixed, paraffin-embedded tissue sections obtained from surgical specimens were stained using appropriate antibodies specific for four markers: ER (1:100 dilution, clone 6F11; Novocastra, Newcastle upon Tyne, UK), PR (clone 16; Novocastra, UK), HER2 (4B5 rabbit monoclonal antibody; Ventana Medical Systems, Tucson, AZ, USA), and Ki-67 (MIB-1; Dako, Glostrup, Denmark). According to the modified Allred system, ER and PR positivity were defined as Allred scores of 3–8, while negativity was defined as Allred scores of 0 and 2, respectively. We considered Allred scores of 7–8 to indicate high expression levels. HER2 status was defined as positive for scores of 3+ and negative for scores of 0 or 1+. Tumors with scores of 2+ were sent for fluorescent in situ hybridization analysis according to the suppliers' protocols (PathVysion kit; Vysis, Downers Grove, IL, USA, or HER2 inform; Ventana). We defined Ki-67 levels $\geq$14% as high.

2.3. 21-Gene RS Assay

The 21-gene RS assay (Oncotype DX, Genomic Health, Redwood City, CA, USA) is based on reverse transcriptase-polymerase chain reaction (RT-PCR) that can be performed on the RNA isolated from formalin-fixed paraffin-embedded (FFPE) tissue [3]. After reviewing the hematoxylin and eosin-stained slides to determine whether sufficient invasive breast cancer was present and whether manual microdissection was indicated, RNA extraction from the unstained sections and the 21-gene RS assay was performed by Genomic Health (Redwood City, CA, USA). This assay evaluates the expression of 16 tumor-associated genes (ER, PGR, BCL2, SCUBE2, GRB7, HER2, Ki-67, STK15, Survivin, CCNB1, MYBL2, MMP11, CTSL2, GSTM1, CD68, BAG1) and 5 reference genes

(ACTB, GAPDH, RPLPO, GUS, TFRC) by using RT-PCR. Based on the expression levels of 21-genes, an algorithm was designed to compute a 21-gene RS for each sample. Quantitative single-gene scores for ER and PR mRNA expression, determined via an RT-PCR, were also provided within the final assay report by Genomic Health.

2.4. Statistical Analysis

Categorical variables were compared by chi-square tests. The chemotherapy rates according to the clinical risk were analyzed by chi-square or Fisher's exact tests. Binary logistic regression analysis was performed to identify independent factors associated with a reduced chemotherapy rate. Variables with $p < 0.10$ in univariable analysis were included in the multivariable analysis. We performed an individual propensity score matching (PSM) analysis in which randomly selected patients with 21-gene RS were paired with comparable patients without 21-gene RS. The one case per one control was selected based on age (≤50 vs. >50 years), histologic type (invasive ductal carcinoma vs. invasive lobular carcinoma vs. others), histologic grade (I or II vs. III), ER (Allred score 0–6 vs. 7–8), PR (Allred score 0–6 vs. 7–8), Ki-67 (<14% vs. ≥14%), pathologic T stage (1 vs. 2), and pathologic *n* stage (0 vs. 1). Recurrence-free survival (RFS) was measured as the period from the date of breast cancer surgery to first breast cancer recurrence, including loco-regional and distant recurrences. The Kaplan–Meier method with a log-rank test was used to calculate the RFS and compare the results between groups. All analyses were performed using IBM SPSS Statistics for Windows, version 23.0 (IBM Corp.; Armonk, NY, USA) and SAS (version 9.3, SAS Inc., Cary, NC, USA). The statistical significance was defined as $p < 0.05$.

3. Results

3.1. Baseline Characteristics

The median age of all patients was 52 years (range, 25–87). Among all patients, 536 (61.0%) and 342 (39.0%) were at low and high clinical risk, respectively (Figure 1). As expected, patients with high clinical risk had more poor prognostic factors such as high HG, Ki-67, pathologic T stage, pathologic *n* stage, LVI, and low PR expression compared to those in patients with low clinical risk. The chemotherapy rate (52.6% vs. 13.2%, $p < 0.001$), and implementation of 21-gene RS (42.1% vs. 32.5%, $p = 0.004$) were significantly higher in patients with high clinical risk. Moreover, patients with high clinical risk and 21-gene RS had favorable clinicopathologic factors, while the reverse trend was observed in patients with low clinical risk (Table S1). Meanwhile, the distributions of categorical 21-gene RS did not differ according to clinical risk (Figure S1); the results were consistent using different 21-gene RS cutoffs used in clinical trials; namely: low (<18 or <11), intermediate (18–30 or 11–25), and high (≥31 or >25).

To minimize the baseline confounders affecting the chemotherapy rate, a one-to-one PSM between patients with or without 21-gene RS was carried out separately in the low and high clinical risk groups. Of 464 patients (median age, 52 years; range, 25–87) in the PSM cohort, 264 (56.9%) showed low clinical risk, while 200 (43.1%) showed high clinical risk. After PSM, all variables were well balanced according to the implementation of 21-gene RS in both clinical risk groups (Table 1).

Table 1. Baseline characteristics according to clinical risk stratified by 21-gene RS use in the propensity-score matched cohort.

Characteristics	Low Clinical Risk (*n* = 264)				High Clinical Risk (*n* = 200)			
	Patients with 21-Gene RS (*n* = 132)	Patients without 21-Gene RS (*n* = 132)	Total (*n* = 264)	*p*-Value	Patients with 21-Gene RS (*n* = 100)	Patients without 21-Gene RS (*n* = 100)	Total (*n* = 200)	*p*-Value
Age (median)	50	50.5	50	0.405	49	55	51	0.198
Age (range)	25-81	32-86	25-86		27-87	33-75	27-87	
Age (y)				0.902				0.777
≤50	70 (53.0%)	71 (53.8%)	141 (53.4%)		49 (49.0%)	47 (47.0%)	96 (48.0%)	
>50	62 (47.0%)	61 (46.2%)	123 (46.6%)		51 (51.0%)	53 (53.0%)	104 (52.0%)	
Histologic type				>0.999				>0.999
IDC	128 (97.0%)	127 (96.2%)	255 (96.6%)		90 (90.0%)	89 (89.0%)	179 (89.5%)	
ILC	2 (1.5%)	2 (1.5%)	4 (1.5%)		8 (8.0%)	9 (9.0%)	17 (8.5%)	
Others *	2 (1.5%)	3 (2.3%)	5 (1.9%)		2 (2.0%)	2 (2.0%)	4 (2.0%)	

Table 1. *Cont.*

Characteristics	Low Clinical Risk (n = 264)				High Clinical Risk (n = 200)			
	Patients with 21-Gene RS (n = 132)	Patients without 21-Gene RS (n = 132)	Total (n = 264)	p-Value	Patients with 21-Gene RS (n = 100)	Patients without 21-Gene RS (n = 100)	Total (n = 200)	p-Value
ER, Allred				0.848				0.010
7–8	117 (88.6%)	116 (87.9%)	233 (88.3%)		90 (90.0%)	96 (96.0%)	186 (93.0%)	
0–6	15 (11.4%)	16 (12.1%)	31 (11.7%)		10 (10.0%)	4 (4.0%)	14 (7.0%)	
PR, Allred				0.318				0.671
7–8	73 (55.3%)	81 (61.4%)	154 (58.3%)		52 (52.0%)	55 (55.0%)	107 (53.5%)	
0–6	59 (44.7%)	51 (38.6%)	110 (41.7%)		48 (48.0%)	45 (45.0%)	93 (46.5%)	
Histologic grade				>0.999				0.732
1 or 2	132 (100%)	132 (100%)	264 (100%)		77 (77.0%)	79 (79.0%)	156 (78.0%)	
3	0	0	0		23 (23.0%)	21 (21.0%)	44 (22.0%)	
LVI †				>0.999				0.884
Yes	12 (9.1%)	12 (9.1%)	24 (9.1%)		37 (37.0%)	38 (38.0%)	75 (37.5%)	
No	120 (90.9%)	120 (90.9%)	240 (90.9%)		63 (63.0%)	62 (62.0%)	125 (62.5%)	
Ki-67				0.295				0.768
≥14	32 (24.2%)	25 (18.9%)	57 (21.6%)		65 (65.0%)	63 (63.0%)	128 (64.0%)	
<14	100 (75.8%)	107 (81.1%)	207 (78.4%)		35 (35.0%)	37 (37.0%)	72 (36.0%)	
T stage				>0.999				0.556
1	129 (97.7%)	128 (97.0%)	257 (97.3%)		38 (38.0%)	34 (34.0%)	72 (36.0%)	
2	3 (2.3%)	4 (3.0%)	7 (2.7%)		62 (62.0%)	66 (66.0%)	128 (64.0%)	
n stage				>0.999				0.888
0	122 (92.4%)	122 (92.4%)	244 (92.4%)		52 (52.0%)	51 (51.0%)	103 (51.5%)	
1	10 (7.6%)	10 (7.6%)	20 (7.6%)		48 (48.0%)	49 (49.0%)	97 (48.5%)	

* Others (n = 9) included mucinous (n = 5), tubular (n = 2), and papillary (n = 2) breast cancers. † Missing values. Abbreviations: RS, recurrence score; IDC, invasive ductal carcinoma; ILC, invasive lobular carcinoma; ER, estrogen receptor; PR, progesterone receptor; LVI, lymphovascular invasion.

3.2. *Chemotherapy Rates*

Among the 536 patients with low clinical risk, 41 of 362 (11.3%) without 21-gene RS and 30 of 174 (17.2%) with 21-gene RS received chemotherapy (p = 0.059). Among patients with node-negative and low clinical risk, 27 of 344 (7.8%) without 21-gene RS and 30 of 161 (18.6%) with 21-gene RS received chemotherapy (p < 0.001). Among patients with node-positive and low clinical risk, 14 of 18 (77.8%) without 21-gene RS and none of the patients with 21-gene RS received chemotherapy (p < 0.001, Figure 2A). Meanwhile, among the 342 patients with high clinical risk, 137 of 198 (69.2%) without 21-gene RS and 43 of 144 (29.9%) with 21-gene RS received chemotherapy (p < 0.001). Among patients with the node-negative disease and high clinical risk, 51 of 91 (56.0%) without 21-gene RS and 30 of 91 (33.0%) with 21-gene RS received chemotherapy (p = 0.002). Among patients with node-positive disease and high clinical risk, 86 of 107 (80.4%) without 21-gene RS and 13 of 53 (24.5%) with 21-gene RS received chemotherapy (p < 0.001, Figure 2B). In the multivariable analysis, the implementation of the 21-gene RS was an independent factor associated with a reduced chemotherapy rate in the high clinical risk group (odds ratio (OR) 0.196; 95% confidence interval (CI), 0.115–0.334; p < 0.001, Table 2). Furthermore, the implementation of 21-gene RS was significantly associated with a reduced chemotherapy rate in both N0 (OR 0.357; 95% CI, 0.176–0.724; p = 0.004) and N1 (OR 0.085; 95% CIs, 0.036–0.200; p < 0.001) disease.

After PSM, the chemotherapy rates did not differ significantly according to 21-gene RS status in women with low clinical risk (15.2% (20 of 132) in patients without 21-gene RS vs. 13.6% (18 of 132) in patients with 21-gene RS, p = 0.726) and those with low clinical risk and node-negative disease (11.5% (14 of 122)in patients without 21-gene RS vs. 14.8% (18 of 122) in patients with 21-gene RS, p = 0.448, Figure 3A). Otherwise, use of the 21-gene RS was associated with significantly reduced chemotherapy rates in women with low clinical risk and node-positive disease (60.0% (6 of 10)in patients without 21-gene RS vs. none in patients with 21-gene RS, p = 0.011). Likewise, use of the 21-gene RS was associated with a significantly decreased chemotherapy rate in women with high clinical risk (66.0% (66 of 100) in patients without 21-gene RS vs. 32.0% (32 of 100) in patients with 21-gene RS, p < 0.001), high clinical risk and node-negative disease (60.8% (31 of 51) in patients without 21-gene RS vs. 38.5% (20 of 52) in patients with 21-gene RS, p = 0.023), and high clinical risk and node-positive disease (71.4% (35 of 49) in patients without 21-gene RS vs. 25.0% (12 of 48) in patients with 21-gene RS, $p < 0.001$, Figure 3B).

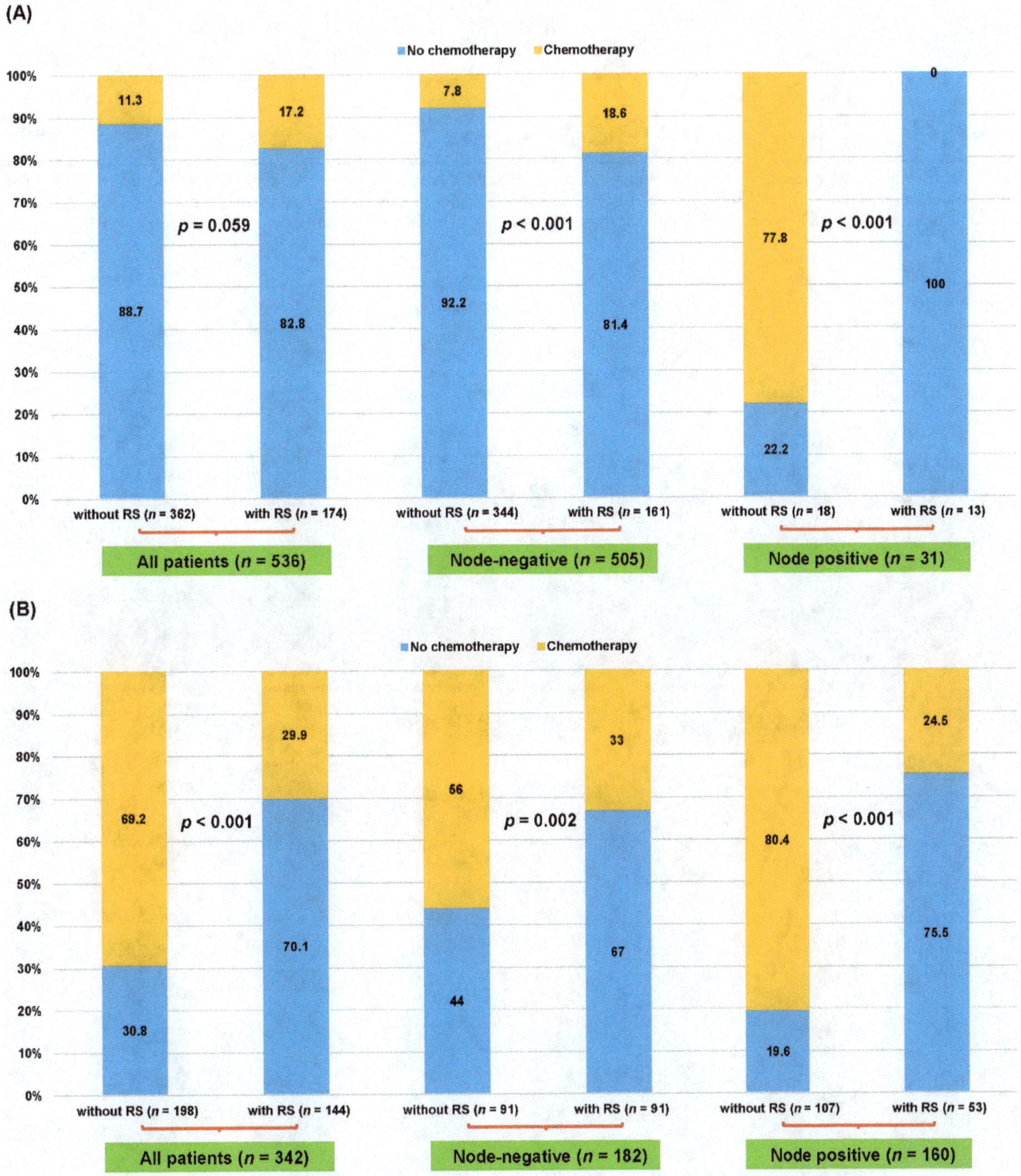

Figure 2. Chemotherapy rates according to the application of the 21-gene Recurrence Score (RS) assay in the entire cohort. Chemotherapy rates according to the application of the 21-gene RS assay stratified by clinical risk in patients with (**A**) low clinical risk and (**B**) high clinical risk. Chi-square test, significance level of 0.05.

Table 2. Adjusted odds ratios (ORs) and 95% confidential intervals (CIs) of 21-gene RS for the implementation of chemotherapy in patients with high clinical risk among the entire cohort.

21-Gene RS	Multivariable Analysis					
	All Patients		Node-Negative		Node-Positive	
	Odds Ratio (95% CIs)	p-Value *	Odds Ratio (95% CIs)	p-Value †	Odds Ratio (95% CIs)	p-Value ‡
No	Ref.		Ref.		Ref.	
Yes	0.196 (0.115–0.334)	<0.001	0.357 (0.176–0.724)	0.004	0.085 (0.036–0.200)	<0.001

Abbreviations: ER, estrogen receptor; PR, progesterone receptor; LVI, lymphovascular invasion; RS, recurrence score. * Covariates for multivariable models were histologic type, ER, PR, histologic grade, LVI, Ki-67, and n stage. † Covariates for multivariable models were histologic type, ER, PR, histologic grade, Ki-67, and T stage. ‡ Covariates for multivariable models were ER, PR, Ki-67, and T stage.

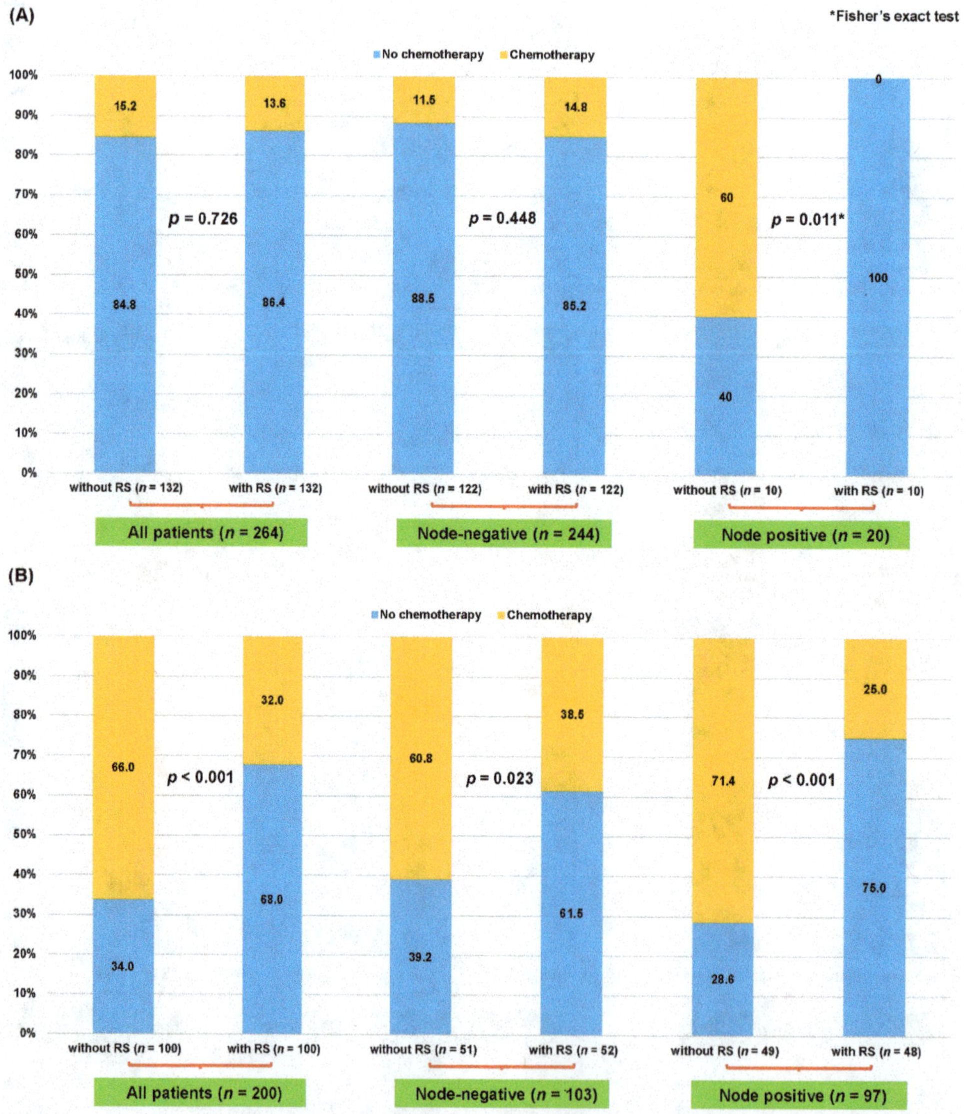

Figure 3. Chemotherapy rates according to the application of the 21-gene Recurrence Score (RS) assay in the propensity-Scheme 21-gene RS assay stratified by clinical risk in patients with **(A)** low clinical risk and **(B)** high clinical risk. Chi-square test, significance level 0.05. * Fisher's exact test, significance level of 0.05.

3.3. Clinical Outcomes

In the entire cohort, there were 14 recurrence events and no deaths during the median follow-up of 42 months (range, 1–83 months). There was no significant difference in RFS according to 21-gene RS status (log-rank test, $p = 0.363$; Figure 4A). In addition, RFS did not differ according to 21-gene RS status in both groups stratified by clinical risk ($p = 0.489$ in the low clinical risk group and $p = 0.736$ in the high clinical risk group, Figure 4B,C). In the PSM cohort, there were eight recurrence events and no deaths during the median follow-up of 45 months (range, 1–83 months). Likewise, there was no significant difference in RFS according to 21-gene RS status (log-rank test, $p = 0.850$ in the PSM cohort, log-rank test, $p = 0.583$ in the PSM cohort with low clinical risk, and $p = 0.467$ in the PSM cohort with high clinical risk; Figure 4D,F).

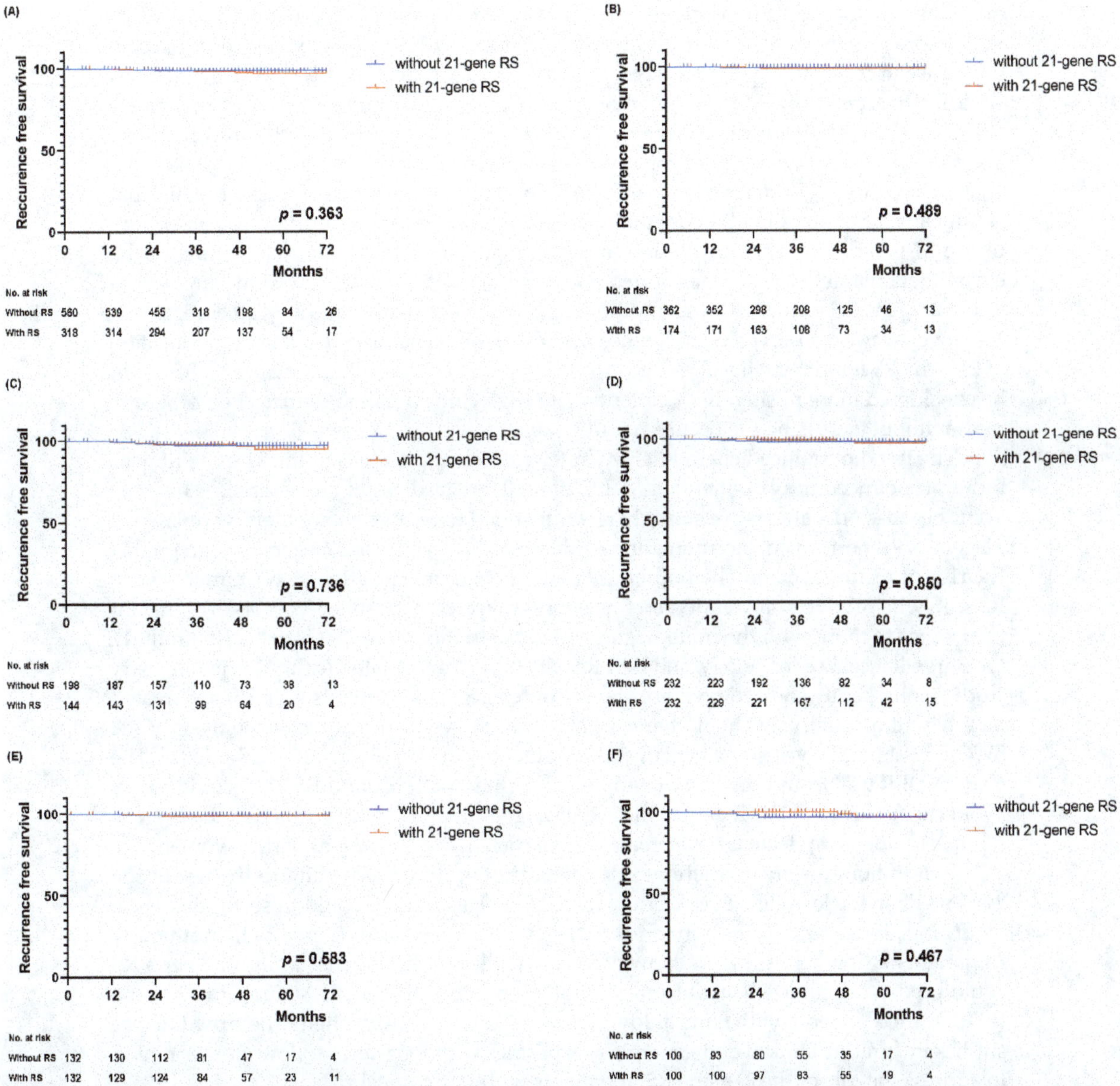

Figure 4. Recurrence-free survival (RFS) according to the application of the 21-gene Recurrence Score (RS) assay. Kaplan–Meier curves of RFS according to the application of the 21-gene RS (**A**) in all patients, (**B**) in all patients with low clinical risk, and (**C**) in all patients with high clinical risk, as well as (**D**) in the entire propensity-score matching (PSM) cohort, (**E**) in the PSM cohort with low clinical risk, and (**F**) in the PSM cohort with high clinical risk. Log-rank test, significance level of 0.05.

4. Discussion

Before the era of genomic assays, aggressive chemotherapy was considered for patients at a high clinical risk. However, within node-positive, HR+ breast cancer, several multigene assays revealed that tumors with favorable genomic profiles showed a good prognosis despite a high clinical risk [9,23]. Thus, many investigators wondered assessed whether chemotherapy could be spared in patients with discordant clinical and genomic risk profiles. Concerning this issue, the MINDACT investigators reported no substantial benefit of chemotherapy in patients with clinical high/genomic low risk in terms of distant RFS [12,19]. Moreover, secondary analysis of the TAILOR-X trial showed that the addition of chemotherapy was associated with lower rates of distant recurrence among women with RS of 21–25 and low clinical risk [11].

In this context, it is important to address the influence of 21-gene RS on chemotherapy decision-making according to clinical risk stratification. First, we speculated that 21-gene RS is more helpful in patients with high clinical risk. Although there was no significant difference in chemotherapy rates according to the application of the 21-gene RS in the low clinical risk group, use of the 21-gene RS reduced the chemotherapy rate by approximately 30–40% in the high clinical risk group. Furthermore, the results of the multivariable analysis showed that the application of 21-gene RS was an independent factor for reduced chemotherapy rate in patients at high clinical risk. However, the concerns remain that significant differences in clinicopathologic factors associated with prognosis according to the 21-gene RS in each of the low and high clinical risk groups may influence the chemotherapy rate. Thus, we performed PSM analysis, with similar results: the application of the 21-gene RS reduced the chemotherapy rate by 34% in patients at high clinical risk. Moreover, we also observed no difference in survival outcomes according to the application of 21-gene RS for either clinical risk group. These results suggest that the 21-gene RS could be considered more positively in patients with high clinical risk to reduce chemotherapy rates without increasing the occurrence of relapse.

The trend of reduced chemotherapy rate with the application of the 21-gene RS was more pronounced in N1 patients than N0 patients, regardless of clinical risk. This may occur because N1 patients are strongly recommended to receive chemotherapy unless the 21-gene RS is performed. Accumulating evidence indicates that the 21-gene RS can predict the risk of recurrence and chemotherapy benefit even in N1 patients. N1 patients with RS < 18 who received only endocrine therapy showed comparable 9-year risks of distant recurrence to those with the node-negative disease in the transATAC trial [24]. Similarly, the Surveillance, Epidemiology, and End Results (SEER) and Clalit Health Services registry studies consistently showed favorable 5-year outcomes in N1 patients with RS <18 treated largely without adjuvant chemotherapy [25,26]. Moreover, a retrospective analysis of the SWOG S8814 trial revealed no benefit of chemotherapy in N1 patients with RS < 18 [9]. The RxPONDER trial found that postmenopausal women with N1 and RS $\leq$ 25 could safely avoid chemotherapy [27]. Together, these data suggest that it is worth applying the 21-gene RS in N1 patients to decrease overtreatment, particularly in postmenopausal women.

In addition, the chemotherapy rates also did not differ according to the use of the 21-gene RS in the low clinical risk group after PSM. This finding could raise another issue regarding the necessity of applying the 21-gene RS assay to determine chemotherapy in patients at low clinical risk. However, it is well established that a high 21-gene RS could predict the clinical benefit from chemotherapy: in the TAILOR-X study, the 21-gene RS identified patients with clinical low risk who benefited from chemotherapy. Further studies integrating clinical and genomic risk profiles with long-term follow are warranted to address the role of the 21-gene RS in patients with low clinical risk.

Our study has a major limitation inherent in retrospective analysis from a single institution with a small proportion of patients who received Oncotype DX assay. In addition, the median follow-up period was relatively short (42 months and 45 months in the PSM cohort), considering that disease-related events occur steadily 5 years after diagnosis in HR+/HER2- breast cancer [28]. Few studies have assessed the survival benefit according to the implementation of the 21-gene RS. To our best knowledge, only one recent study analyzing SEER registry data reported that the application of the 21-gene RS was associated with better breast cancer-specific and overall survivals [29]. However, that study also has limitations, including a median follow-up period of only 36 months and the fact that chemotherapy tended to be underreported in SEER data [30]. Another limitation of the present study was that the chemotherapy decision in our cohort may differ from those made in clinical practice in the future because most patients in our study received treatment before the results of the TAILORx and RxPONDER trials were presented. Lastly, in that era, the guideline for adjuvant treatment was unclear in patients with intermediate RS; thus, the adjuvant treatments may have differed depending on the physicians, which may have affected the clinical outcomes. Therefore, further studies with accurate data collection for adjuvant treatment guided by 21-gene RS and a sufficient follow-up period are needed to clarify whether the application of 21-gene RS influences survival benefits.

5. Conclusions

In summary, this is the first study to analyze the usefulness of the 21-gene RS according to clinical risk in the subset of patients with tumor size 1–5 cm, N0-1, HR+/HER2- breast cancer, in terms of chemotherapy rate and survival. The application of the 21-gene RS reduced chemotherapy rates, particularly in patients with high clinical risk. In contrast, it did not alter the chemotherapy rate in patients with low clinical risk in the case-matched cohort. Furthermore, the survival outcomes according to implementation of the 21-gene RS did not differ, even in patients at high clinical risk. These data suggest that the 21-gene RS should be considered positively to reduce overtreatment without adverse prognosis in patients with high clinical risk. For the patients with low clinical risk, further studies with long-term follow-up data are warranted to address the role of the 21-gene RS, which could offer chemotherapy for patients with high genomic risk.

Author Contributions: Study concept and design: S.J.B., S.G.A., J.J. Acquisition, analysis or interpretation of data: S.J.B., S.G.A., J.H.J., C.C., D.K., J.L., Y.J.C., statistical analysis: S.J.B., S.G.A., Y.J.C., drafting of the manuscript: S.J.B., S.G.A., J.J. Co-first author: S.J.B., S.G.A. All authors have read and agreed to the published version of the manuscript.

References

1. Győrffy, B.; Hatzis, C.; Sanft, T.; Hofstatter, E.; Aktas, B.; Pusztai, L. Multigene prognostic tests in breast cancer: Past, present, future. *Breast Cancer Res.* **2015**, *17*, 11. [CrossRef] [PubMed]
2. Choi, I.S.; Jung, J.; Kim, B.H.; Oh, S.; Kim, J.; Park, J.H.; Park, J.H.; Hwang, K.T. The 21-gene recurrence score assay and prediction of chemotherapy benefit: A propensity score-matched analysis of the seer database. *Cancers* **2020**, *12*, 1829. [CrossRef] [PubMed]
3. Paik, S.; Shak, S.; Tang, G.; Kim, C.; Baker, J.; Cronin, M.; Baehner, F.L.; Walker, M.G.; Watson, D.; Park, T.; et al. A multigene assay to predict recurrence of tamoxifen-treated, node-negative breast cancer. *N. Engl. J. Med.* **2004**, *351*, 2817–2826. [CrossRef] [PubMed]
4. Kwa, M.; Makris, A.; Esteva, F.J. Clinical utility of gene-expression signatures in early stage breast cancer. *Nat. Rev. Clin. Oncol.* **2017**, *14*, 595–610. [CrossRef]
5. Fisher, B.; Dignam, J.; Wolmark, N.; DeCillis, A.; Emir, B.; Wickerham, D.L.; Bryant, J.; Dimitrov, N.V.; Abramson, N.; Atkins, J.N.; et al. Tamoxifen and chemotherapy for lymph node-negative, estrogen receptor-positive breast cancer. *J. Natl. Cancer Inst.* **1997**, *89*, 1673–1682. [CrossRef]
6. Early Breast Cancer Trialists' Collaborative Group (EBCTCG). Effects of chemotherapy and hormonal therapy for early breast cancer on recurrence and 15-year survival: An overview of the randomised trials. *Lancet* **2005**, *365*, 1687–1717. [CrossRef]
7. Peto, R.; Davies, C.; Godwin, J.; Gray, R.; Pan, H.C.; Clarke, M.; Cutter, D.; Darby, S.; McGale, P.; Taylor, C.; et al. Comparisons between different polychemotherapy regimens for early breast cancer: Meta-analyses of long-term outcome among 100,000 women in 123 randomised trials. *Lancet* **2012**, *379*, 432–444.

8. Paik, S.; Tang, G.; Shak, S.; Kim, C.; Baker, J.; Kim, W.; Cronin, M.; Baehner, F.L.; Watson, D.; Bryant, J.; et al. Gene expression and benefit of chemotherapy in women with node-negative, estrogen receptor-positive breast cancer. *J. Clin. Oncol.* **2006**, *24*, 3726–3734. [CrossRef]
9. Albain, K.S.; Barlow, W.E.; Shak, S.; Hortobagyi, G.N.; Livingston, R.B.; Yeh, I.T.; Ravdin, P.; Bugarini, R.; Baehner, F.L.; Davidson, N.E.; et al. Prognostic and predictive value of the 21-gene recurrence score assay in postmenopausal women with node- positive, oestrogen-receptor-positive breast cancer on chemotherapy: A retrospective analysis of a randomised trial. *Lancet Oncol.* **2010**, *11*, 55–65. [CrossRef]
10. Sparano, J.A.; Paik, S. Development of the 21-gene assay and its application in clinical practice and clinical trials. *J. Clin. Oncol.* **2008**, *26*, 721–728. [CrossRef]
11. Sparano, J.A.; Gray, R.J.; Makower, D.F.; Pritchard, K.I.; Albain, K.S.; Hayes, D.F.; Geyer, C.E., Jr.; Dees, E.C.; Goetz, M.P.; Olson, J.A., Jr.; et al. Adjuvant chemotherapy guided by a 21-gene expression assay in breast cancer. *N. Engl. J. Med.* **2018**, *379*, 111–121. [CrossRef]
12. Telli, M.L.; Gradishar, W.J.; Ward, J.H. Nccn guidelines updates: Breast cancer. *J. Natl. Compr. Cancer Netw.* **2019**, *17*, 552–555.
13. Hassett, M.J.; Silver, S.M.; Hughes, M.E.; Blayney, D.W.; Edge, S.B.; Herman, J.G.; Hudis, C.A.; Marcom, P.K.; Pettinga, J.E.; Share, D.; et al. Adoption of gene expression profile testing and association with use of chemotherapy among women with breast cancer. *J. Clin. Oncol.* **2012**, *30*, 2218–2226. [CrossRef]
14. Kurian, A.W.; Bondarenko, I.; Jagsi, R.; Friese, C.R.; McLeod, M.C.; Hawley, S.T.; Hamilton, A.S.; Ward, K.C.; Hofer, T.P.; Katz, S.J. Recent trends in chemotherapy use and oncologists' treatment recommendations for early-stage breast cancer. *J. Natl. Cancer Inst.* **2018**, *110*, 493–500. [CrossRef]
15. Cognetti, F.; Masetti, R.; Fabi, A.; Bianchi, G.; Santini, D.; Rognone, A.; Catania, G.; Angelucci, D.; Naso, G.; Giuliano, M.; et al. Pondx: Real-life utilization and decision impact of the 21-gene assay on clinical practice in italy. *NPJ Breast Cancer* **2021**, *7*, 47. [CrossRef]
16. Curtit, E.; Vannetzel, J.M.; Darmon, J.C.; Roche, S.; Bourgeois, H.; Dewas, S.; Catala, S.; Mereb, E.; Fanget, Ç.F.; Genet, D.; et al. Results of pondx, a prospective multicenter study of the oncotype dx breast cancer assay: Real-life utilization and decision impact in french clinical practice. *Breast* **2019**, *44*, 39–45. [CrossRef]
17. Sparano, J.A.; Gray, R.J.; Ravdin, P.M.; Makower, D.F.; Pritchard, K.I.; Albain, K.S.; Hayes, D.F.; Geyer, C.E., Jr.; Dees, E.C.; Goetz, M.P.; et al. Clinical and genomic risk to guide the use of adjuvant therapy for breast cancer. *N. Engl. J. Med.* **2019**, *380*, 2395–2405. [CrossRef]
18. Mook, S.; Schmidt, M.K.; Rutgers, E.J.; van de Velde, A.O.; Visser, O.; Rutgers, S.M.; Armstrong, N.; van't Veer, L.J.; Ravdin, P.M. Calibration and discriminatory accuracy of prognosis calculation for breast cancer with the online adjuvant! Program: A hospital-based retrospective cohort study. *Lancet Oncol.* **2009**, *10*, 1070–1076. [CrossRef]
19. Cardoso, F.; van't Veer, L.J.; Bogaerts, J.; Slaets, L.; Viale, G.; Delaloge, S.; Pierga, J.Y.; Brain, E.; Causeret, S.; DeLorenzi, M.; et al. 70-gene signature as an aid to treatment decisions in early-stage breast cancer. *N. Engl. J. Med.* **2016**, *375*, 717–729. [CrossRef]
20. Allison, K.H.; Kandalaft, P.L.; Sitlani, C.M.; Dintzis, S.M.; Gown, A.M. Routine pathologic parameters can predict oncotype dx recurrence scores in subsets of er positive patients: Who does not always need testing? *Breast Cancer Res. Treat.* **2012**, *131*, 413–424. [CrossRef]
21. Orucevic, A.; Bell, J.L.; McNabb, A.P.; Heidel, R.E. Oncotype dx breast cancer recurrence score can be predicted with a novel nomogram using clinicopathologic data. *Breast Cancer Res. Treat.* **2017**, *163*, 51–61. [CrossRef]
22. Yoo, S.H.; Kim, T.Y.; Kim, M.; Lee, K.H.; Lee, E.; Lee, H.B.; Moon, H.G.; Han, W.; Noh, D.Y.; Han, S.W.; et al. Development of a nomogram to predict the recurrence score of 21-gene prediction assay in hormone receptor-positive early breast cancer. *Clin. Breast Cancer* **2020**, *20*, 98–107.e101. [CrossRef]
23. Mook, S.; Schmidt, M.K.; Viale, G.; Pruneri, G.; Eekhout, I.; Floore, A.; Glas, A.M.; Bogaerts, J.; Cardoso, F.; Piccart- Gebhart, M.J.; et al. The 70-gene prognosis-signature predicts disease outcome in breast cancer patients with 1-3 positive lymph nodes in an independent validation study. *Breast Cancer Res. Treat.* **2009**, *116*, 295–302. [CrossRef]
24. Dowsett, M.; Cuzick, J.; Wale, C.; Forbes, J.; Mallon, E.A.; Salter, J.; Quinn, E.; Dunbier, A.; Baum, M.; Buzdar, A.; et al. Prediction of risk of distant recurrence using the 21-gene recurrence score in node-negative and node-positive postmenopausal patients with breast cancer treated with anastrozole or tamoxifen: A transatac study. *J. Clin. Oncol.* **2010**, *28*, 1829–1834. [CrossRef]
25. Roberts, M.C.; Miller, D.P.; Shak, S.; Petkov, V.I. Breast cancer-specific survival in patients with lymph node-positive hormone receptor-positive invasive breast cancer and oncotype dx recurrence score results in the seer database. *Breast Cancer Res. Treat.* **2017**, *163*, 303–310. [CrossRef]

26. Stemmer, S.M.; Steiner, M.; Rizel, S.; Geffen, D.B.; Nisenbaum, B.; Peretz, T.; Soussan-Gutman, L.; Bareket-Samish, A.; Isaacs, K.; Rosengarten, O.; et al. Clinical outcomes in er+ her2- node-positive breast cancer patients who were treated according to the recurrence score results: Evidence from a large prospectively designed registry. *NPJ Breast Cancer* **2017**, *3*, 32. [CrossRef]
27. Mamounas, E.P.; Russell, C.A.; Lau, A.; Turner, M.P.; Albain, K.S. Clinical relevance of the 21-gene recurrence score((r)) assay in treatment decisions for patients with node-positive breast cancer in the genomic era. *NPJ Breast Cancer* **2018**, *4*, 27. [CrossRef]
28. Pan, H.; Gray, R.; Braybrooke, J.; Davies, C.; Taylor, C.; McGale, P.; Peto, R.; Pritchard, K.I.; Bergh, J.; Dowsett, M.; et al. 20-year risks of breast-cancer recurrence after stopping endocrine therapy at 5 years. *N. Engl. J. Med.* **2017**, *377*, 1836–1846. [CrossRef]
29. Zhang, L.; Hsieh, M.C.; Petkov, V.; Yu, Q.; Chiu, Y.W.; Wu, X.C. Trend and survival benefit of oncotype dx use among female hormone receptor-positive breast cancer patients in 17 seer registries, 2004–2015. *Breast Cancer Res. Treat.* **2020**, *180*, 491–501. [CrossRef]
30. Noone, A.M.; Lund, J.L.; Mariotto, A.; Cronin, K.; McNeel, T.; Deapen, D.; Warren, J.L. Comparison of seer treatment data with medicare claims. *Med. Care* **2016**, *54*, e55–e64. [CrossRef]

3

Invasion and Metastasis as a Central Hallmark of Breast Cancer

Trishna Saha [1,2], Jonathan Solomon [1], Abraham O. Samson [2,*] and Hava Gil-Henn [1,*]

[1] Cell Migration and Invasion Laboratory, The Azrieli Faculty of Medicine, Bar-Ilan University, Safed 1311502, Israel; trishna.saha27@gmail.com (T.S.); yhontn@gmail.com (J.S.)
[2] Drug Discovery Laboratory, The Azrieli Faculty of Medicine, Bar-Ilan University, Safed 1311502, Israel
* Correspondence: Avraham.Samson@biu.ac.il (A.O.S.); Hava.Henn@biu.ac.il (H.G.-H.)

Abstract: Hanahan and Weinberg introduced the "hallmarks of cancer" and typified essential biological abilities acquired by human cancer. Since then, a growing understanding of hallmark principles associated with breast cancer has assisted knowledge-based therapeutics development; however, despite the rapidly increasing number of targeted therapeutics, enduring disease-free responses for most forms of breast cancer is rare. Invasion and metastasis are the most defining feature of breast cancer malignancy and the leading cause of patient mortality. Hence, we propose a modified hallmarks model adapted to breast cancer, in which invasion and metastasis are shifted to the center of attention, thereby emphasizing it as a potentially superior therapeutic target. Although the scientific community highly appreciates the importance of the invasion and metastasis hallmark, as can be demonstrated by the growing number of publications on breast cancer metastasis, very few clinical trials concentrate on testing anti-metastasis inhibitors and even fewer trials focus on inhibitors for breast cancer metastasis. Here, we discuss the obstacles of applying research on invasion and metastasis therapeutics into the clinic and present current developments that could provide a potential solution to this dilemma.

Keywords: breast cancer; hallmarks; invasion and metastasis; therapeutics; association score

---

1. Introduction

Breast cancer is the most common neoplasm and the second leading cause of death in women [1,2].

It is a complex and highly heterogeneous disease, encompassing multiple tumor subtypes, each characterized by a different morphology, histopathological features and cellular markers, gene expression profiles, outcomes and response to systemic therapies [3–5]. Because of its complexity, immunohistochemical markers, together with clinicopathological criteria such as tumor size and grade, lymph node involvement and histological type, are commonly used for prognosis, recurrence prediction and therapeutic strategy selection [6,7].

Breast tumor subtypes are classically defined according to hormonal and growth factor responsiveness. The main clinically relevant receptors in this regard are estrogen receptor (ER), progesterone receptor (PR) and human epidermal growth factor receptor 2 (HER2). Breast tumors are thus divided into four main subtypes based on immunohistochemical properties and hormone receptor (HR) status [3]: (1) $HR^+/HER2^+$, tumors which are sensitive to either estrogen or progesterone and present HER2 receptors, (2) $HR^+ \backslash HER2^-$, tumors which are sensitive to either estrogen or progesterone but lack HER2 receptors, (3) $HR^- \backslash HER2^+$, tumors which express HER2 receptors, but lack hormone receptors and (4) $HR^- \backslash HER2^-$, also known as triple-negative breast cancer (TNBC).

In 2000, Weinberg and Hanahan defined six hallmarks of cancer: sustaining proliferative signaling, evading growth suppressors, resisting cell death, enabling replicative immortality, inducing angiogenesis and activating invasion and metastasis [8]. In 2011, the authors defined two additional emerging hallmarks, reprogramming of energy metabolism and evading immune destruction and two enabling hallmarks, genome instability and mutation and tumor-promoting inflammation [9]. Together, these constitute "the ten hallmarks of cancer". Here, we discuss each of these ten hallmarks and their relevance to breast cancer.

2. The Hallmarks of Breast Cancer

2.1. Sustaining Proliferative Signaling

Normal tissues control the production and release of growth signals that regulate proper entry and progression through the cell cycle and regular tissue architecture and function. Cancer cells de-regulate these growth signals and, by doing so, acquire the capability to sustain proliferative signaling in several ways. For example, cancer cells can enhance autocrine stimulation [10,11] or paracrine stimulation [12] with stromal cells. They elevate cell surface receptors' expression and accumulate activating mutations that lead to constitutive activation of cell surface receptors or their downstream signaling pathways.

Several key receptors and their downstream signaling pathways have emerged as critical drivers of breast cancer development and growth, as well as potential therapeutic targets. For example, growth factor receptor pathways, particularly receptor tyrosine kinases (RTKs), play a significant role in initiating proliferative and cell survival pathways that are normally tightly controlled [13,14]. Among these, the ErbB family of RTKs has been studied most extensively in breast cancer [15], but other RTKs such as the insulin-like growth factor 1 receptor (IGF1R) have also been explored [16,17].

HER2 amplification or protein overexpression is found in 20–30% of invasive breast cancers and is associated with accelerated cell growth, proliferation and poor clinical outcomes [18,19]. One of the most common inhibitors of HER2 is trastuzumab, a monoclonal antibody that binds to the extracellular domain of HER2 and inhibits several major downstream signaling pathways that regulate tumor growth, such as the RAS/RAF/MEK/MAPK and the PI3K/AKT pathways [20,21]. In addition to activation by homodimerization, enhanced by overexpression of the receptor in breast cancer, HER2 can dimerize with other ErbB family members such as the epidermal growth factor receptor (EGFR). Indeed, targeting both receptors simultaneously can provide therapeutic synergy, which is achieved by using the tyrosine kinase inhibitor lapatinib. Lapatinib inhibits tyrosine phosphorylation and activation of both EGFR and HER2 and, in turn, inhibits activation of the pro-proliferative kinases ERK1/2 and AKT [20].

Elevated levels of insulin-like growth factor 1 (IGF1) and excessive IGF1R signaling have been implicated in an increased risk of breast cancer [22]. IGF1R inhibitors currently in use include neutralizing antibodies and tyrosine kinase inhibitors. It is now understood that extensive crosstalk of IGF1R downstream signaling pathways with other breast cancer signaling pathways exists. Moreover, up-regulation of IGF1R is used by breast cancer cells as a mechanism of resistance to HER2, EGFR and anti-estrogen inhibitors. These mechanisms suggest combining IGF1R inhibitors with other targeted therapies as an effective therapeutic strategy [20,23].

Determining tumor sensitivity to proliferative signaling is crucial in selecting appropriate breast cancer treatment. Indeed, several targeted therapies which aim to block breast tumor cell proliferation are currently being used at the clinic. Tamoxifen is an ER blocker that inhibits estrogen sensitivity and therefore is tailored for the ER^+ subtypes, luminal A and ER^+ luminal B. Trastuzumab, on the other hand, binds to HER2 and shows a highly beneficial effect in subtypes that overexpress HER2, such as $HER2^+$ luminal B and $HR^-/HER2^+$. TNBC, which is the most aggressive breast cancer with the highest metastatic potential, has no targeted treatment at present and is usually treated by chemotherapy [2]. In addition, ER, PR and HER2, another surface marker worth mentioning is the androgen receptor (AR) [24,25]. AR has been shown to have some predictive value in breast cancer, with an overall mixed effect of increased survival and increased resistance to tamoxifen [26]. Several anti-androgenic drugs have been proposed as candidates for AR targeted treatment [26–29]. This new type of targeted treatment could be beneficial if proven effective, especially in otherwise unresponsive AR^+/$HER2^+$ and AR^+/TNBC [26].

2.2. *Genome Instability and Mutation*

The success of the neoplastic process depends on high mutation rates of the genome of neoplastic cells. One way cancer cells increase their mutation rate is by disrupting one or several components of the genomic maintenance and repair machinery. Such alterations are selectively advantageous for tumor progression because they accelerate the rate at which pre-malignant cells can accumulate mutations and become cancerous [8,9]. Approximately ten percent of all breast cancer cases are related to genetic predisposition or family history, with a variance of geographical region and ethnicity [30]. Familial cancer predisposition is usually correlated with alterations in components of the DNA maintenance and repair machinery. The most common germline mutations associated with breast cancer are in breast cancer susceptibility genes 1 and 2 (BRCA1 and BRCA2), which encode proteins responsible for double-stranded DNA repair. Germinal mutations in these two genes correlate with a high rate of somatic gene mutations and subsequently a risk factor of breast and ovarian cancers [31]. In addition, mutations in BRCA1 are associated with the more aggressive, receptor-negative phenotype, whereas BRCA2 mutated breast cancers are predominantly hormone-sensitive. The latter, nevertheless, demonstrates significantly lower survival rates than $BRCA^-$/HR^+ breast cancer patients [32].

2.3. *Resisting Cell Death*

Disruption of the apoptotic process allows tumor cells to evade their intrinsic self-destruction mechanism. The apoptotic trigger is controlled by counter-balancing pro- and anti-apoptotic members of the B-cell lymphoma 2 (BCL2) family of regulatory proteins. Pro-apoptotic genes are typically known to enhance tumor growth and increase resistance to breast cancer therapy [33]. *BCL2*, a well-recognized prognostic factor, is an anti-apoptotic (pro-survival) gene. Specifically, BCL2 is an estrogen-responsive gene and therefore tends to be overexpressed in primary ER^+ tumors [34]. The correlation of BCL2 with estrogen sensitivity may be the underlying reason for the relatively high survival rates of $BCL2^+$ breast cancer patients. In other words, the overall better prognosis of ER^+ tumors outweighs the prospective damage promoted by BCL2. In recent studies, BCL2 inhibitors have been suggested as a possible therapeutic approach to breast cancer, both due to their apoptosis-enabling effect and their potential synergistic effect with tamoxifen as an ER inhibitor. One such inhibiting drug, venetoclax, is a selective BCL2 inhibitor used to treat leukemia but has not yet been evaluated in solid tumors. It has now undergone a phase Ib clinical trial in breast cancer patients to determine safety preparation for further clinical trials [33]. Therefore, resistance to cell death is a possible effectual target for new breast cancer therapies.

2.4. *Enabling Replicative Immortality*

Telomers which protect the ends of chromosomes are essential for the capability of unlimited proliferation of cancer cells. Telomerase is almost absent in non-immortalized and normal cells but is highly expressed in most human cancer cells. Overexpression and high activation of telomerase in pre-malignant cells enable the maintenance of their telomeric DNA at lengths that are sufficient to avoid the triggering of senescence or apoptosis, leading to their immortalization and transformation into malignant cells. Telomerase is activated in 85% of all human cancers [35] and nearly all breast cancer cases [36].

Breast cancer cell telomeres are much shorter than those of normal cells [37], suggesting that tumor cells need to undergo several replication cycles before reaching a lower limit that induces telomerase activity and consequent replication immortality. Therefore, it is thought that telomerase inhibitors may serve as a viable anti-cancer treatment that will cause the tumor to enter senescence and die of old age. Furthermore, such an approach should be relatively safe, as telomerase activity is absent from most healthy cells [36]. However, no telomerase-targeting therapy has been approved so far for clinical use [38].

A recent study examined the inhibition of telomerase by small interference RNA (RNAi) combined with chemotherapy (doxorubicin) on breast cancer cell lines of three types: luminal A (MCF-7), TNBC (MDA-MB-468) and $HER2^+$ (SKBR-3). The combined treatment resulted in an over 90% reduction in telomerase activity and a decrease of more than 60% in cell viability, demonstrating a cumulative effect of chemotherapy. These promising findings may offer a potential new strategy for the inhibition of breast cancer [39].

2.5. Evading Growth Suppressors

One of the mechanisms by which cancer cells maintain a high proliferation rate is by evading programs that negatively regulate cell proliferation. These programs, which exist in every normal cell, mainly depend on tumor suppressor genes. *TP53* is a prototypical tumor suppressor gene that governs a wide range of cellular functions such as cell proliferation, apoptosis, DNA repair, gene expression and metabolism. The TP53 protein receives input from stress and abnormality sensors within the cell and decides, based on the levels of DNA damage caused in the cell genome, whether to halt the cell cycle and enable repair or to trigger apoptosis in cases where excessive damage that cannot be repaired exists [40].

Inactivating mutations in *TP53* are observed in nearly 50% of all cancers and 25–30% of the basal-like subtype of breast cancer [41]. Moreover, women who carry a *TP53* germline mutation have an 85% chance of developing breast cancer by the age of 60 [42]. Thus, in addition to being a prognostic factor, the *TP53* mutation profile may influence the effectiveness of chemotherapy and hormonal therapy, which are used to treat breast cancer and are therefore examined before administration of such treatments [41,43–45].

2.6. Reprogramming Energy Metabolism

The uncontrolled cell proliferation that represents neoplastic disease involves, in addition to de-regulated control of cell proliferation, corresponding adjustments of energy metabolism to fuel cell growth and division. Thus, a common observation in neoplastic disease is a sharp increase in glucose consumption that accompanies a shift to anaerobic glycolysis instead of a more efficient aerobic mitochondria-mediated oxidative phosphorylation utilized by healthy nucleated cells. These changes are usually related to activation of RAS and MYC and inactivating mutations in *TP53* [46], enhancing the continuous proliferation of cancer cells.

In breast cancer, there is a difference in metabolic activity between the different subtypes, as both hormones and growth factors regulate glucose consumption and energy metabolism, leading to slightly different enzymatic profiles of ER^+, HR^+ and TNBC tumors [47]. Furthermore, blocking proliferation signaling, a preferred strategy for treating receptor-positive breast cancer subtypes, leads to downstream metabolic changes, further disrupting overall tumor growth [47].

2.7. Inducing Angiogenesis

Like normal tissues, tumors require nutrients and oxygen and the ability to evacuate metabolic waste and carbon dioxide. These needs are emphasized in tumors due to the rise in glucose consumption and the ever-increasing energy demands of the growing tumor. Tumor-associated neo-vasculature, generated by the process of angiogenesis, addresses these needs. Angiogenesis is a process that is transiently activated during embryogenesis and in normal physiological processes such as wound healing and the female reproductive cycle in the adult. During tumor progression, an angiogenic switch is activated and remains constitutively on, leading to continuous sprouting of new vessels which help to sustain expanding neoplastic growth [8,9].

Bevacizumab (Avastin) is a monoclonal antibody that targets the vascular endothelial growth factor (VEGF), a prototypical promoter of angiogenesis. Bevacizumab is used to treat many types of cancer, such as non-small-cell lung cancer, glioblastoma, renal cell carcinoma, ovarian cancer and cervical cancer [48]. Similarly, bevacizumab was approved by the federal drug and use administration (FDA) for use in metastatic breast cancer in 2008. However, this approval was reversed two years later due to a lack of supporting evidence from clinical observations and safety concerns [48,49]. The assessment of the FDA regarding the use of bevacizumab in breast cancer was considered controversial, especially in cases of $HER2^-$ breast cancer and TNBC, which are highly resistant to standard breast cancer therapy [48]. Today, bevacizumab is used to treat breast cancer in Europe and other countries parallel to its continuous examination in clinical trials [48,49]. The efficacy variation of bevacizumab between breast cancer and other cancers may be explained by differences in the underlying angiogenesis-related mechanisms of these distinct cancer types.

2.8. Tumor Promoting Inflammation

It has long been recognized that some tumors are densely infiltrated by immune cells, thereby mirroring inflammatory conditions in non-neoplastic tissues. Such tumor-associated immune responses were initially thought to reflect an attempt of the immune system to eradicate tumors. However, it is now known that inflammation can also contribute to multiple hallmark capabilities by supplying bioactive molecules such as growth and survival factors, pro-angiogenic factors and extracellular matrix modifying enzymes to the tumor microenvironment, which supports tumor progression and metastasis. Inflammatory cells can also release reactive oxygen species mutagenic for nearby cancer cells, accelerating their genetic evolution towards malignancy [8,9].

2.9. Evading Immune Destruction

According to the immune surveillance theory, cells and tissues are constantly monitored by the immune system, which recognizes and eliminates most developing cancer cells and immature tumors that accidentally develop [50]. According to this logic, the tumors that succeed developing have somehow managed to avoid detection by the immune system or limit the extent of targeted killing by the immune system, thereby evading eradication. Immunogenic cancer cells may escape immune destruction by disabling components of the immune system addressed to eliminate them. They do so by secreting immunosuppressive factors and recruiting immunosuppressive cells such as regulatory T cells and myeloid-derived suppressor cells that can suppress the actions of cytotoxic lymphocytes [8,9].

Understanding the mechanisms used by cancer cells to evade immune destruction has led to the development of immunotherapy, which is based on stimulating a patient's immune system to recognize and destroy cancer cells more effectively. An essential part of the immune system is its ability to keep itself from attacking normal cells in the body. To do so, it uses "checkpoints," proteins on immune cells that need to be turned on or off to start an immune response. Breast cancer cells often use these checkpoints to avoid being attacked by the immune system. Therapies that target these checkpoint proteins assist in restoring the immune response against breast cancer cells. Today, immunotherapy is used to treat some types of breast cancer. Pembrolizumab (Keytruda) is a drug that targets programmed cell death 1 protein (PD-1), a protein on T cells that normally help keeps these cells from attacking other cells in the body. By blocking PD-1, this drug boosts the immune response against breast cancer cells and often leads to tumor shrinkage. Pembrolizumab is used in combination with chemotherapy to treat TNBC which expresses programmed cell death protein ligand 1 (PD-L1). Atezolizumab targets PD-L1, the ligand of PD-1, which is found on some tumor cells and immune cells. Blocking this protein can help boost the immune response against breast cancer cells and consequently shrink some tumors or slow their growth. Atezolizumab is used in combination with paclitaxel for advanced TNBC when the tumor expresses the PD-L1 protein [51].

The immunogenicity of breast cancer is heterogeneous and depends mainly on the specific subtype of breast cancer. Although ER^- and $HER2^+$ tumors have shown evidence of immunogenicity, these types of inflammatory breast tumors are rare when compared to TNBC tumors, which are unique among breast cancer subtypes in having strong antigen expression and high stromal and tumor-infiltrating lymphocytes, parameters with a vital prognostic and predictive significance to immunotherapy and chemotherapy. Except for these immunogenic subtypes, breast tumors are usually considered immunologically silent or "cold" tumors, characterized by the presence of low mutation and neoantigen burden and few tumor-infiltrating lymphocytes. In addition, resistance to cancer immunotherapies often develops in breast cancer due to alternative immunosuppressive checkpoint pathways. Therefore, despite the use of combination immunotherapy in metastatic TNBC patients today, the immunologic treatment of breast cancer remains a significant challenge [52].

2.10. *Invasion and Metastasis*

Metastatic dissemination of tumor cells, also known as the invasion-metastasis cascade [9], is a multi-step process that starts with local invasion of tumor cells into the surrounding stroma, followed by intravasation into the vasculature, endurance of shear stress in the vasculature, extravasation to distant sites and organs and, finally, adaptation to a new microenvironment and the formation of micro-metastases that will develop into a detectable secondary tumor. Metastatic dissemination of breast cancer cells from the primary tumor and their spread into distant sites in the body is the leading cause of mortality in breast cancer patients. Moreover, while primary breast tumors can arise from various genetic causes and hallmarks, metastasis is a common stage and should serve as a primary target for therapeutic intervention. Current therapeutic standards for breast cancer involve surgical resection of the primary tumor accompanied by radiation therapy or chemotherapy. Cytotoxic drugs and hormone-blocking therapeutics are often used in breast cancer; however, they do not prevent metastasis as they mainly affect proliferation, cell cycle and apoptosis. Despite the importance and centrality of the invasion and metastasis hallmark in breast cancer, no treatment to permanently eradicate metastatic breast cancer exists at present.

Fundamental understanding of the cancer hallmarks has facilitated the development of knowledge-based therapeutics. Regardless of the rapidly growing number of targeted therapies, their effectiveness is usually transient and prolonged progression-free survival and remedy are rare; the chances of survival usually increase if the tumor is detected early and surgically excised [53]. Two major reasons explain the failure of current targeted therapies to cure breast cancer patients. First, the metastatic process, which is the leading cause of disease recurrence and mortality in breast cancer patients, can arise during the early stages of pre-malignant cancer, while current therapeutics target all other hallmarks of breast cancer excluding invasion and metastasis. Second, breast cancer cells undergo Darwinian evolution and natural selection in response to therapies that target hallmarks such as proliferation, apoptosis and cell survival. This process leads to the development of tumor cells resistant to therapy. Notably, while treatments for most cancer hallmarks are currently available, no cure for invasion and metastasis in general and breast cancer in particular currently exists.

Gene expression profiling of breast tumors has yielded signatures from which prognostic tests could be derived to facilitate clinical and therapeutic decision-making in breast cancer patients. Interestingly, although intended to predict the metastatic potential of breast tumors, most of these tests gain predictive and prognostic power from the quantification of genes that are involved in proliferation and are efficient for only specific subtypes of breast cancer [54]. Using the needle collection technique, which enables isolation of the invasive population of cancer cells from a tumor, it was previously demonstrated that proliferation and cell cycle genes are down-regulated, while the expression of motility and invasion and DNA-repair genes is up-regulated in invasive breast cancer cells within the primary tumor [55]. Today's predictive tests are based on whole tumor tissue, which includes a heterogeneous population of tumor cells and various stromal cells. Considering that in every given moment only a small fraction of cancer cells invades the surrounding tissue and intravasates into blood vessels and due to the transient, rare and short-lived nature of the metastatic process, gene expression changes which regulate invasiveness and metastasis in breast tumor cells within the primary tumor would be missed by profiling whole tumor chunks.

Within primary breast tumors, tumor cell intravasation occurs at micro-anatomical doorways on blood vessels of the tumors, called Tumor Micro Environment of Metastasis (TMEM). Each functional TMEM doorway comprises three different cell types in direct and stable physical contact: a tumor cell highly expressing the actin-regulatory protein Mammalian-enabled (MENA), a tumor-associated macrophage expressing high levels of perivascular tyrosine kinase with immunoglobulin-like loops and epidermal growth factor homology domains 2 (TIE2) and VEGF ($TIE2^{hi}/VEGF^{hi}$) macrophage and an angiopoietin 2 (ANG2) secreting endothelial cell [56,57]. TMEM doorways have been identified in mouse and human mammary carcinomas and their density correlates with metastatic outcomes in breast cancer patients [58–60]. Because intravasation of tumor cells into blood vessels is a critical step in the systemic spread of tumor cells and a general mechanism that metastatic cells use, which does not directly depend on changes in gene expression or natural selection within the primary tumor, TMEM may be preferable as a method for predicting the metastatic potential of breast tumor cells.

3. Scientific Research and Therapeutic Applications

To gain an insight into research efforts invested on each of the hallmarks, we analyzed the association between each of the ten hallmarks and relevant scientific research publications. As demonstrated in Figure 1, the invasion and metastasis hallmark is associated with the most significant number of publications (association score 0.107), implying that this hallmark is highly explored. Not surprisingly, the second highly studied hallmark is sustaining proliferative signaling (association score 0.052), demonstrating that significant effort is still invested in the proliferation of the primary tumor. We next compared research publications related to anti-metastasis inhibitors versus all research publications associated with breast cancer therapeutics. Surprisingly, only a small fraction (<3%) of publications was related to anti-metastasis inhibitors, while most publications on breast cancer therapeutics address the other hallmarks (Figure 2). Moreover, although the importance of the invasion and metastasis hallmark is highly appreciated in the scientific community and as can be demonstrated by the constantly growing number of publications on breast cancer metastasis and therapeutics, very few clinical trials concentrate on testing anti-metastasis inhibitors at present and even less of them focus on inhibitors of breast cancer metastasis. These data suggest that while the invasion and metastasis hallmark is highly appreciated and widely researched in the laboratory, a significant gap exists between research performed in the laboratory and its clinical and therapeutic applications.

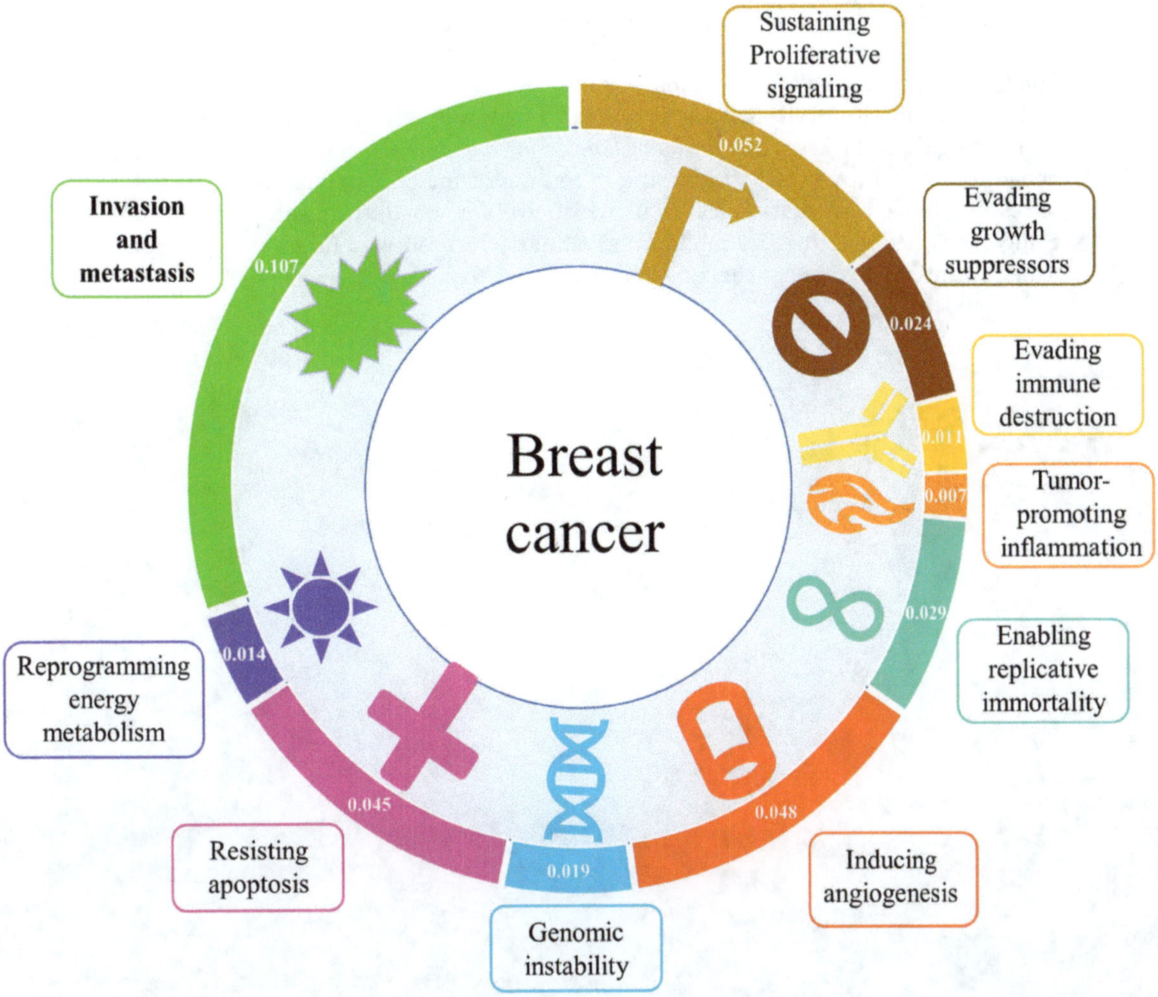

Figure 1. Outline of the ten hallmarks of cancer with PubMed association score for each hallmark keyword with breast cancer. The association score of each of the hallmarks, represented by one of the keywords: "proliferation", "growth", "immune", "inflammation", "immortality", "angiogenesis", "mutation", "apoptosis", "metabolism", "metastasis", AND "breast cancer" was calculated using PubMed citations. The number of citations for each hallmark with breast cancer was then divided by the number of each query term alone according to the following equation: association score = (citations of "keyword" for each hallmark AND "breast cancer")/(citations of "keyword" for each hallmark). Note that the association score of invasion and metastasis is significantly higher than the other hallmarks, suggesting that this hallmark is highly explored and should be considered a prime therapeutic target.

Translating research findings in invasion and metastasis into clinical applications is challenging for two major reasons. First, tumor size, which is affected by all other hallmarks of cancer besides invasion and metastasis, is considered an indicator for cancer progression mainly because it is a measurable endpoint and is constantly used in clinical trials. However, tumor size does not usually correlate with the invasion and metastasis potential of tumor cells and can sometimes even have an opposite correlation [61]. Second, as metastatic dissemination is a prolonged process, which can sometimes even appear after a decade or two after initial diagnosis and treatment, considerations such as time frame of the experiment, treatment period with the inhibitor which is meant to prevent metastasis, the starting point of the experiment and selection of correct experimental groups, become relevant. Several recent developments could offer a solution to this dilemma. First, an FDA draft guidance defined metastasis-free survival (MFS) as a valid endpoint in clinical trials was recently published [62]. Defining MFS as an endpoint instead of overall survival enables earlier evaluation of prognostic criteria in general and metastatic dissemination.

Second, it was previously published that cytotoxic treatment of breast cancer such as neoadjuvant therapy can potentially induce cell invasiveness and metastatic dissemination due to its ability to result in cell damage and wound healing-like inflammatory processes which recruit immune cells that are manipulated by tumor cells to become pro-metastatic. Performing clinical trials with anti-metastatic drugs on breast cancer patients who receive neoadjuvant therapy could shorten the experiment time and enable faster evaluation of results. Indeed, several clinical trials which use the neoadjuvant setup are currently being performed with the Tie2 inhibitor rebastinib, which is tested for its ability to inhibit neoadjuvant-induced breast cancer metastasis.

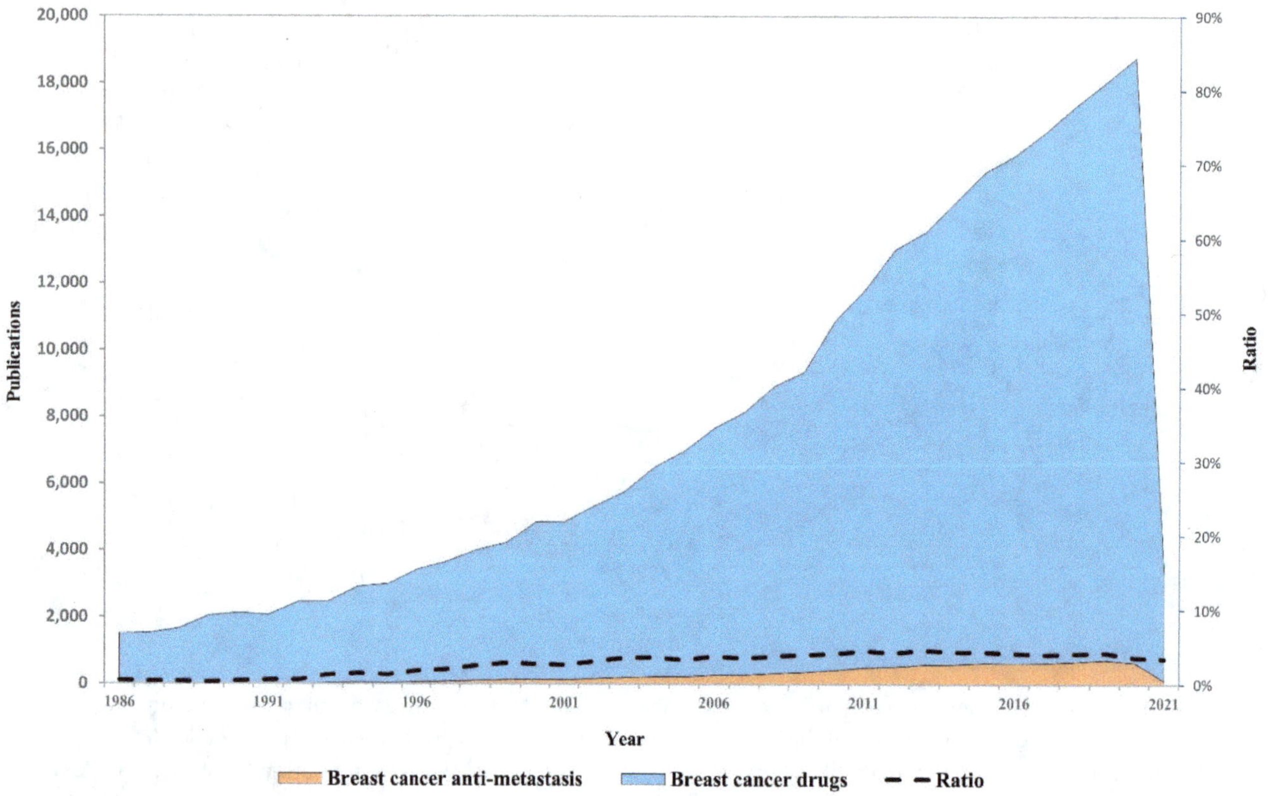

Figure 2. Annual publications associated with breast cancer drugs versus breast cancer anti-metastatic drugs. Total annual publications among breast cancer-related research in the years 1986–2021 as obtained by PubMed search. The search query used to retrieve drug-associated publications was: ("drug" | "drugs" | " treatment" | "treatments" | "therapy" | "therapies") AND ("breast"). The search query used to retrieve antimetastatic-associated publications was: ("anti-metastatic" | "antimetastatic" | "anti-metastasis" | "antimetastasis" | "anti-invasive" | "anti-invasion" | "anti-migratory" | "anti-migration" | "anti-degradation" | "antiproteolytic" | "antiproteolysis" | "anti-MMP" | "anti-matrix metalloproteinase" | "metastasis prevention" | "metastatic prevention" | "anti-invadopodia") OR ("invasion" | "invadopodia" | "migration" | "degradation" | "proteolysis" | "proteolytic" | "MMP" | "matrix metalloproteinase") AND ("inhibitor" | "inhibitors" | "antagonist" | "antagonists") AND ("breast"). The ratio between the queries is represented by a dashed line.

4. Concluding Remarks

Even though the hallmarks model excellently illustrates what goes wrong in breast cancer cells, it fails to interrogate the hierarchy of the hallmarks in the broader aspect of therapeutic approaches. Being the most defining characteristic of malignancy, the invasion and metastasis hallmark should be placed in the center of attention and considered a potentially superior therapeutic target. Our analysis demonstrates that, while it is well recognized that invasion and metastasis is the most important hallmark of breast cancer, its prevention receives very little attention in the literature compared to preventing other hallmarks in primary or secondary breast tumors. These observations justify the necessity of shifting both scientific and clinical attention towards the invasion and metastasis hallmark as a potential therapeutic target in breast cancer. With new developments such as defining MFS as an endpoint in clinical trials and recognizing neoadjuvant treatment as a possible accelerator of breast cancer metastasis, this strategy becomes feasible. A successful application of this concept will depend on a collaborative effort of researchers, physicians and pharmaceutical scientists.

Author Contributions: Conceptualization, H.G.-H. and A.O.S.; data curation, T.S.; funding acquisition, H.G.-H. and A.O.S.; supervision, H.G.-H. and A.O.S.; writing—H.G.-H., J.S., T.S. and A.O.S. All authors have read and agreed to the published version of the manuscript.

References

1. Azamjah, N.; Soltan-Zadeh, Y.; Zayeri, F. Global Trend of Breast Cancer Mortality Rate: A 25-Year Study. *Asian Pac. J. Cancer Prev.* **2019**, *20*, 2015–2020. [CrossRef]
2. Loibl, S.; Poortmans, P.; Morrow, M.; Denkert, C.; Curigliano, G. Breast cancer. *Lancet* **2021**. [CrossRef]
3. Dai, X.; Xiang, L.; Li, T.; Bai, Z. Cancer Hallmarks, Biomarkers and Breast Cancer Molecular Subtypes. *J. Cancer* **2016**, *7*, 1281–1294. [CrossRef] [PubMed]
4. Davey, M.G.; Ryan, E.J.; Davey, M.S.; Lowery, A.J.; Miller, N.; Kerin, M.J. Clinicopathological and prognostic significance of programmed cell death ligand 1 expression in patients diagnosed with breast cancer: Meta-analysis. *Br. J. Surg.* **2021**. [CrossRef]
5. Tang, P.; Tse, G.M. Immunohistochemical Surrogates for Molecular Classification of Breast Carcinoma: A 2015 Update. *Arch. Pathol. Lab. Med.* **2016**, *140*, 806–814. [CrossRef]
6. Jurikova, M.; Danihel, L.; Polak, S.; Varga, I. Ki67, PCNA, and MCM proteins: Markers of proliferation in the diagnosis of breast cancer. *Acta Histochem.* **2016**, *118*, 544–552. [CrossRef] [PubMed]
7. Kondov, B.; Milenkovikj, Z.; Kondov, G.; Petrushevska, G.; Basheska, N.; Bogdanovska-Todorovska, M.; Tolevska, N.; Ivkovski, L. Presentation of the Molecular Subtypes of Breast Cancer Detected By Immunohistochemistry in Surgically Treated Patients. *Open Access Maced J. Med. Sci* **2018**, *6*, 961–967. [CrossRef] [PubMed]
8. Hanahan, D.; Weinberg, R.A. The hallmarks of cancer. *Cell* **2000**, *100*, 57–70. [CrossRef]
9. Hanahan, D.; Weinberg, R.A. Hallmarks of cancer: The next generation. *Cell* **2011**, *144*, 646–674. [CrossRef]
10. Du, Z.; Lovly, C.M. Mechanisms of receptor tyrosine kinase activation in cancer. *Mol. Cancer* **2018**, *17*, 58. [CrossRef]
11. Walsh, J.H.; Karnes, W.E.; Cuttitta, F.; Walker, A. Autocrine growth factors and solid tumor malignancy. *West. J. Med.* **1991**, *155*, 152–163. [PubMed]
12. Maacha, S.; Bhat, A.A.; Jimenez, L.; Raza, A.; Haris, M.; Uddin, S.; Grivel, J.C. Extracellular vesicles-mediated intercellular communication: Roles in the tumor microenvironment and anti-cancer drug resistance. *Mol. Cancer* **2019**, *18*, 55. [CrossRef] [PubMed]
13. Perona, R. Cell signalling: Growth factors and tyrosine kinase receptors. *Clin. Transl. Oncol.* **2006**, *8*, 77–82. [CrossRef]
14. Witsch, E.; Sela, M.; Yarden, Y. Roles for growth factors in cancer progression. *Physiology* **2010**, *25*, 85–101. [CrossRef] [PubMed]
15. Hynes, N.E.; MacDonald, G. ErbB receptors and signaling pathways in cancer. *Curr. Opin. Cell Biol.* **2009**, *21*, 177–184. [CrossRef] [PubMed]
16. Cardillo, M.R.; Monti, S.; Di Silverio, F.; Gentile, V.; Sciarra, F.; Toscano, V. Insulin-like growth factor (IGF)-I, IGF-II and IGF type I receptor (IGFR-I) expression in prostatic cancer. *Anticancer. Res.* **2003**, *23*, 3825–3835. [PubMed]
17. Papa, V.; Gliozzo, B.; Clark, G.M.; McGuire, W.L.; Moore, D.; Fujita-Yamaguchi, Y.; Vigneri, R.; Goldfine, I.D.; Pezzino, V. Insulin-like growth factor-I receptors are overexpressed and predict a low risk in human breast cancer. *Cancer Res.* **1993**, *53*, 3736–3740. [PubMed]
18. Moasser, M.M. The oncogene HER2: Its signaling and transforming functions and its role in human cancer pathogenesis. *Oncogene* **2007**, *26*, 6469–6487. [CrossRef] [PubMed]

19. Slamon, D.J.; Godolphin, W.; Jones, L.A.; Holt, J.A.; Wong, S.G.; Keith, D.E.; Levin, W.J.; Stuart, S.G.; Udove, J.; Ullrich, A.; et al. Studies of the HER-2/neu proto-oncogene in human breast and ovarian cancer. *Science* **1989**, *244*, 707–712. [CrossRef]
20. Butti, R.; Das, S.; Gunasekaran, V.P.; Yadav, A.S.; Kumar, D.; Kundu, G.C. Receptor tyrosine kinases (RTKs) in breast cancer: Signaling, therapeutic implications and challenges. *Mol. Cancer* **2018**, *17*, 34. [CrossRef]
21. Cordover, E.; Minden, A. Signaling pathways downstream to receptor tyrosine kinases: Targets for cancer treatment. *J. Cancer Metastasis Treat.* **2020**, *6*, 1–19.
22. Peyrat, J.P.; Bonneterre, J.; Hecquet, B.; Vennin, P.; Louchez, M.M.; Fournier, C.; Lefebvre, J.; Demaille, A. Plasma insulin-like growth factor-1 (IGF-1) concentrations in human breast cancer. *Eur. J. Cancer* **1993**, *29A*, 492–497. [CrossRef]
23. Ianza, A.; Sirico, M.; Bernocchi, O.; Generali, D. Role of the IGF-1 Axis in Overcoming Resistance in Breast Cancer. *Front. Cell Dev. Biol.* **2021**, *9*, 641449. [CrossRef] [PubMed]
24. Niemeier, L.A.; Dabbs, D.J.; Beriwal, S.; Striebel, J.M.; Bhargava, R. Androgen receptor in breast cancer: Expression in estrogen receptor-positive tumors and in estrogen receptor-negative tumors with apocrine differentiation. *Mod. Pathol.* **2010**, *23*, 205–212. [CrossRef]
25. Vera-Badillo, F.E.; Templeton, A.J.; de Gouveia, P.; Diaz-Padilla, I.; Bedard, P.L.; Al-Mubarak, M.; Seruga, B.; Tannock, I.F.; Ocana, A.; Amir, E. Androgen receptor expression and outcomes in early breast cancer: A systematic review and meta-analysis. *J. Natl. Cancer Inst.* **2014**, *106*, djt319. [CrossRef] [PubMed]
26. Rahim, B.; O'Regan, R. AR Signaling in Breast Cancer. *Cancers* **2017**, *9*, 21. [CrossRef]
27. Anestis, A.; Zoi, I.; Papavassiliou, A.G.; Karamouzis, M.V. Androgen Receptor in Breast Cancer-Clinical and Preclinical Research Insights. *Molecules* **2020**, *25*, 358. [CrossRef] [PubMed]
28. Bonnefoi, H.; Grellety, T.; Tredan, O.; Saghatchian, M.; Dalenc, F.; Mailliez, A.; L'Haridon, T.; Cottu, P.; Abadie-Lacourtoisie, S.; You, B.; et al. A phase II trial of abiraterone acetate plus prednisone in patients with triple-negative androgen receptor positive locally advanced or metastatic breast cancer (UCBG 12-1). *Ann. Oncol.* **2016**, *27*, 812–818. [CrossRef]
29. Gerratana, L.; Basile, D.; Buono, G.; De Placido, S.; Giuliano, M.; Minichillo, S.; Coinu, A.; Martorana, F.; De Santo, I.; Del Mastro, L.; et al. Androgen receptor in triple negative breast cancer: A potential target for the targetless subtype. *Cancer Treat. Rev.* **2018**, *68*, 102–110. [CrossRef]
30. Kuchenbaecker, K.B.; Hopper, J.L.; Barnes, D.R.; Phillips, K.A.; Mooij, T.M.; Roos-Blom, M.J.; Jervis, S.; van Leeuwen, F.E.; Milne, R.L.; Andrieu, N.; et al. Risks of Breast, Ovarian, and Contralateral Breast Cancer for BRCA1 and BRCA2 Mutation Carriers. *JAMA* **2017**, *317*, 2402–2416. [CrossRef]
31. Varol, U.; Kucukzeybek, Y.; Alacacioglu, A.; Somali, I.; Altun, Z.; Aktas, S.; Oktay Tarhan, M. BRCA genes: BRCA 1 and BRCA 2. *J. BUON* **2018**, *23*, 862–866.
32. Kotsopoulos, J. BRCA Mutations and Breast Cancer Prevention. *Cancers* **2018**, *10*, 524. [CrossRef]
33. Lok, S.W.; Whittle, J.R.; Vaillant, F.; Teh, C.E.; Lo, L.L.; Policheni, A.N.; Bergin, A.R.T.; Desai, J.; Ftouni, S.; Gandolfo, L.C.; et al. A Phase Ib Dose-Escalation and Expansion Study of the BCL2 Inhibitor Venetoclax Combined with Tamoxifen in ER and BCL2-Positive Metastatic Breast Cancer. *Cancer Discov.* **2019**, *9*, 354–369. [CrossRef] [PubMed]
34. Perillo, B.; Sasso, A.; Abbondanza, C.; Palumbo, G. 17beta-estradiol inhibits apoptosis in MCF-7 cells, inducing bcl-2 expression via two estrogen-responsive elements present in the coding sequence. *Mol. Cell Biol.* **2000**, *20*, 2890–2901. [CrossRef] [PubMed]
35. Akincilar, S.C.; Unal, B.; Tergaonkar, V. Reactivation of telomerase in cancer. *Cell Mol. Life Sci.* **2016**, *73*, 1659–1670. [CrossRef]
36. Holysz, H.; Lipinska, N.; Paszel-Jaworska, A.; Rubis, B. Telomerase as a useful target in cancer fighting-the breast cancer case. *Tumour Biol.* **2013**, *34*, 1371–1380. [CrossRef] [PubMed]
37. Herbert, B.S.; Wright, W.E.; Shay, J.W. Telomerase and breast cancer. *Breast Cancer Res.* **2001**, *3*, 146–149. [CrossRef] [PubMed]
38. Guterres, A.N.; Villanueva, J. Targeting telomerase for cancer therapy. *Oncogene* **2020**, *39*, 5811–5824. [CrossRef]
39. Aboelela, S.; Ashmawy, A.; Shaarawy, S.; El-Hefny, M.; Medhat, A. Telomerase as a Possible Candidate Targeting Therapy in Different Breast Cancer Cell Lines. *Asian Pac. J. Cancer Prev.* **2020**, *21*, 2243–2250. [CrossRef] [PubMed]
40. Varna, M.; Bousquet, G.; Plassa, L.F.; Bertheau, P.; Janin, A. TP53 status and response to treatment in breast cancers. *J. Biomed. Biotechnol.* **2011**, *2011*, 284584. [CrossRef] [PubMed]
41. Silwal-Pandit, L.; Langerod, A.; Borresen-Dale, A.L. TP53 Mutations in Breast and Ovarian Cancer. *Cold Spring Harb Perspect Med.* **2017**, *7*. [CrossRef] [PubMed]

42. Schon, K.; Tischkowitz, M. Clinical implications of germline mutations in breast cancer: TP53. *Breast Cancer Res. Treat.* **2018**, *167*, 417–423. [CrossRef]
43. Berns, E.M.; Foekens, J.A.; Vossen, R.; Look, M.P.; Devilee, P.; Henzen-Logmans, S.C.; van Staveren, I.L.; van Putten, W.L.; Inganas, M.; Meijer-van Gelder, M.E.; et al. Complete sequencing of TP53 predicts poor response to systemic therapy of advanced breast cancer. *Cancer Res.* **2000**, *60*, 2155–2162.
44. Fernandez-Cuesta, L.; Anaganti, S.; Hainaut, P.; Olivier, M. p53 status influences response to tamoxifen but not to fulvestrant in breast cancer cell lines. *Int. J. Cancer* **2011**, *128*, 1813–1821. [CrossRef] [PubMed]
45. Kim, H.S.; Yom, C.K.; Kim, H.J.; Lee, J.W.; Sohn, J.H.; Kim, J.H.; Park, Y.L.; Ahn, S.H. Overexpression of p53 is correlated with poor outcome in premenopausal women with breast cancer treated with tamoxifen after chemotherapy. *Breast Cancer Res. Treat.* **2010**, *121*, 777–788. [CrossRef]
46. Vander Heiden, M.G.; Cantley, L.C.; Thompson, C.B. Understanding the Warburg effect: The metabolic requirements of cell proliferation. *Science* **2009**, *324*, 1029–1033. [CrossRef]
47. Gandhi, N.; Das, G.M. Metabolic Reprogramming in Breast Cancer and Its Therapeutic Implications. *Cells* **2019**, *8*, 89. [CrossRef]
48. Garcia, J.; Hurwitz, H.I.; Sandler, A.B.; Miles, D.; Coleman, R.L.; Deurloo, R.; Chinot, O.L. Bevacizumab (Avastin(R)) in cancer treatment: A review of 15 years of clinical experience and future outlook. *Cancer Treat. Rev.* **2020**, *86*, 102017. [CrossRef]
49. Varella, L.; Abraham, J.; Kruse, M. Revisiting the Role of Bevacizumab in the Treatment of Breast Cancer. *Semin Oncol.* **2017**, *44*, 273–285. [CrossRef]
50. Ribatti, D. The concept of immune surveillance against tumors. The first theories. *Oncotarget* **2017**, *8*, 7175–7180. [CrossRef] [PubMed]
51. Rosato, R.R.; Davila-Gonzalez, D.; Choi, D.S.; Qian, W.; Chen, W.; Kozielski, A.J.; Wong, H.; Dave, B.; Chang, J.C. Evaluation of anti-PD-1-based therapy against triple-negative breast cancer patient-derived xenograft tumors engrafted in humanized mouse models. *Breast Cancer Res.* **2018**, *20*, 108. [CrossRef]
52. Garcia-Aranda, M.; Redondo, M. Immunotherapy: A Challenge of Breast Cancer Treatment. *Cancers* **2019**, *11*, 1822. [CrossRef] [PubMed]
53. Hanahan, D. Rethinking the war on cancer. *Lancet* **2014**, *383*, 558–563. [CrossRef]
54. Weigelt, B.; Baehner, F.L.; Reis-Filho, J.S. The contribution of gene expression profiling to breast cancer classification, prognostica- tion and prediction: A retrospective of the last decade. *J. Pathol.* **2010**, *220*, 263–280. [CrossRef]
55. Patsialou, A.; Wang, Y.; Lin, J.; Whitney, K.; Goswami, S.; Kenny, P.A.; Condeelis, J.S. Selective gene-expression profiling of migratory tumor cells in vivo predicts clinical outcome in breast cancer patients. *Breast Cancer Res.* **2012**, *14*, R139. [CrossRef]
56. Harney, A.S.; Arwert, E.N.; Entenberg, D.; Wang, Y.; Guo, P.; Qian, B.Z.; Oktay, M.H.; Pollard, J.W.; Jones, J.G.; Condeelis, J.S. Real-Time Imaging Reveals Local, Transient Vascular Permeability, and Tumor Cell Intravasation Stimulated by TIE2hi Macrophage-Derived VEGFA. *Cancer Discov.* **2015**, *5*, 932–943. [CrossRef] [PubMed]
57. Karagiannis, G.S.; Goswami, S.; Jones, J.G.; Oktay, M.H.; Condeelis, J.S. Signatures of breast cancer metastasis at a glance. *J. Cell Sci.* **2016**, *129*, 1751–1758. [CrossRef]
58. Oktay, M.H.; Gertler, F.B.; Liu, Y.F.; Rohan, T.E.; Condeelis, J.S.; Jones, J.G. Correlated immunohistochemical and cytological assays for the prediction of hematogenous dissemination of breast cancer. *J. Histochem. Cytochem.* **2012**, *60*, 168–173. [CrossRef]
59. Robinson, B.D.; Sica, G.L.; Liu, Y.F.; Rohan, T.E.; Gertler, F.B.; Condeelis, J.S.; Jones, J.G. Tumor microenvironment of metastasis in human breast carcinoma: A potential prognostic marker linked to hematogenous dissemination. *Clin. Cancer Res.* **2009**, *15*, 2433–2441. [CrossRef]
60. Rohan, T.E.; Xue, X.; Lin, H.M.; D'Alfonso, T.M.; Ginter, P.S.; Oktay, M.H.; Robinson, B.D.; Ginsberg, M.; Gertler, F.B.; Glass, A.G.; et al. Tumor microenvironment of metastasis and risk of distant metastasis of breast cancer. *J. Natl. Cancer Inst.* **2014**, *106*. [CrossRef]
61. Gil-Henn, H.; Patsialou, A.; Wang, Y.; Warren, M.S.; Condeelis, J.S.; Koleske, A.J. Arg/Abl2 promotes invasion and attenuates proliferation of breast cancer in vivo. *Oncogene* **2013**, *32*, 2622–2630. [CrossRef] [PubMed]
62. Beaver, J.A.; Kluetz, P.G.; Pazdur, R. Metastasis-free Survival—A New End Point in Prostate Cancer Trials. *N. Engl. J. Med.* **2018**, *378*, 2458–2460. [CrossRef] [PubMed]

4

Improved Survival after Breast-Conserving Therapy Compared with Mastectomy in Stage I-IIA Breast Cancer

Ivica Ratosa [1,2], Gaber Plavc [1,2], Nina Pislar [3], Tina Zagar [4], Andraz Perhavec [2,3] and Pierfrancesco Franco [5,6,*]

1 Department of Radiation Oncology, Institute of Oncology Ljubljana, 1000 Ljubljana, Slovenia; iratosa@onko-i.si (I.R.); gplavc@onko-i.si (G.P.)
2 Faculty of Medicine, University of Ljubljana, 1000 Ljubljana, Slovenia; aperhavec@onko-i.si
3 Department of Surgery, Institute of Oncology Ljubljana, 1000 Ljubljana, Slovenia; npislar@onko-i.si
4 Department of Epidemiology and Cancer Registry, Institute of Oncology Ljubljana, 1000 Ljubljana, Slovenia; tzagar@onko-i.si
5 Department of Translational Medicine, University of Eastern Piedmont, 28100 Novara, Italy
6 Radiation Oncology Unit, AOU "Maggiore della Carità", 28100 Novara, Italy
* Correspondence: pierfrancesco.franco@uniupo.it;

Simple Summary: The majority of patients with breast cancer are suitable for either breast-conserving therapy, consisting of breast-conserving surgery and radiation therapy, or mastectomy alone. In the present study, we compared survival outcomes in 1360 patients affected with early-stage breast cancer (stage I-IIA) according to the type of local treatment. We confirmed that patients treated with breast-conserving therapy had a lower rate of local, regional, and distant disease recurrences, and at least equivalent overall survival compared to those treated with mastectomy alone. Our results add to previous research showing a potential benefit of breast-conserving therapy when compared to mastectomy in patients suitable for both treatments at baseline.

Abstract: In the current study, we sought to compare survival outcomes after breast-conserving therapy (BCT) or mastectomy alone in patients with stage I-IIA breast cancer, whose tumors are typically suitable for both locoregional treatments. The study cohort consisted of 1360 patients with stage I-IIA (T1–2N0 or T0–1N1) breast cancer diagnosed between 2001 and 2013 and treated with either BCT (n = 1021, 75.1%) or mastectomy alone (n = 339, 24.9%). Median follow-ups for disease-free survival (DFS) and overall survival (OS) were 6.9 years (range, 0.3–15.9) and 7.5 years (range, 0.2–25.9), respectively. Fifteen (1.1%), 14 (1.0%) and 48 (3.5%) patients experienced local, regional, and distant relapse, respectively. For the whole cohort of patients, the estimated 5-year DFS and OS were 96% and 97%, respectively. After stratification based on the type of local treatment, the estimated 5-year DFS for BCT was 97%, while it was 91% ($p < 0.001$) for mastectomy-only treatment. Inverse probability of treatment weighting matching based on confounding confirmed that mastectomy was associated with worse DFS (HR 2.839, 95% CI 1.760–4.579, $p < 0.0001$), but not with OS (HR 1.455, 95% CI 0.844–2.511, $p = 0.177$). In our study, BCT was shown to have improved disease-specific outcomes compared to mastectomy alone, emphasizing the important role of adjuvant treatments, including postoperative radiation therapy, in patients with early-stage breast cancer at diagnosis.

Keywords: early-stage breast cancer; breast-conserving therapy; mastectomy; radiation therapy; outcome

1. Introduction

Long-term follow-up data from several randomized controlled trials undertaken to compare the efficacy of mastectomy with that of breast-conserving therapy (BCT) consisting of lumpectomy or quadrantectomy followed by postoperative radiotherapy showed no differences in terms of disease-free survival (DFS), distant-disease-free survival, and overall survival (OS) among the treatment groups [1–5]. The trials, conducted in the 1970s and

1980s, paved the way for the increased utilization of BCT for patients with stage I-II breast cancer [6]. Retrospective studies based on the analysis of large patient populations with early-stage breast cancer (EBC) treated in modern contexts indicate that BCT is at least comparable or even better in terms of breast-cancer-specific survival (BCSS) and OS compared to mastectomy without radiation therapy for early-stage breast cancer [7–13]. Improved DFS and OS rates were recently confirmed in smaller cohort studies [14–20] and were also observed in young women with EBC [21–23]. Based on older research, local recurrence is considered to be more common after BCT than after mastectomy. However, over the last 20 years, local recurrence rates after BCT have decreased substantially and are now shown to be as low as after mastectomy, most likely due to better understanding of breast cancer heterogeneity and consequently tailored systemic and radiation treatments [24,25].

For patients with breast cancer who are potentially suitable for both local treatments, BCT is suggested as the evidence-based primary local treatment [26]. Breast-conserving surgery is one of the major advances in the management of breast cancer. Nevertheless, breast-conserving surgery rates, as commonly reported, have reached a plateau in the last decade. In 2010–2011, breast-conserving surgery rates for the general population with unilateral EBC were 64.5–69% in the US [27–29], 73.3% in Europe [30], and 36.5–49.4% for patients younger than 50 years [28,31]. However, in some countries, the overall rate of breast-conserving surgery is lower than 50% [32,33].

The aim of BCT, as compared to mastectomy, is to achieve oncological safety with less extensive surgery, minimizing the psychosocial sequelae, and to obtain favorable cosmetic results with the use of oncoplastic techniques whenever possible. Most women feel negatively impacted by the scars resulting from breast cancer surgery, a consequence that particularly affects patients undergoing mastectomy [34]. When comparing long-term quality of life amongst patients treated with BCT or mastectomy, significantly lower scores for body image, role, and physical and sexual functioning, and more lifestyle disruptions were found for those treated with mastectomy. Conversely, psychosocial functioning slowly increased over time for women who underwent BCT, regardless of their age [35,36]. For patients undergoing mastectomy, access to breast reconstruction procedures is essential to increase positive body image and overall satisfaction and to maintain health-related quality of life [26,37]. However, barriers to immediate or delayed breast reconstruction exist on many levels, depending on the type of hospital (teaching vs. private), geographic location, reimbursement by insurance companies, lack of patient awareness, and the acceptability of the procedures by both physicians and patients [38]. In the past decade, the use of breast reconstruction has increased globally together with the indications for the use of postmastectomy irradiation for EBC [39,40]. It has been documented that the use of postmastectomy radiation therapy may be a negative outcome predictor for breast reconstruction [39]. On the other hand, opting for breast reconstruction may also influence clinical decision making in recommending postoperative radiation therapy due to the impact of radiation on long-term cosmetic results [39,41].

In the current study, we aimed to compare the outcomes of BCT and mastectomy-only treatment performed in the modern era in patients with stage I-IIA breast cancer, whose tumors are typically suitable for either BCT or mastectomy. The primary outcomes were DFS and OS, and secondary outcomes included any breast cancer recurrence (local, regional, and/or distant).

2. Materials and Methods

2.1. Study Cohort and Data Collection

For the present study, data were retrospectively collected and retrieved. The study cohort consisted of patients with stage I-IIA (T1–2N0 or T0–1N1) breast cancer diagnosed between 2001 and 2013 and treated with upfront BCT or mastectomy only with or without reconstruction, achieving clear resection margins in both cases. General patient demographic, histological characteristic, systemic therapy (chemotherapy, endocrine, or anti-HER2 therapies), and local treatment (surgery, radiotherapy) data were collected from individual clinical records. Clinical follow-up information for all patients was updated until 31 March 2021. For the purpose of this study, patient disease stage was classified based on medical records, according to breast carcinoma *TNM Classification of Malignant Tumours* (7th edition) [42]. Intrinsic subtypes of BC were defined as luminal A-like (estrogen-receptor positive, ER+; human epidermal growth factor receptor 2 negative, HER2−; Ki67 < 20%, progesterone receptor positive (PR+) with a cut-point of ≥20%); luminal B-like HER2-negative (ER+, HER2−, Ki67 ≥ 20%, or low PR+); luminal B-like HER2-positive (ER+, HER2+, any PR, any Ki67); HER2-positive (HER2+, PR−, ER−); and 'Basal-like' (ER−, PR−, HER2−) according to clinicopathological surrogate definitions as defined in the St Gallen International Expert Consensus on the primary therapy of EBC in 2013 [43].

2.2. Statistical Analysis

To compare clinical and tumor characteristics between the two groups (patients treated with BCT vs. those treated with mastectomy) we used independent-sample t-tests for continuous variables and Pearson's χ^2 or Fisher's exact tests for categorical variables. Data were expressed as median with a sample range for continuous variables, and as counts with frequencies for categorical data. The Kaplan–Meier method was used to calculate estimated survival curves, and the log-rank test was used to compare the two groups. Univariate and multivariate Cox's proportional hazards models were used to assess the effects of covariates on survival. The effect sizes were given as hazard ratios (HR) with 95% confidence intervals (CI). Overall survival (OS) was specified as the time of BC diagnosis to the date of death or last follow-up. Disease-free survival (DFS) was defined as time to disease recurrence (any type; local and/or regional and/or distant) after surgery. All tests were two-sided, and the statistical level of significance was set to $p < 0.05$. In addition, to reduce bias in our observational study and to analyze the cohort with a representative distribution of matching factors, we used a propensity-score-matched analysis with an inverse probability of treatment weighting (IPTW), calculating the reciprocal of the probability of receiving the treatment that the patient in fact received. We performed adjusted analyses using a multiple linear regression model and IPTW using the propensity score estimated via logistic regression. The outcome model used in the IPTW analysis was a linear regression of outcome on BCT or mastectomy, weighted by the estimated propensity score [44,45]. Covariate adjustment was based on age at diagnosis, pathological tumor and nodal stage, overall breast cancer stage group, tumor grade, type of axillary surgery, and the receipt of chemotherapy and/or endocrine therapy. Data were analyzed using IBM SPSS Statistics software version 26 (Statistical package for the Social Sciences Statistical Software, SPSS Inc, IBM Corporation, Armonk, NY, USA).

3. Results

In total, 1360 patients with stage I-IIA breast cancer treated with either BCT (n = 1021, 75.1%) or mastectomy only (n = 339, 24.9%) were included in the study. The median age at breast cancer diagnosis was 61 years in both groups (BCT range 23–87 and mastectomy range 27–91). The majority of breast tumors were sized ≤2 cm (n = 1100, 81.5%) and had positive estrogen or progesterone receptors (n = 1241, 92.3%). More than half of the patients had left-sided breast cancer (n = 729; 54.2%). Compared with patients receiving mastectomy only as local therapy, patients undergoing BCT were less likely to be younger than 50 or older than 70 years, less likely to have had more extensive axillary surgery, and more likely to have stage I breast cancer. We observed no differences in the two groups with respect to tumor grade, intrinsic subtype, and administration of endocrine or targeted therapy. However, more patients in the mastectomy group received adjuvant chemotherapy (Table 1).

Table 1. Patients' clinical, pathological, and treatment characteristics.

Variable	All Patients n = 1360 (100.0%)	BCT n = 1021 (75.1%)	Mastectomy n = 339 (24.9%)	p Value
Age at diagnosis				<0.0005
<50 years	246 (18.1)	159 (15.6)	87 (25.7)	
50–70 years	880 (64.7)	710 (69.5)	170 (50.1)	
>70 years	234 (17.2)	152 (14.9)	82 (24.2)	
Year of treatment				<0.0005
2001–2007	243 (17.9)	212 (20.8)	31 (9.10)	
2008–2013	1117 (82.1)	809 (79.2)	308 (90.9)	
Pathological tumor stage				<0.0005
T1	1100 (81.5)	873 (86.0)	227 (67.8)	
T2	240 (17.8)	139 (13.7)	101 (30.1)	
≤T2, details unavailable	10 (0.7)	3 (0.3)	7 (2.1)	
Pathological node stage				0.324
Nx	18 (1.3)	13 (1.3)	5 (1.5)	
N0	1085 (79.8)	822 (80.5)	263 (77.6)	
N0	1043 (76.7)	793 (77.7)	250 (73.7)	
N0 (ITC)	42 (3.1)	29 (2.8)	13 (3.8)	
N1	240 (17.6)	177 (17.3)	63 (18.6)	
N1 (NOS)	140 (10.3)	101 (9.9)	39 (11.5)	
N1mic	26 (1.9)	21 (2.1)	5 (1.5)	
N1a	74 (5.4)	55 (5.4)	19 (5.6)	
≤TN1, details unavailable	17 (1.3)	9 (0.9)	8 (2.4)	
Overall stage group				<0.0005
Stage IA	560 (41.2)	464 (45.4)	96 (28.3)	
Stage IB	331 (24.3)	255 (25.0)	76 (22.4)	
Stage IIA	469 (34.5)	302 (29.6)	167 (49.3)	
Grade				0.143
G1	443 (32.6)	340 (33.3)	103 (30.4)	
G2	652 (47.9)	496 (48.6)	156 (46.0)	
G3	264 (19.4)	184 (18.0)	80 (23.6)	
Unknown	1 (0.1)	1 (0.1)	0	
Molecular subtype				0.065
Luminal A	864 (63.5)	667 (65.3)	197 (58.1)	
Luminal B HER2−	390 (28.7)	279 (27.3)	111 (32.7)	
Luminal B HER2+	55 (4.0)	35 (3.4)	20 (5.9)	
HR−/HER2+	13 (1.0)	10 (1.0)	3 (0.9)	
HR−/HER2−	38 (2.8)	30 (2.9)	8 (2.4)	
Axillary surgery				<0.0005
Omitted	39 (2.9)	28 (2.7)	11 (3.2)	
SNB only	1067 (78.5)	839 (82.2)	228 (67.3)	
Axillary dissection	254 (18.7)	154 (15.1)	100 (29.5)	
Endocrine therapy				0.947
Yes	1239 (91.1)	929 (91.0)	310 (91.4)	
No	116 (8.5)	88 (8.6)	28 (8.3)	
Unknown	5 (0.4)	4 (0.4)	1 (0.3)	
Chemotherapy				0.001
Yes	411 (30.2)	271 (26.5)	140 (41,7)	
No	947 (69.7)	748 (73.3)	199 (58.3)	
Unknown	2 (0.1)	2 (0.2)	0	
Anti-HER2 therapy				0.256
Yes	55 (4.0)	37 (3.6)	18 (5.3)	
No	513 (37.7)	384 (37.6)	129 (38.1)	
Unknown	792 (58.3)	600 (58.8)	192 (56.6)	

Abbreviations: n = number; BCT = breast-conserving therapy; T = tumor; N = node; G = grade; HR = hormone receptor; HER2 = human epidermal growth receptor 2; NOS = not otherwise specified; mic = micrometastases; ITC = isolated tumor cells; SNB = sentinel node biopsy. Type of variable in bold.

3.1. Surgery

Most patients received a limited axillary surgery ($n = 1360$, 81.3%). Data regarding breast reconstruction were known for 557 (41.0%) patients. Among the 62 patients receiving breast reconstruction, 4 had stage IA, 31 had stage IB, and 27 had stage IIA breast cancer.

3.2. Radiation Therapy

Out of the 1021 patients receiving radiotherapy, all following breast-conserving surgery, 495 (48.5%) were treated with conventional fractionation (median dose 50 Gy; range 28–50.4 Gy), 489 (47.9%) with moderate hypofractionated schedules (median dose 45 Gy; range 34.5–47.5), and 37 (3.6%) received one of the ultra-hypofractionated schedules (median dose 31.5 Gy; range 20–50 Gy). Additional dose to the tumor bed was received by 661 (64.7%) patients. Almost all patients received whole-breast radiotherapy only, excluding axillary or supraclavicular nodal volumes ($n = 1014$; 99.3%).

3.3. Systemic Treatment

Timing (preoperative versus postoperative) and type of systemic treatment are presented separately for both groups in Table 2. The receipt of taxane-based chemotherapy was more frequently observed in the mastectomy group, as compared to the BCT group (32.8% versus 24.7%; $p < 0.0005$).

Table 2. Type and sequence of systemic treatment.

Variable	All Patients	BCT	Mastectomy	*p* Value
	n = 411 (100%)	*n* = 271 (65.9%)	*n* = 140 (34.1%)	
Chemotherapy				
Neoadjuvant systemic therapy	17 (4.1)	7 (2.6)	10 (7.1)	
Adjuvant systemic therapy	383 (93.2)	253 (93.4)	130 (92.9)	0.016
Unknown sequence	11 (2.7)	11 (4.0)	0	
Type of systemic chemotherapy				
Anthracyclines/Cyclophosphamide	236 (57.4)	172 (63.5)	64 (45.7)	
Taxanes/Cyclophosphamide	33 (8.0)	21 (7.7)	12 (8.6)	
Anthracyclines/Taxanes	80 (19.5)	46 (17.0)	34 (24.3)	<0.0005
CMF	27 (6.6)	8 (3.0)	19 (13.6)	
Other drugs and combinations	13 (3.2)	9 (3.3)	4 (2.9)	
Unknown	22 (5.4)	15 (5.5)	7 (5.0)	

In total, 578 (45.1%) evaluated patients received endocrine therapy with aromatase inhibitors, 539 (42.0%) with tamoxifen, and 122 (12.9%) with treatment combinations (i.e., tamoxifen and aromatase inhibitors). Compared with patients treated with mastectomy only, patients undergoing BCT more often received adjuvant endocrine therapy with aromatase inhibitors ($n = 141$; 40.3% versus $n = 437$; 46.9%) and were less likely to receive adjuvant therapy with tamoxifen (152; 43.4% versus 387; 41.5%). The observed differences were statistically significant ($p < 0.0005$).

3.4. Outcome

Median follow-up for DFS and OS was 6.9 years (range: 0.3–15.9) and 7.5 years (range: 0.2–25.9), respectively. Overall, 86 (6.3%) patients experienced local (LR), regional (RR), or distant recurrence. We observed statistically meaningful differences across all recurrence types (Table 3). The cumulative incidences of 5-year LR and 10-year LR were 2.0% and 3.0% for the whole group, respectively. For the BCT group, the cumulative incidences of 5-year and 10-year LR were 1.0% and 3.0%; the corresponding cumulative incidences for the mastectomy group were 4% for both observed intervals. Observed absolute differences in cumulative incidence of recurrences between BCT and mastectomy groups were small, although statistically significant.

Table 3. Cumulative incidence of local, regional, and distant recurrence for patients treated with breast-conserving therapy or with mastectomy.

Site of Recurrence	All Patients	BCT	Mastectomy	p Value
	n = 1360 (100%)	n = 1021 (75.1%)	n = 339 (24.9%)	
No recurrence	1275 (93.8)	969 (94.9)	306 (90.3)	<0.0001
Any recurrence	85 (6.2)	52 (5.1)	33 (9.7)	
Local recurrence	15 (1.1)	10 (1.0)	5 (1.5)	0.001
Regional nodes or adjacent tissues/organs	14 (1.0)	8 (0.8)	6 (1.8)	0.002
Distant metastasis	48 (3.5)	34 (3.3)	14 (4.1)	<0.0001
Unknown recurrence type	8 (0.6)	0	8 (2.4)	0.018
Second primary cancer	47 (3.5)	29 (2.8)	18 (5.3)	0.039

Abbreviations: n = number; BCT = breast-conserving therapy. Type of variable in bold.

For the whole cohort, the estimated 5-year and 10-year DFS were 96% and 95%, respectively. After stratification according to the type of local treatment, the estimated 5-year and 10-year DFS for the BCT group were 97% and 96%, and the estimated 5-year and 10-year DFS for the mastectomy-only group were 91% and 90% (log-rank; $p < 0.001$). In a univariate analysis, the following factors were associated with a decreased DFS: not receiving BCT, age > 70 years, tumor size ≥ 2 cm, stage IIA, tumor grade ≥ 2, and omission of endocrine adjuvant therapy. Upon multivariate Cox analysis, type of local treatment and tumor grade maintained statistical significance (Table 4).

Table 4. Univariate and multivariate Cox regression analysis for 5-year disease-free survival.

Variable	5-Year DFS	Univariate Analysis HR (95% CI)	p Value	Multivariate Analysis HR (95% CI)	p Value
Local treatment					
BCT	97%	1	<0.0005	1	0.006
Mastectomy	91%	2.883 (1.868–4.449)		2.291 (1.106–4.771)	
Age at diagnosis					
<50 years	95%	1	0.032	1	0.099
50–70 years	97%	0.932 (0.491–1.768)		0.863 (0.479–1.556)	
>70 years	93%	1.878 (0.911–3.873)		1.424 (0.708–2.864)	
Pathological tumor stage					
T1	97%	1	<0.0005	1	0.679
T2	90%	3.537 (2.279–5.489)		1.628 (0.769–3.444)	
≤T2, details unavailable	88%	3.759 (0.909–15.551)		1.823 (0.411–8.088)	
Pathological node stage					
N0	96%	1	0.267	1	0.354
N1	96%	1.105 (0.648–1.886)		0.075 (0.003–1.701)	
N status unknown	90%	2.584 (0.936–7.138)		5.103 (0.083–313.368)	
Overall stage group					
Stage IA	98%	1	<0.0005	1	0.269
Stage IB	98%	0.714 (0.330–1.544)		0.558 (0.251–1.241)	
Stage IIA	93%	2.545 (1.588–4.081)		1.479 (0.653–3.346)	
Grade					
G1	98%	1	<0.0005	1	<0.0005
G2	97%	1.168 (0.676–2.019)		1.164 (0.651–2.082)	
G3	91%	3.144 (1.786–5.536)		2.284 (1.124–4.641)	
Axillary surgery					
SNB only	97%	1	0.093	1	0.823
Axillary dissection	95%	1.370 (0.840–2.235)		1.043 (0.540–2.012)	
Omitted	89%	2.564 (1.103–5.960)		3.494 (1.442–8.463)	
Endocrine therapy					
Yes	97%	1	<0.0005	1	0.25
No	87%	3.430 (2.059–5.715)		2.974 (1.648–5.368)	

Table 4. *Cont.*

Variable	5-Year DFS	Univariate Analysis HR (95% CI)	Univariate Analysis *p* Value	Multivariate Analysis HR (95% CI)	Multivariate Analysis *p* Value
Chemotherapy					
Yes	93%	1	0.064	1	0.143
No	97%	0.600 (0.389–0.924)		1.445 (0.781–2.674)	
Anti-HER2 therapy					
Yes	96%	1	0.482	1	0.21
No	95%	1.614 (0.386–6.752)		2.991 (0.673–13.302)	

Abbreviations: HR = hazard ratio; CI = confidence interval; BCT = breast-conserving therapy; T = tumor; N = node; G = grade; HR = hormone receptor; HER2 = human epidermal growth receptor 2; SNB = sentinel node biopsy. Type of variable in bold.

The estimated 5-year and 10-year OS, calculated for the whole cohort, were 97% and 92%, respectively. Among patients treated with BCT, 5-year and 10-year OS estimates were 97% and 93%, and for those treated with mastectomy-only, 95% and 89%, respectively (log-rank; $p = 0.045$). Univariate and multivariate analyses were performed to analyze factors associated with worse survival outcomes. The use of mastectomy as the only local treatment was found to be correlated with worse OS in univariate analysis, but this finding was not confirmed in the multivariate Cox regression analysis (Table 5).

Table 5. Univariate and multivariate Cox regression analysis for 5-year overall survival.

Variable	5-Year OS	Univariate Analysis HR (95% CI)	Univariate Analysis *p* Value	Multivariate Analysis HR (95% CI)	Multivariate Analysis *p* Value
Local treatment					
BCT	97%	1	0.047	1	0.689
Mastectomy	95%	1.660 (1.006–2.738)		1.060 (0.564–1.994)	
Age at diagnosis					
<50 years	96%	1	0.066	1	0.691
50–70 years	98%	0.932 (0.491–1.768)		0.778 (0.365–1.657)	
>70 years	93%	1.878 (0.911–3.873)		1.151 (0.469–2.824)	
Pathological tumor stage					
T1	97%	1	0.037	1	0.573
T2	94%	2.013 (1.212–3.344)		0.488 (0.020–11.894)	
≤T2, details unavailable	94%	1.510 (0.208–10.950)		0.701 (0.006–81.144)	
Pathological node stage					
N0	97%	1	0.705	1	0.573
N1	97%	0.777 (0.409–1.477)		0.271 (0.009–7.817)	
N status unknown	94%	1.169 (0.285–4.789)		0.724 (0.012–42.111)	
Overall stage group					
Stage IA	99%	1	0.001	1	0.804
Stage IB	95%	2.966 (1.576–5.582)		0.186 (0.005–6.430)	
Stage IIA	95%	2.338 (1.270–4.304)		0.567 (0.116–2.774)	
Grade					
G1	99%	1	0.029	1	0.022
G2	97%	1.780 (0.980–3.232)		1.454 (0.623–3.395)	
G3	95%	1.982 (0.992–3.959)		1.310 (0.420–4.086)	
Axillary surgery					
SNB only	97%	1	0.43	1	0.686
Axillary dissection	97%	0.688 (0.361–1.311)		1.204 (0.441–3.286)	
Omitted	92%	1.296 (0.406–4.139)		0.784 (0.013–47.085)	
Endocrine therapy					
Yes	97%	1	0.665	1	0.582
No	95%	1.243 (0.596–2.589)		0.928 (0.321–2.682)	
Chemotherapy					
Yes	97%	1	0.554	1	0.042
No	97%	1.294 (0.760–2.202)		1.858 (0.744–4.638)	

Table 5. *Cont.*

		Univariate Analysis		Multivariate Analysis	
Variable	**5-Year OS**	**HR (95% CI)**	***p* Value**	**HR (95% CI)**	***p* Value**
Anti-HER2 therapy					
Yes	91%	1	0.931	1	0.452
No	95%	0.960 (0.382–2.413)		0.667 (0.239–1.864)	

Abbreviations: HR = hazard ratio; CI = confidence interval; BCT = breast-conserving therapy; T = Tumor; N = node; G = grade; HR = hormone receptor; HER2 = human epidermal growth receptor 2; SNB = sentinel node biopsy. Type of variable in bold.

High tumor grade and the omission of systemic chemotherapy were the only two factors associated with poorer OS. The type of local treatment was not associated with improved OS using multivariable Cox regression. Kaplan–Meier survival curves for all included patients representing DFS and OS with respect to breast cancer stage group are presented in Figure 1.

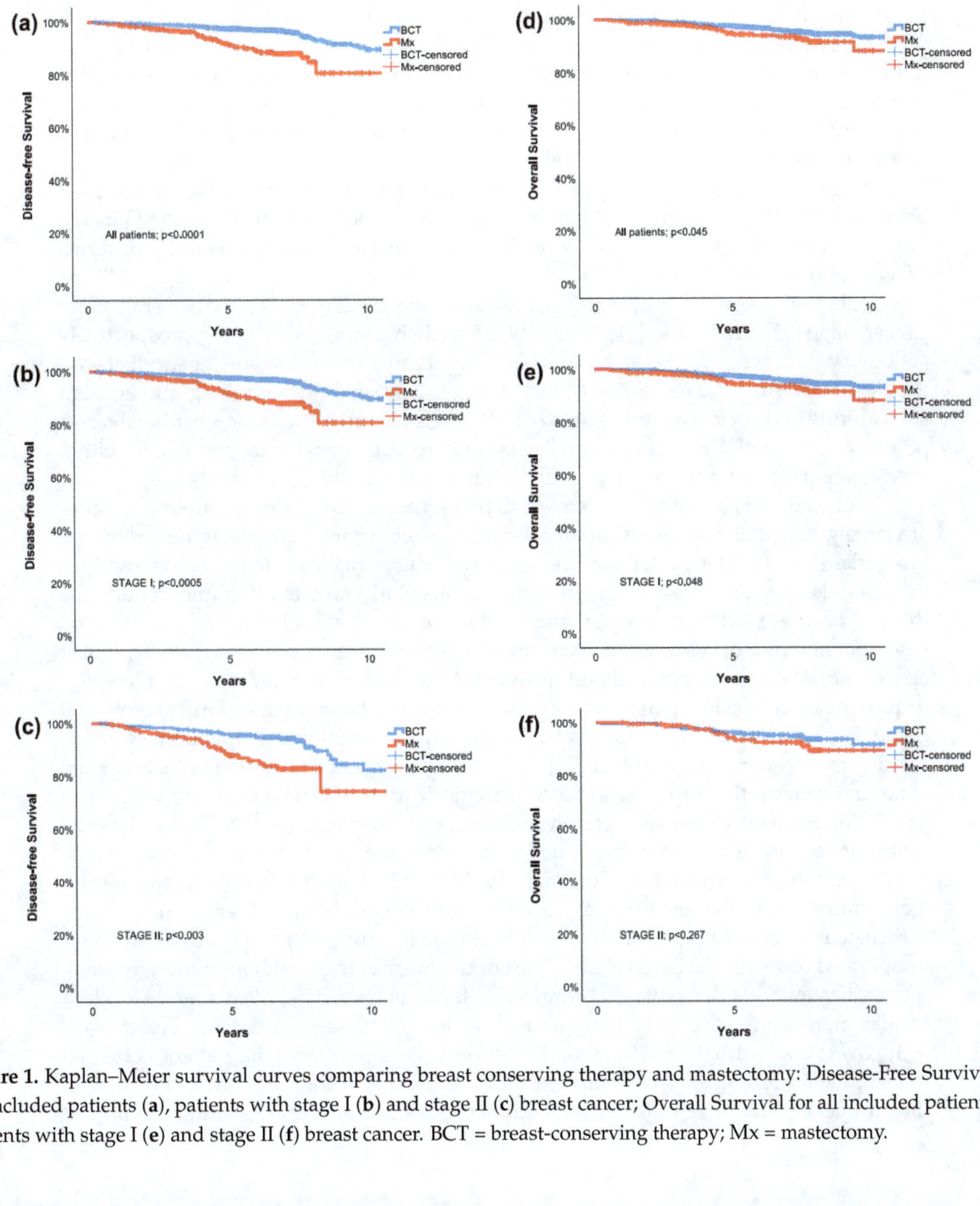

Figure 1. Kaplan–Meier survival curves comparing breast conserving therapy and mastectomy: Disease-Free Survival for all included patients (**a**), patients with stage I (**b**) and stage II (**c**) breast cancer; Overall Survival for all included patients (**d**), patients with stage I (**e**) and stage II (**f**) breast cancer. BCT = breast-conserving therapy; Mx = mastectomy.

After IPTW matching based on confounding variables (age at diagnosis, pathological tumor and nodal stage, overall breast cancer stage group, tumor grade, type of axillary surgery, and the receipt of chemotherapy or endocrine therapy), and after excluding study subjects with extreme weights, 1343 patients were available for the analysis. Mastectomy was associated with worse DFS (HR 2.839, 95% CI 1.760–4.579, $p < 0.0001$). This finding was not confirmed for OS (HR 1.455, 95% CI 0.844–2.511, $p = 0.177$).

4. Discussion

In our patient cohort treated in the contemporary era, we evaluated the therapeutic outcomes in patients with stage I-IIA breast cancer treated with either conservative surgery combined with postoperative radiation therapy or with mastectomy alone. We demonstrated an outcome improvement associated with BCT in terms of both 5-year DFS and 5-year OS, with absolute differences of 6% and 2%, respectively. The observed differences were also consistent at 10 years. However, using multivariable Cox regression and after IPTW matching, the only outcome that was found to be significantly impacted by the type of local treatment (BCT compared to mastectomy) was DFS.

In our study, we observed very low LR, RR, and distant metastasis rates within the whole cohort. The cumulative in-breast/chest-wall failure rates at 10 years after treatment were 3.0% for the BCT group and 4.0% for the mastectomy group. Compared to historical series, reporting approximately 5–10% in-breast failures after 10 years from treatment, our results compare favorably [46,47]. This finding is in agreement with the reports of other studies, which are all convincing and uniformly show DFS and/or OS benefits for BCT compared to mastectomy in patients with stage I-II breast cancer (Table 6). Equivalent or improved outcomes with BCT as compared with mastectomy in terms of locoregional control, BCSS, DFS, or OS have been reported regardless of age [14,15], intrinsic breast cancer subtype [48–51], pathological tumor stage [11,14,15,51], overall breast cancer stage [52], and grade [51]. Recently, a Swedish cohort study using prospectively collected data of women with stage T1-2 N0-2 breast cancer confirmed better survival with BCT vs. mastectomy (irrespective of radiation therapy) even when taking into account comorbidity and socioeconomic status in both node-negative and node-positive disease, pointing out that offering more extensive surgery to patients who are suitable for either breast-conserving surgery or mastectomy is not saving lives [51].

Improved survival rates in patients with breast cancer over the past couple of decades are largely attributable to the use of breast cancer screening and better imaging, predictive biomarkers, and better understanding of breast cancer heterogeneity. New advances in the field of systemic treatments, including molecularly targeted therapies, endocrine therapy, taxane-based chemotherapy, and bisphosphonates have all effectively contributed to reduce the risk of distant and local breast cancer recurrence. Consequently, breast cancer mortality rates have declined in recent decades even in patients with a low risk of recurrence at baseline [53]. However, the contributions of a particular type of local treatment and new developments related to both surgical techniques and modern radiation therapy are frequently overlooked [54]. It is well known that prevention of locoregional recurrence reduces the risk of breast-cancer-specific death and is related to improvements in OS [55,56]. Many possible reasons for the better outcomes observed for patients with breast cancer undergoing lumpectomy combined with postoperative radiotherapy compared with mastectomy have been already elucidated [46,54,57,58]. Surgery does provide superior local control within resected tissue; however, with tangential radiotherapy techniques, the treated volume is larger (as compared to simple mastectomy) and typically includes unoperated breast tissue in its entirety, part of the muscle, regional lymphatics, draining lymphatics towards the axillary region, subcutaneous lymphatic plexus, and skin [46]. Incidental irradiation may potentially sterilize microscopic disease outside the breast tissue as it covers approximately 85% of axillary level I lymph nodes if the patient is treated in a supine position [59]. At the same time, radiotherapy techniques have improved in the past years, with three-dimensional treatment planning and heart-sparing techniques, including deep-inspiration breath-hold, prone-positioning, and partial breast irradiation substantially decreasing the dose to the heart and subsequently reducing mortality rate from the cardiac events [60].

Table 6. Published studies comparing breast-conserving therapy with mastectomy for patients with stage I-II breast cancer.

Study	Years of Treatment	Stage	Number of Included Patients	Measured Outcome	BCT	Mastectomy	*p* Value
Hartman-Johnsen et al., 2015 [14]	1998–2008	T1–2 N0–1	BCT: 8065 Mastectomy: 4950	5-year BCSS	97%	88%	NA
Hartman-Johnsen et al., 2017 [15]	1998–2009	T1–2 N0–1	All: 6387	10-year BCSS	97% (T1N0) 98% (T1N1)	96% (T1N0) 89% (T1N1)	NA
Wang et al., 2018 [16]	1999–2014	T1 N0–1mi	BCT: 1296 Mastectomy: 4841	5-year DFS 5-year DMFS 5-year OS	95.30% 97% 99.10%	90.20% 92.20% 96.10%	0.001 <0.001 0.001
de Boniface et al., [20]	2000–2004	T1–2 N0–2 *	BCT: 2338 Mastectomy: 429	13-year OS 13-year BCSS	79.50% 90.50%	64.30% 84%	<0.001 <0.001
Corradini et al., 2019 [17]	1998–2014	T1–2 N0–1	BCT: 6412 Mastectomy: 1153	10-year DMFS 10-year OS	89.40% 85.30%	85.50% 79.30%	0.013 0.011
Lan et al., 2019 [18]	1998–2016	T1–2 N0–1	BCT: 410 Mastectomy: 1406	5-year LRFS	89%	85.30%	0.012
Sun et al., 2020 [19]	2009–2014	T1–2 N0–1	BCT: 404 Mastectomy (±RT): 3858	5-year DFS 5-year OS	96.50% 92.90%	92.70% 84%	0.001 <0.001
Almahariq et al., 2020 [13]	2006–2014	T1–2 N0	BCT: 144,263 Mastectomy: 87,379	5-year OS 7-year OS	94.40% 90%	91.80% 85.20%	<0.001 <0.001
Current study	2001–2013	T1–2 N0–1	BCT: 1021 Mastectomy: 339	5-year DFS 10-year DFS 5-year OS 10-year OS	97% 96% 97% 96%	91% 90% 95% 94%	<0.0005 0.045

* The cohort included up to 5% of patients with N2 disease. Abbreviations: BCT = breast-conserving therapy; BCSS = breast-cancer-specific survival; DFS = disease-free survival; DMFS = distant-metastasis-free survival; OS = overall survival; LRFS = locoregional relapse-free survival; RT = radiation therapy; NA = not available.

The possibility of an anticancer immune response that can be elicited by radiotherapy outside of the radiation field, targeting micro- or macro-metastases, is also one of the postulated mechanisms of action. Abscopal effects have been demonstrated not only at higher doses per fraction but also at the lower dose per fraction (2.0–2.5 Gy) typically used in breast cancer postoperative radiotherapy [61]. Moreover, it is well known that postoperative radiotherapy not only reduces local recurrence, but also diminishes the risk of any recurrence type, including distant relapse, which could be explained by mechanisms such as the abscopal effect [62].

Omitting postoperative radiation therapy after mastectomy in patients undergoing breast reconstruction or in those with N1 disease may be a partial culprit of higher disease recurrence in these patients. In our study, 17.6% of patients had pathological N1 disease and the percentage of patients with pathological N1 disease did not differ between the groups. None of the patients with pathological N1 disease in the mastectomy group received postoperative radiation therapy. In a study by Sun et al., the authors analyzed the treatment outcomes of 4262 patients with clinical stage T1-2N1M0 breast cancer, and 832 (21.6%) of them received mastectomy and postoperative radiation therapy. In multivariate and propensity-score matching analyses, radiation therapy, but not type of surgical treatment, appeared to be an independent prognostic factor for improved OS, DFS, and loco-regional recurrence [19]. Although results from the meta-analysis of individual patient data clearly demonstrated a benefit in reducing both recurrence and breast cancer mortality in women with one to three positive lymph nodes, postmastectomy radiotherapy is less often routinely recommended than radiotherapy following breast-conserving surgery in patients with pathological N1 disease [46,62]. Patients who require post-mastectomy radiation therapy following immediate breast reconstruction are exposed to a detectably higher risk of post-reconstruction complications, including infection, implant removal, and capsular contracture in patients receiving implant-based reconstruction, and fat necrosis in those receiving autologous-tissue-based reconstruction [63]. Factors influencing the final cosmetic outcome and patients' preferences may all affect the final decision to undergo postoperative chest-wall radiation therapy.

Despite the many benefits observed with BCT, the rates of unilateral or bilateral mastectomies for patients with unilateral breast cancer, who are candidates for BCT, are on the rise [29,64]. Perceived risks such as a fear of developing a second breast cancer, a historical belief that mastectomy is a safer option, possible avoidance of long-term breast cancer surveillance imaging, and the inconvenience of daily radiotherapy treatments may all have contributed to increasing mastectomy rates, which is of concern [53,65–67]. Nevertheless, it is important to note that different mastectomy and reconstruction techniques may lead to various amounts of remaining breast glandular tissue, potentially increasing the risk of breast cancer residual disease or recurrence [68].

As pointed out by Dodwell et al., women with screen-detected breast cancer are more likely to undergo BCT and mammographic screening confers a survival advantage compared to symptomatic presentation [69]. In our study, in which two-thirds of patients were aged between 50 and 70 years (n = 880, 64.7%) and a similar proportion had stage I disease (n = 891, 65.5%), individual data regarding screening status were missing.

The strengths of our study include a large patient cohort and thorough analysis with adjustments for confounding factors. Nevertheless, we acknowledge the limitations of our study and the difficulties in bias elimination in observational research. Our results may have been influenced by the retrospective nature of the study, as the quality of our data depend on reliable data collection. Additionally, follow-up was short and some of the data were not available at the time of the analysis. In our study, the impact of specific patient and tumor characteristics (e.g., age, tumor grade or size, lymph node status, and the receipt of endocrine therapy and systemic therapy) were adjusted with the use of a rigorous approach to reduce the effects of confounding in the estimation of the type of local treatment effect. However, we acknowledge the limitations of the propensity score analysis and IPTW-matching method, especially that there was no adjustment for the impact of all baseline characteristics [45]. In addition, a comparison of the results of patients with stage I-IIA EBC and treated with mastectomy followed by postoperative radiation therapy would certainly add value to our research.

5. Conclusions

Breast-conserving surgery followed by postoperative radiotherapy was shown in our study to have superior outcomes, including local, regional, and distant recurrence of the disease, and at least equivalent OS compared to mastectomy alone in patients with early-stage I-IIA breast cancer. The observed differences were statistically significant, but the clinical differences were relatively small. Nevertheless, it is essential that patients with EBC who are suitable for either BCT or mastectomy are well informed throughout the shared decision-making process about each locoregional treatment option and the corresponding long-term outcomes.

Author Contributions: Contributions are as follows for each author on this manuscript: Conceptualization, I.R. and P.F.; methodology, I.R., G.P., T.Z., P.F.; software, I.R., P.F., N.P.; validation, I.R., P.F., and A.P.; formal analysis, I.R. and P.F.; investigation, I.R. and P.F.; resources, I.R., P.F., N.P., A.P. and T.Z.; data curation, G.P., I.R., P.F., N.P. and T.Z.; writing—original draft preparation, I.R. and P.F.; writing—review and editing, I.R., P.F., G.P., N.P., T.Z. and A.P.; visualization, I.R. and P.F; supervision,

P.F.; project administration, G.P., I.R., P.F., N.P., T.Z. and A.P. All authors have read and agreed to the published version of the manuscript.

References

1. Veronesi, U.; Cascinelli, N.; Mariani, L.; Greco, M.; Saccozzi, R.; Luini, A.; Aguilar, M.; Marubini, E. Twenty-year follow-up of a randomized study comparing breast-conserving surgery with radical mastectomy for early breast cancer. *N. Engl. J. Med.* **2002**, *347*, 1227–1232. [CrossRef]
2. Fisher, B.; Anderson, S.; Bryant, J.; Margolese, R.G.; Deutsch, M.; Fisher, E.R.; Jeong, J.H.; Wolmark, N. Twenty-year follow-up of a randomized trial comparing total mastectomy, lumpectomy, and lumpectomy plus irradiation for the treatment of invasive breast cancer. *N. Engl. J. Med.* **2002**, *347*, 1233–1241. [CrossRef]
3. Poggi, M.M.; Danforth, D.N.; Sciuto, L.C.; Smith, S.L.; Steinberg, S.M.; Liewehr, D.J.; Menard, C.; Lippman, M.E.; Lichter, A.S.; Altemus, R.M. Eighteen-year results in the treatment of early breast carcinoma with mastectomy versus breast conservation therapy: The National Cancer Institute randomized trial. *Cancer* **2003**, *98*, 697–702. [CrossRef]
4. Blichert-Toft, M.; Nielsen, M.; Düring, M.; Møller, S.; Rank, F.; Overgaard, M.; Mouridsen, H.T. Long-term results of breast conserving surgery vs. mastectomy for early stage invasive breast cancer: 20-year follow-up of the Danish randomized DBCG- 82TM protocol. *Acta Oncol.* **2008**, *47*, 672–681. [CrossRef]
5. Litière, S.; Werutsky, G.; Fentiman, I.S.; Rutgers, E.; Christiaens, M.R.; Van Limbergen, E.; Baaijens, M.H.; Bogaerts, J.; Bartelink, H. Breast conserving therapy versus mastectomy for stage I-II breast cancer: 20-year follow-up of the EORTC 10801 phase 3 randomised trial. *Lancet Oncol.* **2012**, *13*, 412–419. [CrossRef]
6. Lazovich, D.; Solomon, C.C.; Thomas, D.B.; Moe, R.E.; White, E. Breast conservation therapy in the United States following the 1990 National Institutes of Health Consensus Development Conference on the treatment of patients with early stage invasive breast carcinoma. *Cancer* **1999**, *86*, 628–637. [CrossRef]
7. Lagendijk, M.; van Maaren, M.C.; Saadatmand, S.; Strobbe, L.J.A.; Poortmans, P.M.P.; Koppert, L.B.; Tilanus-Linthorst, M.M.A.; Siesling, S. Breast conserving therapy and mastectomy revisited: Breast cancer-specific survival and the influence of prognostic factors in 129,692 patients. *Int. J. Cancer* **2018**, *142*, 165–175. [CrossRef] [PubMed]
8. Van Maaren, M.C.; de Munck, L.; Jobsen, J.J.; Poortmans, P.; de Bock, G.H.; Siesling, S.; Strobbe, L.J.A. Breast-conserving therapy versus mastectomy in T1-2N2 stage breast cancer: A population-based study on 10-year overall, relative, and distant metastasis-free survival in 3071 patients. *Breast Cancer Res. Treat.* **2016**, *160*, 511–521. [CrossRef]
9. Van Maaren, M.C.; de Munck, L.; de Bock, G.H.; Jobsen, J.J.; van Dalen, T.; Linn, S.C.; Poortmans, P.; Strobbe, L.J.A.; Siesling, S. 10-year survival after breast-conserving surgery plus radiotherapy compared with mastectomy in early breast cancer in The Netherlands: A population-based study. *Lancet Oncol.* **2016**, *17*, 1158–1170. [CrossRef]
10. De Boniface, J.; Szulkin, R.; Johansson, A. Survival after breast conservation versus mastectomy adjusted for comorbidity and socioeconomic status: National 6-year follow-up on 48986 women. *Breast* **2021**, *56*, S69. [CrossRef]
11. Agarwal, S.; Pappas, L.; Neumayer, L.; Kokeny, K.; Agarwal, J. Effect of breast conservation therapy vs mastectomy on disease- specific survival for early-stage breast cancer. *JAMA Surg.* **2014**, *149*, 267–274. [CrossRef] [PubMed]
12. Wrubel, E.; Natwick, R.; Wright, G.P. Breast-Conserving Therapy is Associated with Improved Survival Compared with Mastectomy for Early-Stage Breast Cancer: A Propensity Score Matched Comparison Using the National Cancer Database. *Ann. Surg. Oncol.* **2021**, *28*, 914–919. [CrossRef]
13. Almahariq, M.F.; Quinn, T.J.; Siddiqui, Z.; Jawad, M.S.; Chen, P.Y.; Gustafson, G.S.; Dilworth, J.T. Breast conserving therapy is associated with improved overall survival compared to mastectomy in early-stage, lymph node-negative breast cancer. *Radiother Oncol.* **2020**, *142*, 186–194. [CrossRef]
14. Hartmann-Johnsen, O.J.; Kåresen, R.; Schlichting, E.; Nygård, J.F. Survival is Better after Breast Conserving Therapy than Mastectomy for Early Stage Breast Cancer: A Registry-Based Follow-up Study of Norwegian Women Primary Operated Between 1998 and 2008. *Ann. Surg. Oncol.* **2015**, *22*, 3836–3845. [CrossRef] [PubMed]
15. Hartmann-Johnsen, O.J.; Kåresen, R.; Schlichting, E.; Nygård, J.F. Better survival after breast-conserving therapy compared to mastectomy when axillary node status is positive in early-stage breast cancer: A registry-based follow-up study of 6387 Norwegian women participating in screening, primarily operated between 1998 and 2009. *World J. Surg. Oncol.* **2017**, *15*, 118. [CrossRef] [PubMed]

16. Wang, J.; Wang, S.; Tang, Y.; Jing, H.; Sun, G.; Jin, J.; Liu, Y.; Song, Y.; Wang, W.; Fang, H.; et al. Comparison of Treatment Outcomes With Breast-conserving Surgery Plus Radiotherapy Versus Mastectomy for Patients with Stage I Breast Cancer: A Propensity Score-matched Analysis. *Clin. Breast Cancer* **2018**, *18*, e975–e984. [CrossRef] [PubMed]
17. Corradini, S.; Reitz, D.; Pazos, M.; Schönecker, S.; Braun, M.; Harbeck, N.; Matuschek, C.; Bölke, E.; Ganswindt, U.; Alongi, F.; et al. Mastectomy or breast-conserving therapy for early breast cancer in real-life clinical practice: Outcome comparison of 7565 cases. *Cancers* **2019**, *11*, 160. [CrossRef] [PubMed]
18. Lan, X.W.; Wen, G.; He, Z.; Huang, J.H.; Zou, X.B.; Lin, X.; Tan, Y.T.; Huang, X.B. Comparison of long-term results between radiotherapy after breast-conserving surgery and postmastectomy radiotherapy in stage T1-2N1M0 breast cancer. *Cancer Manag Res.* **2019**, *11*, 6477–6487. [CrossRef] [PubMed]
19. Sun, G.Y.; Wen, G.; Zhang, Y.J.; Tang, Y.; Jing, H.; Wang, J.Y.; Zhang, J.H.; Yang, Y.; Zhao, X.R.; Chen, S.Y.; et al. Radiotherapy plays an important role in improving the survival outcome in patients with T1–2N1M0 breast cancer—A joint analysis of 4262 real world cases from two institutions. *BMC Cancer* **2020**, *20*, 1155. [CrossRef]
20. De Boniface, J.; Frisell, J.; Bergkvist, L.; Andersson, Y. Breast-conserving surgery followed by whole-breast irradiation offers survival benefits over mastectomy without irradiation. *Br. J. Surg.* **2018**, *105*, 1607–1614. [CrossRef]
21. Mahmood, U.; Morris, C.; Neuner, G.; Koshy, M.; Kesmodel, S.; Buras, R.; Chumsri, S.; Bao, T.; Tkaczuk, K.; Feigenberg, S. Similar survival with breast conservation therapy or mastectomy in the management of young women with early-stage breast cancer. *Int. J. Radiat. Oncol. Biol. Phys.* **2012**, *83*, 1387–1393. [CrossRef]
22. Frandsen, J.; Ly, D.; Cannon, G.; Suneja, G.; Matsen, C.; Gaffney, D.K.; Wright, M.; Kokeny, K.E.; Poppe, M.M. In the Modern Treatment Era, Is Breast Conservation Equivalent to Mastectomy in Women Younger Than 40 Years of Age? A Multi-Institution Study. *Int. J. Radiat. Oncol. Biol. Phys.* **2015**, *93*, 1096–1103. [CrossRef] [PubMed]
23. Cao, J.Q.; Truong, P.T.; Olivotto, I.A.; Olson, R.; Coulombe, G.; Keyes, M.; Weir, L.; Gelmon, K.; Bernstein, V.; Woods, R.; et al. Should women younger than 40 years of age with invasive breast cancer have a mastectomy? 15-year outcomes in a population-based cohort. *Int. J. Radiat. Oncol. Biol. Phys.* **2014**, *90*, 509–517. [CrossRef]
24. Mamtani, A.; Morrow, M. Why Are There So Many Mastectomies in the United States? *Annu. Rev. Med.* **2017**, *68*, 229–241. [CrossRef] [PubMed]
25. Riedel, F.; Hennigs, A.; Hug, S.; Schaefgen, B.; Sohn, C.; Schuetz, F.; Golatta, M.; Heil, J. Is Mastectomy Oncologically Safer than Breast-Conserving Treatment in Early Breast Cancer. *Breast Care* **2017**, *12*, 385–390. [CrossRef]
26. Cardoso, F.; Kyriakides, S.; Ohno, S.; Penault-Llorca, F.; Poortmans, P.; Rubio, I.T.; Zackrisson, S.; Senkus, E.; ESMO Guidelines Committee. Early breast cancer: ESMO Clinical Practice Guidelines for diagnosis, treatment and follow-up. *Ann. Oncol.* **2019**, *30*, 1194–1220. [CrossRef]
27. Kummerow, K.L.; Du, L.; Penson, D.F.; Shyr, Y.; Hooks, M.A. Nationwide trends in mastectomy for early-stage breast cancer. *JAMA Surg.* **2015**, *150*, 9–16. [CrossRef]
28. Pesce, C.E.; Liederbach, E.; Czechura, T.; Winchester, D.J.; Yao, K. Changing surgical trends in young patients with early stage breast cancer, 2003 to 2010: A report from the National Cancer Data Base. *J. Am. Coll. Surg.* **2014**, *219*, 19–28. [CrossRef]
29. Baskin, A.S.; Wang, T.; Bredbeck, B.C.; Sinco, B.R.; Berlin, N.L.; Dossett, L.A. Trends in Contralateral Prophylactic Mastectomy Utilization for Small Unilateral Breast Cancer. *J. Surg. Res.* **2021**, *262*, 71–84. [CrossRef] [PubMed]
30. Garcia-Etienne, C.A.; Tomatis, M.; Heil, J.; Friedrichs, K.; Kreienberg, R.; Denk, A.; Kiechle, M.; Lorenz-Salehi, F.; Kimmig, R.; Emons, G.; et al. Mastectomy trends for early-stage breast cancer: A report from the EUSOMA multi-institutional European database. *Eur. J. Cancer* **2012**, *48*, 1947–1956. [CrossRef] [PubMed]
31. Sinnadurai, S.; Kwong, A.; Hartman, M.; Tan, E.Y.; Bhoo-Pathy, N.T.; Dahlui, M.; See, M.H.; Yip, C.H.; Taib, N.A.; Bhoo-Pathy, N. Breast-conserving surgery versus mastectomy in young women with breast cancer in Asian settings. *BJS Open* **2019**, *3*, 48–55. [CrossRef]
32. Yu, L.-X.; Shi, P.; Tian, X.-S.; Yu, Z.-G. A multi-center investigation of breast-conserving surgery based on data from the Chinese Society of Breast Surgery (CSBrS-005). *Chin. Med. J.* **2020**, *133*, 2660–2664. [CrossRef]
33. Hassan Ali, S.; Somashekhar, S.P.; Arun, K.N. Rate of Breast-Conserving Surgery vs Mastectomy in Breast Cancer: A Tertiary Care Centre Experience from South India. *Indian J. Surg. Oncol.* **2019**, *10*, 72–76. [CrossRef]
34. Gass, J.; Mitchell, S.; Hanna, M. How do breast cancer surgery scars impact survivorship? Findings from a nationwide survey in the United States. *BMC Cancer* **2019**, *19*, 342. [CrossRef]
35. Arndt, V.; Stegmaier, C.; Ziegler, H.; Brenner, H. Quality of life over 5 years in women with breast cancer after breast-conserving therapy versus mastectomy: A population-based study. *J. Cancer Res. Clin. Oncol.* **2008**, *134*, 1311–1318. [CrossRef]

36. Engel, J.; Kerr, J.; Schlesinger-Raab, A.; Sauer, H.; Hölzel, D. Quality of life following breast-conserving therapy or mastectomy: Results of a 5-year prospective study. *Breast J.* **2004**, *10*, 223–231. [CrossRef]
37. Zehra, S.; Doyle, F.; Barry, M.; Walsh, S.; Kell, M.R. Health-related quality of life following breast reconstruction compared to total mastectomy and breast-conserving surgery among breast cancer survivors: A systematic review and meta-analysis. *Breast Cancer* **2020**, *27*, 534–566. [CrossRef]
38. Retrouvey, H.; Solaja, O.; Gagliardi, A.R.; Webster, F.; Zhong, T. Barriers of Access to Breast Reconstruction: A Systematic Review. *Plast. Reconstr. Surg.* **2019**, *143*, 465e–476e. [CrossRef] [PubMed]
39. Frasier, L.L.; Holden, S.; Holden, T.; Schumacher, J.R.; Leverson, G.; Anderson, B.; Greenberg, C.C.; Neuman, H.B. Temporal trends in postmastectomy radiation therapy and breast reconstruction associated with changes in national comprehensive cancer network guidelines. *JAMA Oncol.* **2016**, *2*, 95–101. [CrossRef] [PubMed]
40. Yang, R.L.; Newman, A.S.; Lin, I.C.; Reinke, C.E.; Karakousis, G.C.; Czerniecki, B.J.; Wu, L.C.; Kelz, R.R. Trends in immediate breast reconstruction across insurance groups after enactment of breast cancer legislation. *Cancer* **2013**, *119*, 2462–2468. [CrossRef] [PubMed]
41. Jagsi, R.; Abrahamse, P.; Hawley, S.T.; Graff, J.J.; Hamilton, A.S.; Katz, S.J. Underascertainment of radiotherapy receipt in Surveillance, Epidemiology, and End Results registry data. *Cancer* **2012**, *118*, 333–341. [CrossRef] [PubMed]
42. Sobin, L.H.; Gospodarowicz, M.K.; Wittekind, C. *TNM Classification of Malignant Tumours*, 7th ed.; International Union Against Cancer; John Wiley and Sons: Hoboken, NJ, USA, 2009.
43. Goldhirsch, A.; Winer, E.P.; Coates, A.S.; Gelber, R.D.; Piccart-Gebhart, M.; Thürlimann, B.; Senn, H.J.; Panel Members. Personaliz- ing the treatment of women with early breast cancer: Highlights of the St Gallen International Expert Consensus on the Primary Therapy of Early Breast Cancer 2013. *Ann. Oncol.* **2013**, *24*, 2206–2223. [CrossRef]
44. Austin, P.C. Goodness-of-fit diagnostics for the propensity score model when estimating treatment effects using covariate adjustment with the propensity score. *Pharmacoepidemiol. Drug Saf.* **2008**, *17*, 1202–1217. [CrossRef]
45. Lalani, N.; Jimenez, R.B.; Yeap, B. Understanding Propensity Score Analyses. *Int. J. Radiat. Oncol. Biol. Phys.* **2020**, *107*, 404–407. [CrossRef]
46. Marks, L.B.; Gupta, G.P.; Muss, H.B.; Ollila, D.W. Mastectomy May Be an Inferior Oncologic Approach Compared to Breast Preservation. *Int. J. Radiat. Oncol. Biol. Phys.* **2019**, *103*, 78–80. [CrossRef] [PubMed]
47. Early Breast Cancer Trialists' Collaborative Group. Effects of Radiotherapy and Surgery in Early Breast Cancer. An Overview of the Randomized Trials. *N. Engl. J. Med.* **1995**, *333*, 1444–1455. [CrossRef]
48. Zhang, J.; Yang, C.; Lei, C.; Zhang, Y.; Ji, F.; Gao, H.; Yang, M.; Zhang, L.; Li, J.; Zhu, T.; et al. Survival outcomes after breast- conserving therapy compared with mastectomy for patients with early-stage metaplastic breast cancer: A population-based study of 2412 patients. *Breast* **2021**, *58*, 10–17. [CrossRef] [PubMed]
49. Abdulkarim, B.S.; Cuartero, J.; Hanson, J.; Deschênes, J.; Lesniak, D.; Sabri, S. Increased risk of locoregional recurrence for women with T1-2N0 triple-negative breast cancer treated with modified radical mastectomy without adjuvant radiation therapy compared with breast-conserving therapy. *J. Clin. Oncol.* **2011**, *29*, 2852–2858. [CrossRef]
50. Zumsteg, Z.S.; Morrow, M.; Arnold, B.; Zheng, J.; Zhang, Z.; Robson, M.; Traina, T.; McCormick, B.; Powell, S.; Ho, A.Y. Breast-conserving therapy achieves locoregional outcomes comparable to mastectomy in women with T1-2N0 triple-negative breast cancer. *Ann. Surg. Oncol.* **2013**, *20*, 3469–3476. [CrossRef]
51. De Boniface, J.; Szulkin, R.; Johansson, A.L.V. Survival after Breast Conservation vs Mastectomy Adjusted for Comorbidity and Socioeconomic Status: A Swedish National 6-Year Follow-up of 48986 Women. *JAMA Surg* **2021**, *156*, 628–637. [CrossRef]
52. van Maaren, M.C.; le Cessie, S.; Strobbe, L.J.A.; Groothuis-Oudshoorn, C.G.M.; Poortmans, P.M.P.; Siesling, S. Different statis- tical techniques dealing with confounding in observational research: Measuring the effect of breast-conserving therapy and mastectomy on survival. *J. Cancer Res. Clin. Oncol.* **2019**, *145*, 1485–1493. [CrossRef]
53. Anampa, J.; Makower, D.; Sparano, J.A. Progress in adjuvant chemotherapy for breast cancer: An overview. *BMC Med.* **2015**, *13*, 195. [CrossRef] [PubMed]
54. Murphy, J.; Gandhi, A. Does Mastectomy Reduce Overall Survival in Early Stage Breast Cancer? *Clin. Oncol. R. Coll. Radiol.* **2021**, *33*, 440–447. [CrossRef]
55. Clarke, M.; Collins, R.; Darby, S.; Davies, C.; Elphinstone, P.; Evans, V.; Godwin, J.; Gray, R.; Hicks, C.; James, S.; et al. Early Breast Cancer Trialists' Collaborative Group (EBCTCG). Effects of radiotherapy and of differences in the extent of surgery for early breast cancer on local recurrence and 15-year survival: An overview of the randomised trials. *Lancet* **2005**, *366*, 2087–2106. [CrossRef]

56. Sautter-Bihl, M.L.; Sedlmayer, F.; Budach, W.; Dunst, J.; Feyer, P.; Fietkau, R.; Haase, W.; Harms, W.; Rödel, C.; Souchon, R.; et al. One life saved by four prevented recurrences? *Strahlenther. Onkol.* **2012**, *188*, 461–463. [CrossRef] [PubMed]
57. Gentilini, O.D.; Cardoso, M.-J.; Poortmans, P. Less is more. Breast conservation might be even better than mastectomy in early breast cancer patients. *Breast* **2017**, *35*, 32–33. [CrossRef]
58. Van Maaren, M.C.; Poortmans, P.; Siesling, S. Breast-conserving therapy versus mastectomy. *Oncoscience* **2016**, *3*, 304–305. [CrossRef]
59. Park, S.-H.; Kim, J.-C.; Lee, J.E.; Park, I.-K. Virtual lymph node analysis to evaluate axillary lymph node coverage provided by tangential breast irradiation. *Radiat. Oncol. J.* **2015**, *33*, 50–56. [CrossRef]
60. Haussmann, J.; Corradini, S.; Nestle-Kraemling, C.; Bölke, E.; Njanang, F.J.D.; Tamaskovics, B.; Orth, K.; Ruckhaeberle, E.; Fehm, T.; Mohrmann, S.; et al. Recent advances in radiotherapy of breast cancer. *Radiat. Oncol.* **2020**, *15*, 71. [CrossRef] [PubMed]
61. Deutsch, E.; Chargari, C.; Galluzzi, L.; Kroemer, G. Optimising efficacy and reducing toxicity of anticancer radioimmunotherapy. *Lancet Oncol.* **2019**, *20*, e452–e463. [CrossRef]
62. EBCTCG (Early Breast Cancer Trialists' Collaborative Group); McGale, P.; Taylor, C.; Correa, C.; Cutter, D.; Duane, F.; Ewertz, M.; Gray, R.; Mannu, G.; Peto, R.; et al. Effect of radiotherapy after mastectomy and axillary surgery on 10-year recurrence and 20-year breast cancer mortality: Meta-analysis of individual patient data for 8135 women in 22 randomised trials. *Lancet* **2014**, *383*, 2127–2135. [CrossRef]
63. Jagsi, R.; Jiang, J.; Momoh, A.O.; Alderman, A.; Giordano, S.H.; Buchholz, T.A.; Pierce, L.J.; Kronowitz, S.J.; Smith, B.D. Complications After Mastectomy and Immediate Breast Reconstruction for Breast Cancer: A Claims-Based Analysis. *Ann. Surg.* **2016**, *263*, 219–227. [CrossRef]
64. Findlay-Shirras, L.; Lima, I.; Smith, G.; Clemons, M.; Arnaout, A. Canada follows the US in the rise of bilateral mastectomies for unilateral breast cancer: A 23-year population cohort study. *Breast Cancer Res. Treat.* **2021**, *185*, 517–525. [CrossRef]
65. Wang, T.; Mott, N.; Miller, J.; Berlin, N.L.; Hawley, S.; Jagsi, R.; Dossett, L.A. Patient Perspectives on Treatment Options for Older Women with Hormone Receptor-Positive Breast Cancer: A Qualitative Study. *JAMA Netw. Open* **2020**, *3*, e2017129. [CrossRef] [PubMed]
66. Nash, R.; Goodman, M.; Lin, C.C.; Freedman, R.A.; Dominici, L.S.; Ward, K.; Jemal, A. State Variation in the Receipt of a Contralateral Prophylactic Mastectomy Among Women Who Received a Diagnosis of Invasive Unilateral Early-Stage Breast Cancer in the United States, 2004–2012. *JAMA Surg.* **2017**, *152*, 648–657. [CrossRef]
67. Hawley, S.T.; Jagsi, R.; Morrow, M.; Janz, N.K.; Hamilton, A.; Graff, J.J.; Katz, S.J. Social and Clinical Determinants of Contralateral Prophylactic Mastectomy. *JAMA Surg.* **2014**, *149*, 582–589. [CrossRef] [PubMed]
68. Kaidar-Person, O.; Offersen, B.V.; Boersma, L.J.; de Ruysscher, D.; Tramm, T.; Kühn, T.; Gentilini, O.; Mátrai, Z.; Poortmans, P. A multidisciplinary view of mastectomy and breast reconstruction: Understanding the challenges. *Breast* **2021**, *56*, 42–52. [CrossRef]
69. Dodwell, D.; Wheatley, D. Counterpoint: Does Mastectomy Reduce Overall Survival in Early Stage Breast Cancer? *Clin. Oncol.* **2021**, *33*, 448–450. [CrossRef] [PubMed]

5

LightSpot®-FL-1 Fluorescent Probe: An Innovative Tool for Cancer Drug Resistance Analysis by Direct Detection and Quantification of the P-glycoprotein (P-gp) on Monolayer Culture and Spheroid Triple Negative Breast Cancer Models

Antoine Goisnard [1,†], Pierre Daumar [1,†], Clémence Dubois [1,2], Corinne Aubel [3], Manon Roux [2], Marie Depresle [2], Jean Gauthier [2,4], Bernard Vidalinc [2,4], Frédérique Penault-Llorca [5], Emmanuelle Mounetou [1] and Mahchid Bamdad [1,*]

1 Institut Universitaire de Technologie, Université Clermont Auvergne, UMR INSERM-UCA, U1240, Imagerie Moléculaire et Stratégies Théranostiques, 63000 Clermont Ferrand, France; antoine.goisnard@uca.fr (A.G.); pierre.daumar@uca.fr (P.D.); clemence.dubois@uca.fr (C.D.); emmanuelle.mounetou@inserm.fr (E.M.)

2 BIOMARQUEURS Company, 5 Avenue Blaise Pascal, 63178 Aubière, France; manon.roux@uca.fr (M.R.); marie.depresle@uca.fr (M.D.); jean.gauthier@uca.fr (J.G.); bernard.vidalinc@uca.fr (B.V.)

3 Faculté de Médecine, Université Clermont Auvergne, UMR INSERM-UCA, U1240, Imagerie Moléculaire et Stratégies Théranostiques, 63000 Clermont Ferrand, France; corinne.aubel@uca.fr

4 BIOPASS Company, 5 Avenue Blaise Pascal, 63178 Aubière, France

5 Centre de Lutte Contre le Cancer Jean Perrin, Université Clermont Auvergne, UMR INSERM-UCA, U1240, Imagerie Moléculaire et Stratégies Théranostiques, 63000 Clermont Ferrand, France; frederique.penault-llorca@clermont.unicancer.fr

* Correspondence: mahchid.bamdad@uca.fr;

† These authors contributed equally to this work.

Simple Summary: Tumoral drug resistance is mainly caused by multidrug resistance transporters (MDR), such as the P-gp, which presents high clinical interest. For this reason, the P-gp-mediated drug resistance diagnosis may be very relevant for optimizing anticancer treatment efficacy. However, the lack of effective analytical tools limits this clinical diagnostic approach. Therefore, our group has developed LightSpot®-FL-1, a new cell-permeant fluorescent probe able to specifically localize and quantify the P-gp inside unicellular, monolayer, and cellular mass models. The application of this innovative tool was firstly demonstrated in the preclinical field, using five triple-negative breast cancer (TNBC) cell models. The comparison between classical anti-P-gp immunostaining and LightSpot®-FL-1 P-gp staining highlighted a strong similarity with P-gp localization and expression level quantification. LightSpot®-FL-1 P-gp detection and quantification, using several fluorescence imaging methods, are easy, direct, and cost-effective and are, therefore, very promising for future clinical diagnosis development.

Abstract: P-gp is the most widely studied MDR protein conferring cellular resistance to many standard or targeted therapeutic agents. For this reason, P-gp chemoresistance evaluation, established before or during chemotherapy, can be very relevant in order to optimize the efficacy of treatments, particularly for aggressive tumoral subtypes such as triple-negative breast cancer (TNBC). In this context, our team developed an innovative cell-permeant fluorescent probe called the LightSpot®-FL-1, which is able to specifically localize and quantify the P-gp in cells or cell masses, as evidenced on different TNBC cell models. First, flow cytometry analysis showed LightSpot®-FL-1 cell penetration and persistence in time, in TNBC cells. Then, LightSpot®-FL-1 staining was compared to anti-P-gp immunostaining by fluorescence microscopy on five TNBC cell lines. Results showed a clear similarity of P-gp localization and expression level, confirmed by Pearson's and Mander's colocalization coefficients with 92.1% and 100.0%, and a strong correlation coefficient of $R^2 = 0.99$. In addition, the LightSpot®-FL-1 staining allowed the quantification of a P-gp induction (33% expression increase) following a 6-hour spheroid model exposure to the anti-PARP Olaparib. Thus, the new LightSpot®-FL-1 cell-permeant probe, targeting P-gp, appears to be an effective tool for drug resistance evaluation in preclinical models and shows promising possibilities for future use in clinical diagnosis.

Keywords: multidrug resistance; P-gp staining; LightSpot®-FL-1 cell-permeant fluorescent probe; triple-negative breast cancer

1. Introduction

The permeability-glycoprotein (P-gp) was discovered about forty years ago, initially as a membrane transporter at the origin of chemoresistance in cancer [1]. In reality, P-gp is part of a wide class of "ATP-binding cassette" (ABC) superfamily transporter proteins, called "multidrug resistance" (MDR). MDR proteins, and the P-gp in particular, were highly conserved during the evolutionary process and are ubiquitous. In fact, they are naturally expressed in a wide variety of living organisms from prokaryotes to eukaryotes, such as bacteria, protozoa, fish, *Drosophila* and mammals [2–6]. In humans, MDR proteins are commonly studied because of their involvement in tumoral multidrug resistance mechanisms [7,8]. Indeed, MDR proteins act as xenobiotic transmembrane efflux pumps, recognizing a large panel of substrates with different structures and properties, such as various pollutants and drugs [9–11]. These pumps establish a veritable cellular defense network, exhibiting a protective role against external aggressions. At present, MDR transporters are considered to be an essential part of the innate cellular defense system, also called the "chemoimmunity" network, that presents various characteristics reminiscent of classical immunology [12]. This system is particularly complex because a single MDR transporter can recognize a wide variety of substrates, and one anticancer agent can also be the target of several transporters. Thus, MDR proteins have been identified as one of the main causes of tumoral cell cross-resistance against anticancer drugs. Indeed, many conventional chemotherapeutic agents, such as anthracyclines, taxanes or vinca-alkaloids, and/or targeted therapeutics such as tyrosine kinase inhibitors or poly-ADP ribose polymerase inhibitors (anti-PARPs) are expelled from cells by MDR transporters [13–15], and many tumoral types overexpress several MDR transporters. The main identified MDR proteins presenting a clinical involvement are (i) the P-gp encoded by *ABCB1*, (ii) the MDR-associated proteins (MRP) encoded by *ABCC* genes, such as MRP1 (*ABCC1*) or MRP7 (*ABCC10*), and (iii) the breast cancer resistance protein (BCRP) encoded by the *ABCG2* gene [8,16].

Numerous biological mechanisms can lead to the development of chemoresistance, among which MDR-mediated drug efflux is the most frequently described [17]. Likewise, high expression of MDR proteins is often associated with aggressive subtypes and low disease-free survival rates in breast tumors [18]. Thereby, their clinical relevance resides in their predictive value on tumoral drug resistance, which is directly linked to the prognosis of the disease [19,20]. Thus, the importance of considering the P-gp expression level in tumors to optimize patients' treatment orientation was highlighted in several studies [19,21,22]. However, the P-gp expression level is not frequently evaluated in clinical practice, which can in part be attributed to one specific issue, namely the lack of relevant analytical tools [8].

Triple-negative breast cancer (TNBC) is a breast cancer subtype that is immunohistochemically negative for the estrogen receptor (ER) and for the progesterone receptor (PR), and is also associated with the absence of HER2 protein overexpression and/or *HER2* gene amplification [23]. This heterogeneous and aggressive disease accounts for 15 to 20% of breast cancers and is associated with poor prognosis and drug resistance [17,24,25]. Despite colossal efforts made regarding TNBC treatments, only 20% of patients present a pathologically complete response after treatment, while others are most likely to present an early recurrence or develop a metastatic disease [26]. As a matter of fact, TNBC tumors are, at first, particularly sensitive to chemotherapy, but a high proportion becomes resistant during treatment and presents difficulties for achieving a complete pathological response. This phenomenon is called the "triple-negative paradox" and explains why TNBC represents a relevant study model for cancer-cell drug resistance [17,27].

In the last few years, the works of our research group were focused on optimizing TNBC treatment, in correlation with resistance mechanisms mediated by MDR proteins. Indeed, we highlighted the relay overexpression of BCRP and P-gp MDR proteins on SUM1315 monolayer TNBC cell cultures, after exposure to the PARP inhibitor Olaparib [28]. Our group has developed various in vitro preclinical tools, e.g., TNBC cancer spheroids mimicking avascular small-size micro-tumors [29–32], notably for realizing high-throughput drug screening or modeling the distribution of small molecules of interest inside these cell masses [33]. In parallel, through pharmaco-modulation approaches, we designed bio-active fluorescent compounds such as LightSpot® fluorescent tracers targeting P-gp [34].

In these present works, we report on the validation of the LightSpot®-FL-1 tracer as an innovative fluorescent probe for selective and sensitive detection, localization, and quantification of the P-gp in cells or cell masses. The proof of concept was established on several unicellular, monolayer or spheroid TNBC models and a microscopy-based methodology was performed to explore native or induced P-gp expression on those models.

2. Experimental Section

2.1. *LightSpot®-FL-1 Chemical Synthesis Achievement*

Commercially available reagents and solvents were used without further purification for the synthesis and characterization of LightSpot®-FL-1, as previously described [34]. Briefly, LightSpot®-FL-1 was obtained by coupling an amine-bearing P-gp inhibitor derivative with the commercial amine-reactive *N*-hydroxysuccinimidyl ester of the BODIPY-FL fluorophore (CAS 146616-66-2, Interchim, Montluçon, France). After the coupling reaction proceeded, a preparative High-Performance Liquid Chromatography (HPLC) purification system (Shimadzu Inc., Kyoto, Japan) was performed to afford LightSpot®-FL-1 in good yield (>70%). LightSpot®-FL-1 was isolated at > 96% purity based on HPLC-UV-DAD analysis, and fully characterized by ^{1}H NMR, ^{13}C NMR, 2-dimensional COSY and HSQC NMR, and high-resolution mass spectrometry. Excitation and emission maxima were determined from LightSpot®-FL-1 solutions in ethanol at 505 and 510 nm, respectively. Pure dry aliquots of LightSpot®-FL-1 were stored at −20 °C and were used to prepare 1.0 mM stock solutions in DMSO for biological experiments.

2.2. *Monolayer Cell Culture and Spheroid Formation*

Triple-negative breast cancer SUM1315 (MO2, ASTERAND), MDA-MB-231 (ATCC®, HTB-26™), HCC1937 (ATCC® CRL-2336™), SW527 (ATCC® CRL-7940™) and DU4475 (ATCC®, HTB-123™) cell lines were stored in the Biological Resource Center of the Jean Perrin Comprehensive Cancer Center, identified under No. BB-0033-00075 (Clermont-Ferrand, France). Each cell line was checked for the absence of mycoplasma contamination (Mycoplasmacheck® test, Eurofins Genomics, Luxembourg, Luxembourg) and maintained in their recommended cell culture media at 37 °C under 5% CO_2 in a humidified incubator. For monolayer cell culture, SUM1315 cells were cultured in Ham's F-12 medium (Gibco, Dublin, Ireland), supplemented with 5% FCS (fetal calf serum, Eurobio Scientific, Paris, France), 10 mM HEPES buffer (Sigma, Darmstadt, Germany), 4 µg/mL insulin (Novo Nordisk, Bagsværd, Denmark), 10 ng/mL epidermal growth factor (EGF, Sigma, Darmstadt, Germany) and 20 µg/mL gentamicin (Panpharma, Paris, France). MDA-MB-231, HCC1937 and DU4475 cells were cultured in RPMI 1640 medium (Gibco, Dublin, Ireland) supplemented with 10% decomplemented fetal calf serum and 20 µg/mL gentamicin. SW527 cells were cultures in DMEM high-glucose medium (Gibco, Dublin, Ireland) supplemented with 10% decomplemented fetal calf serum and 20 µg/mL gentamycin.

Spheroids were formed with the SUM1315 TNBC cell line, according to our previous works [29]. Briefly, cells in suspension were seeded in ultra-low-attachment round-bottom microplates in a prepared culture medium (Corning, New York, NY, USA, catalog #4520) at a concentration of 1000 cells/well. After 24 h, Geltrex® reduced growth factor basement membrane matrix (Gibco, Dublin, Ireland), diluted with cold medium, was dispensed in each well for a final concentration of 2%. Microplates were then horizontally shacked for 20 min at 200 rpm, before being replaced in the incubator.

2.3. *Lightspot®-Fl-1 Cellular Uptake and Outtake Analysis by Flow Cytometry*

Suspension DU4475 and monolayer SUM1315 cell cultures were used, according to the culture conditions described above. For SUM1315, cell detachment was achieved by trypsinization. Then, cellular suspensions containing 800,000 cells/mL were prepared in a culture medium for both cell lines. Cells maintained at 37 °C in the culture medium were then incubated with 1 μM fluorescent LightSpot®-FL-1 compound, dissolved in DMSO and diluted in the culture medium. The final DMSO concentration in all cell culture conditions was at 0.1%. Fluorescence intensity in cells was measured after 5, 15, 30, 45 and 60 min using a flow cytometer LSRII (Becton Dickinson, Franklin Lakes, NJ, USA) with a blue excitation laser (488 nm, 20 mW) and FITC filter (530/30 nm). Cells were then centrifuged (125× *g* for 5 min) in order to be washed. For this process, the cell pellet was resuspended in the cell culture medium at 37 °C. Fluorescence intensity was then monitored after 5, 15, 60 and 120 min, following the washing step.

2.4. *LightSpot®-FL-1 Fluorescent Staining on Monolayer and Suspension Cell Cultures*

For the adherent SUM1315 cell line, cells were seeded in IbiTreat 8-well μ-Slides (Ibidi®, Gräfelfing, Germany) at a concentration of 50,000 cells per well. Slides were maintained at 37 °C under 5% CO_2 in a humidified incubator until the cell carpet reached 60% of confluence. For the suspension DU4475 cell line, cells were directly harvested from the culture flask. In both cases, cells were either fixed with a 4% paraformaldehyde (PFA) solution or were maintained unfixed in culture conditions. For both fixed and unfixed cells, all subsequent experimental and imaging steps were achieved in the same experimental conditions. Cells were then incubated in a 1 μM LightSpot®-FL-1 D-PBS solution for one hour. Three successive washes of 20 min were then conducted in D-PBS to remove unspecific cell staining. Nuclear staining was carried out using 1 μg/mL bisbenzimide Hoechst33258 solution (Sigma Aldrich, Darmstadt, Germany, catalog #14530). Cells were finally imaged with a Cytation™3 MV (BioTek®, Winooski, VT, USA) fluorescent microscopy module (M = 40, X-fluorescence filters = GFP, LED = 10, time exposure = 200 ms, gain = 10). The cells' mean fluorescence intensity was calculated with Gen5 3.08 software (BioTek®, cellular analysis, threshold = 4000, minimal size = 5 μm, maximal size = 100 μm).

2.5. *LightSpot®-FL-1 and Anti-P-gp Co-staining Analysis on Monolayer and Suspension Cell Cultures*

LightSpot®-FL-1 staining was conducted as previously described for SUM1315, MDA-MB-231, HCC1937, SW527 and DU4475 cell lines, before completing the anti-P-gp immunostaining. For this, cells were incubated with clone F4 anti-P-gp monoclonal mouse antibody (Invitrogen, Carlsbad, CA, USA, catalog # MA5-13854, diluted at 1/75) for one hour. Three successive washes were then carried out in D-PBS before incubating cells with secondary goat anti-mouse Alexa Fluor™ 647 nm antibody (Invitrogen, Carlsbad, CA, USA, catalog #A21236 diluted at 1/800). Cells were finally imaged with a Cytation™3 MV (BioTek®, Winooski, VT, USA) fluorescent microscopy module (M = 40, X-fluorescence filters = GFP, LED = 10, time exposure = 200 ms, gain = 10/Cy 5, LED = 10, time exposure = 1840 ms, gain = 16). The GFP and Cy5 cells' mean fluorescence intensity were calculated with Gen5 3.08 software (BioTek®, cellular analysis, primary mask set on GFP filter, threshold = 4000, minimal size = 5 μm, maximal size = 100 μm). For DU4475 cells presenting the strongest signals among tested cell lines, a colocalization study was made using the Coloc 2 plugin of ImageJ software (NIH, Bethesda, MD, USA). This allowed us to calculate Pearson's correlation and Mander's overlap coefficients between the GFP- and Cy5-acquired images.

2.6. LightSpot®-FL-1 Fluorescent Staining on SUM1315 Spheroids

After 3 days of culture, the spheroids were harvested and fixed for 12 h in 4% PFA solution. They were then incubated for 90 min in 1 μM LightSpot®-FL-1 solution. Then, spheroids were imaged with the Cytation™3 MV (BioTek®, Winooski, VT, USA) fluorescent microscopy module (M = 4, X-fluorescence filters = GFP, LED = 10, time exposure = 150 ms, gain = 4) 30, 60, 90 and 120 min after the end of LightSpot®-FL-1 incubation. Between each observation, the spheroids were washed in D-PBS. The spheroid global fluorescent intensity was measured with Gen5 3.08 software (BioTek®, cellular analysis on GFP filter, threshold = 5000, minimal size = 100 μm, maximal size = 500 μm).

2.7. P-gp Expression Level Measurement in SUM1315 Monolayer Cell Line and in Spheroid Models after Olaparib Treatment

Olaparib (Carbosynth, Compton, catalog #FO33122) was solubilized in DMSO to prepare a 50 mM stock solution. Dilutions were prepared in Ham's F-12 medium for final treatment concentrations of 0.5, 5 or 50 μM. The final DMSO concentration remained constant at 0.1% in all tested conditions.

For the SUM1315 monolayer culture, cells were seeded in IbiTreat 8-well μ-Slides (Ibidi®, Gräfelfing, Germany) at a concentration of 50,000 cells per well and maintained in a humid incubator until 60% of confluency. Cells were exposed for 3 h to 0.5, 5 or 50 μM of Olaparib and then fixed for 10 min with PFA at 4%. This drug was solubilized in DMSO, and the final DMSO concentration was maintained at 0.1% in both treated and untreated conditions. For each Olaparib concentration, the PFA-fixed cells were then stained with 1 μM LightSpot®-FL-1 or with anti-P-gp immunostaining, as previously described above. For the immunostaining, goat anti-mouse primary antibody (Invitrogen, Carlsbad, CA, USA, catalog #MA5–13854, diluted at 1/75) was coupled with Alexa Fluor™ 568 mn (Invitrogen, Carlsbad, CA, USA). Images were acquired with a Cytation™3 MV (BioTek®, Winooski, VT, USA) fluorescent microscopy module (M = 40, X-fluorescence filters = GFP, LED = 10, time exposure = 200 ms, gain = 10/Texas Red, LED = 10, time exposure = 2200 ms, gain = 16). The fluorescence intensities of GFP and Texas Red signals were calculated using the Gen5 3.08 software (BioTek®, cellular analysis, threshold = 4000 for GFP signal and 3100 for Texas Red signal, minimal size = 50 μm, maximal size = 100 μm).

SUM1315 spheroids were exposed for 3 or 6 h with 0.5, 5 or 50 μM of Olaparib. In parallel, 0.1% DMSO controls were also performed. After treatment, spheroids were fixed in 4%PFA solution and incubated for 90 min with LightSpot®-FL-1 diluted at 1 μM. They were then washed for 90 min in D-PBS and were observed with a Cytation™3 MV (BioTek®, Winooski, VT, USA) fluorescent microscopy module (M = 4, X-fluorescence filter = GFP, LED = 10, time exposure = 150 ms, Gain = 4). Spheroid global fluorescent intensity was measured using Gen5 3.08 software (BioTek®, cellular analysis on GFP filter, threshold = 5000, minimal size = 100 μm, maximal size = 500 μm).

2.8. Statistical Analysis

Results were presented as mean ± standard deviation. All experiments were performed independently on at least three separate occasions. Unpaired 2-sided Student's *t*-test or ANOVA and Tukey's multiple comparison test were used to evaluate statistical significance. Results were considered statistically different when $p < 0.05$ (*). The strongest differences were noted as follows: $p < 0.01$ (**), $p < 0.001$ (***), $p < 0.0001$ (****) and $p < 0.00001$ (*****). Non-significant results were noted as "ns".

3. Results

3.1. Synthesis and Characterization of the LightSpot®-FL-1 Probe

The structure of LightSpot®-FL-1 presents a peptidic moiety that acts as a P-gp ligand, conjugated via an amide bond to the cell-permeant, bright, and photostable BODIPY-FL fluorophore (Figure 1). The amide bond was formed by the reaction of an amine-bearing peptidic P-gp ligand with BODIPY-FL succinimidyl ester. Subsequent HPLC purification led to LightSpot®-FL-1, with a good yield (>70%) and excellent purity (>96%). After full characterization, the excitation and emission maxima were determined from LightSpot®-FL-1 solutions in ethanol at 505 and 510 nm, respectively.

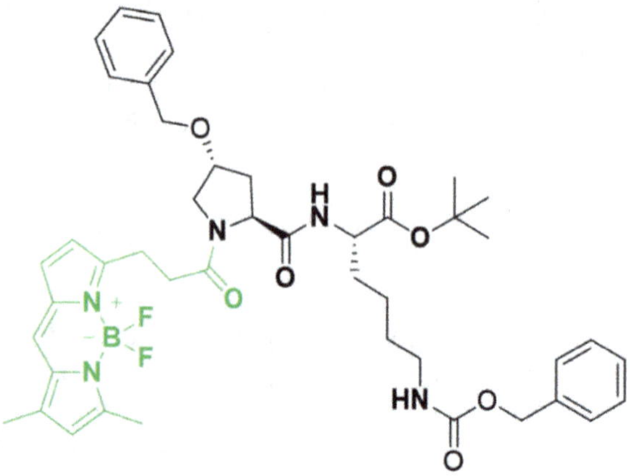

Figure 1. Chemical structure of LightSpot®-FL-1: a peptidic P-gp ligand (black) conjugated to the BODIPY-FL fluorophore (green).

3.2. *LightSpot®-FL-1 Fluorescent Probe Selectively Targets P-gp in the DU4475 and SUM1315 TNBC Cell Line*

3.2.1. LightSpot®-FL-1 Kinetic Uptake by Flow Cytometry

To assess the impact of the BODIPY-FL conjugation on the ligand moiety spatiotemporal cellular distribution, the ability of LightSpot®-FL-1 to penetrate and subsist in cells was evaluated by flow cytometry.

For this, two TNBC cell line models were used, the suspension DU4475 and the monolayer SUM1315 cell cultures in which the P-gp is naturally overexpressed [28,35]. Both cell lines were exposed to 1 μM LightSpot®-FL-1 for 1 h. LightSpot®-FL-1 intracellular fluorescence intensity was measured over time, during cell exposure, and after washes to remove the unbound LightSpot®-F-L1 (Figure 2a,b). In both cell lines, a rapid LightSpot®-FL-1 uptake was detected in the first 15 min, with a mean fluorescence intensity from 127 FU to 5.0×10^3 FU, and from 8 FU to 39.5×10^3 FU for DU4475 and SUM1315 cells, respectively. Then, the intracellular LightSpot®-FL-1 rate was stabilized in both cells, with 4.8×10^3 FU for DU4475 cells (Figure 2a) and 46.4×10^3 FU for SUM1315 after 60 min (Figure 2b). After LightSpot®-FL-1 rate stabilization, cells were washed to eliminate unbound LightSpot®-FL-1. After this step, intracellular LightSpot®-FL-1 fluorescence was again measured in each cell line, corresponding to the intracellular LightSpot®-FL-1 specifically bound on its P-gp target. Thereafter, a clear decrease of LightSpot®-FL-1 fluorescence intensity was detected in both cell lines with 2.9×10^3 FU for DU4475 cells and 23.2×10^3 FU for SUM1315 cells, 5 min after the wash step. The LightSpot®-FL-1 maintenance in the cells was then followed in each cell line. In DU4475 cells, the linked LightSpot®-FL-1 rate remained relatively stable over time, with 1.9×10^3 FU after 1 h and 1.6×10^3 FU after 2 h (Figure 2a). However, for SUM1315 cells, the intracellular LightSpot®-FL-1 rate continued to decrease to 12.9×10^3 FU after 1 h, and to 6.3×10^3 FU after 2 h (Figure 2b). These results showed that the intracellular fluoroprobe LightSpot®-FL-1 was maintained in both cell lines over time.

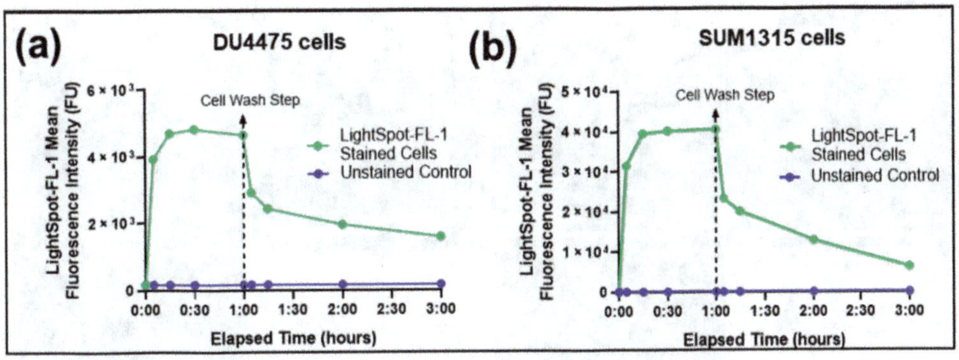

Figure 2. LightSpot®-FL-1 kinetic uptake in DU4475 and SUM1315 TNBC cell lines. DU4475 (**a**) and SUM1315 (**b**) TNBC cells were exposed to a 1 µM LightSpot®-FL-1 fluorescent probe and the cellular fluorescence intensity (fluorescence units: FU) was measured at different times by flow cytometry analysis. After 1 h of exposure, DU4475 (**a**) and SUM1315 (**b**) cells were washed with culture medium (cell wash step) and the cellular fluorescence intensity was again measured at different times by flow cytometry, 2 h after the cell-wash step. During the entire experiment time, unstained cells were analyzed in parallel as control values.

Lightspot®-FL-1 Staining Intensity Comparison between Living or Fixed Cells by Fluorescence Imaging

The LightSpot®-FL-1 staining efficiency was then analyzed and compared between living and fixed cells. For these experiments, living cells or PFA-fixed cells were incubated with 1 µM LightSpot®-FL-1 solution for 1 h before being washed. In the acquired images, DU4475 (Figure 3a–c) and SUM1315 (Figure 3d–f) cells presented the same LightSpot®-FL-1 green fluorescent staining profiles between living or fixed conditions. Moreover, no similarities with blue Hoechst33258 staining were observed (Figure 3c,f) indicating an absence of LightSpot®-FL-1 compound accumulation in the cell nuclei (Figure 3e,f). LightSpot®-FL-1 staining intensity was then quantified and was $20.8 \pm 2.9 \times 10^3$ FU and of $20.7 \pm 3.7 \times 10^3$ FU for living and fixed DU4475 cells, respectively ($p = 0.94$; Figure 3g). For the SUM1315 cell line, the staining intensity was $8.4 \pm 1.3 \times 10^3$ FU and $8.9 \pm 0.8 \times 10^3$ FU for living and fixed cells, respectively ($p = 0.17$; Figure 3g). These results showed that the intensity of the LightSpot®-FL-1 staining was similar on living or fixed cells with similar staining parameters, in terms of distribution and intensity. Therefore, for the following experiments, only fixed-cell models were used.

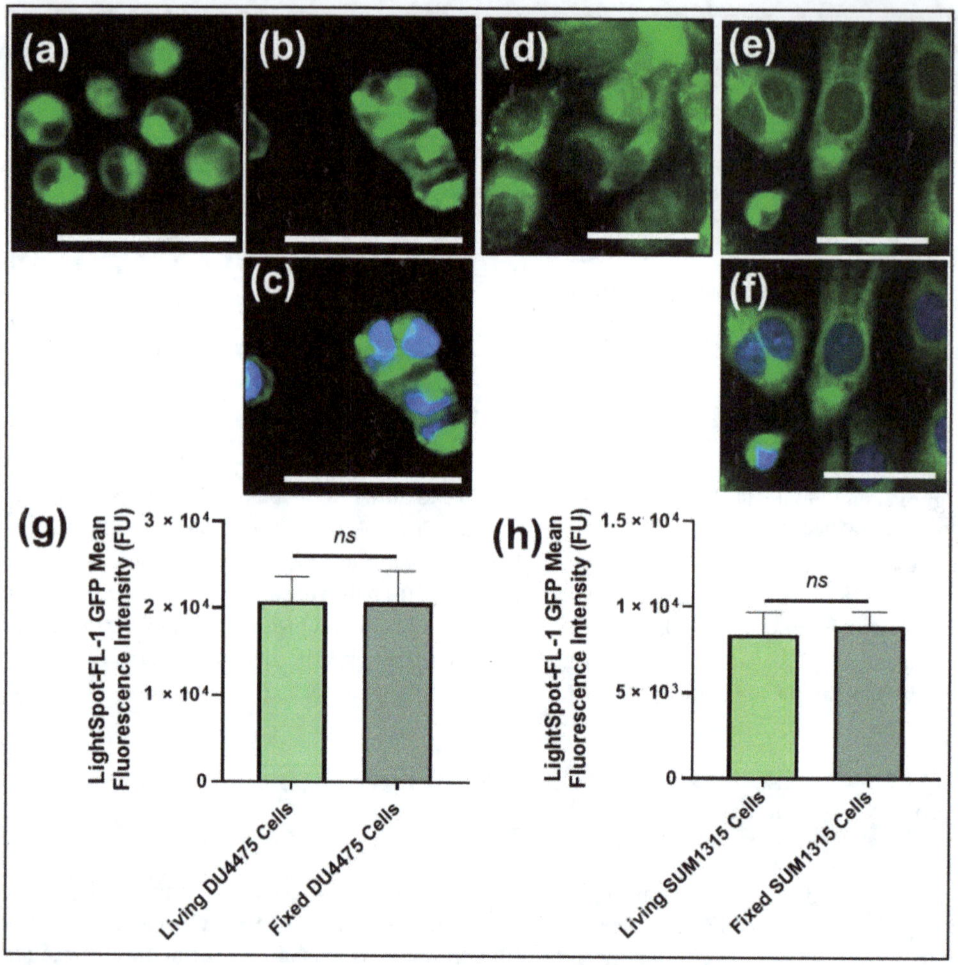

Figure 3. LightSpot®-FL-1 staining comparison between living and fixed DU4475 and SUM1315 TNBC cell lines. Living (**a**) or fixed (**b**) DU4475 cells and living (**d**) or fixed (**e**) SUM1315 cells were stained with the LightSpot®-FL-1 probe at 1 μM (green signal). In parallel, a nuclear counterstaining was also carried out using Hoechst33258 for fixed DU4475 (**c**) and SUM1315 (**f**) cell conditions (merged pictures presenting LightSpot®-FL-1 signal in green and nuclear staining in blue). All pictures were acquired with the Cytation™3 MV (BioTek®, M = 4 X, scale bar = 50 μm). For each experimental condition, LightSpot®-FL-1 global cell fluorescent intensity was measured with Gen5 software (BioTek®) for DU4475 (**g**) and SUM1315 (**h**) cells. Significances between living and fixed conditions were indicated as ns (not significant; $p > 0.05$).

P-gp Co-Staining with LightSpot-FL-1 and Immunostaining

For the analysis of P-gp targeting by the LightSpot®-FL-1 fluorescent probe, the distribution of this intracellular tracer (green signal) was compared to specific immunostaining, combining anti-P-gp mouse antibody (F4 clone) and a goat anti-mouse secondary antibody coupled to Alexa Fluor™ 647 (red signal). For this, co-staining was carried out on both DU4475 and SUM1315 BLTN models. In the unicellular DU4475 cell line (Figure 4a,b,e), a clear similarity of localization was detected between the LightSpot®-FL-1 probe labeling (Figure 4a) and the anti-P-gp immunostaining (Figure 4b). On SUM1315, similar staining profiles were obtained (Figure 4c,d,f). These staining similarities were highlighted by line profiles drawn on the DU4475 and SUM1315 merged picture (Figure 4e,f,g,h). Moreover, the colocalization of LightSpot®-FL-1 and anti-P-gp staining on DU4475 was also confirmed by Pearson's correlation coefficient analysis, reaching 92.1%, and by Mander's overlap coefficient, reaching 100.0%, attesting to similar signal distribution.

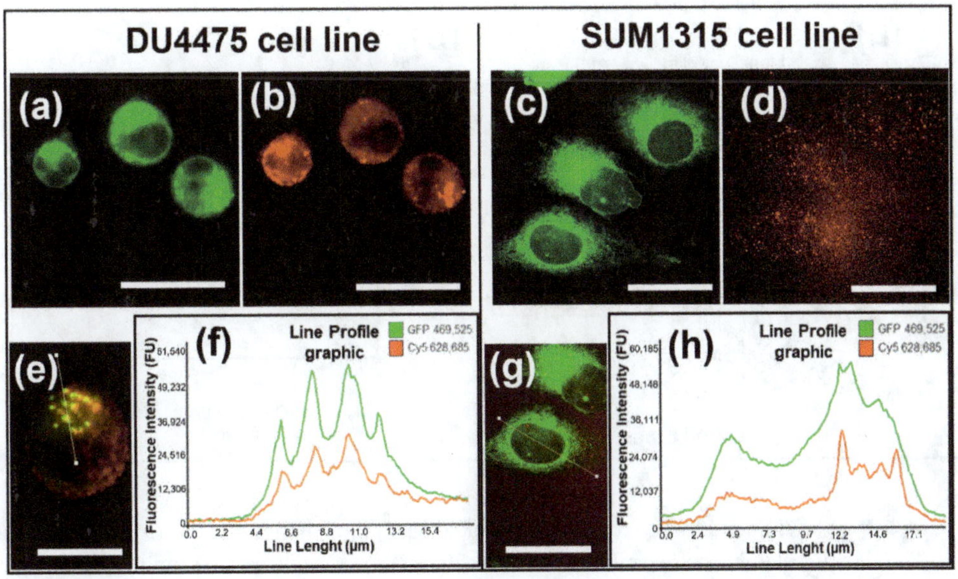

Figure 4. P-gp targeting comparison between LightSpot®-FL-1 staining and anti-P-gp immunostaining on DU4475 and SUM1315 TNBC cell lines. Co-staining was carried out, combining LightSpot®-FL-1 with anti-P-gp immunostaining. Pictures of LightSpot®-FL-1 labeling (green GFP signal) are presented for DU4475 (**a**) and SUM1315 cells (**c**). Similarly, immunostaining pictures (red Cy5 signal) are presented for DU4475 (**b**) and SUM1315 cells (**d**). Merged pictures are presented for DU4475 (**e**) and SUM1315 (**g**) cells. A line profile was drawn on merged pictures, superimposing both LightSpot®-FL-1 and anti-Pgp immunostaining signals. The fluorescence intensity spectra across the line profile are shown with the line profile graphic on DU4475 cells (**f**) and SUM135 cells (**h**). All pictures were acquired with the Cytation™3 MV (BioTek®, M = 4 X, scale bar = 25 µm).

3.3. LightSpot®-FL-1 Allows Sensitive Detection and Quantification of Basal P-gp Expression Level in Various TNBC Cell Lines

The performance of the cell-permeant fluorescent probe LightSpot®-FL-1 was then checked by the quantification of P-gp expression level on five various TNBC cell lines, DU4475, SW527, HCC1937, MDA-MB-231 and SUM1315, in comparison with the anti-P-gp immunostaining reference method (Figure 4).

In all TNBC studied models, P-gp signal quantification was proportional between LightSpot®-FL-1 labeling and anti-P-gp labeling (Figure 5a). Indeed, the fluorescence intensities of LightSpot®-FL-1 labeling were $20.7 \pm 3.1 \times 10^3$ FU, $11.7 \pm 2.9 \times 10^3$ FU, $7.6 \pm 1.7 \times 10^3$ FU, $8.4 \pm 1.1 \times 10^3$ FU, $7.4 \pm 1.1 \times 10^3$ FU for DU4475, SW527, HCC1937, MDA-MB-231 and SUM1315 cell lines, respectively (Figure 5a). Likewise, anti-P-gp immunofluorescence intensities were $19.9 \pm 4.2 \times 10^3$ FU, $10.6 \pm 1.8 \times 10^3$ FU, $8.5 \pm 0.6 \times 10^3$ FU, $6.9 \pm 0.8 \times 10^3$ FU, and $6.9 \pm 0.9 \times 10^3$ FU for DU4475, SW527, HCC1937, MDA-MB-231 and SUM1315 cell lines, respectively (Figure 5a). Moreover, the fluorescence signal intensities correlation was studied for all cell lines, giving an R^2 determination coefficient of 0.9943, attesting to a strong correspondence between the intensities of the LightSpot®-FL-1 tracer and anti-P-gp signals (Figure 5b). These results showed a strong intensity correlation between the LightSpot®-FL-1 staining and the anti-P-gp immunostaining, clearly highlighting the LightSpot®-FL-1 probe performance in terms of detection sensitivity for P-gp expression levels in all TNBC models studied.

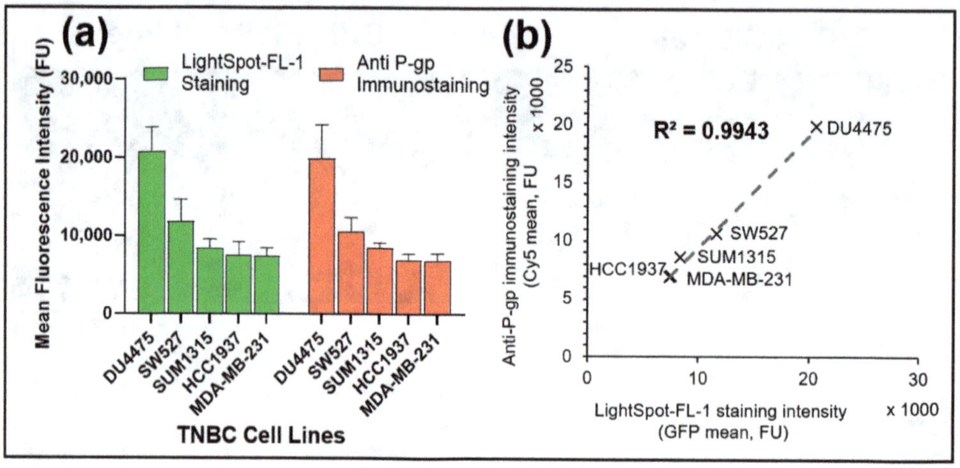

Figure 5. P-gp level quantification comparison after co-staining with LightSpot®-FL-1 staining and anti-P-gp immunostaining on several triple-negative breast cancer cell lines. Co-staining was carried out by combining LightSpot®-FL-1 staining with anti-P-gp immunostaining on five different TNBC cell lines i.e., DU4475, SW527, HCC1937, MDA-MB-231 and SUM1315. For each cell line, (**a**) both LightSpot-FL staining (green bars) and anti-P-gp immunostaining (red bars) fluorescence intensities were measured using the Gen5 software (BioTek®). Correlation between both stainings was evaluated (**b**) with the correlation line and the R^2 coefficient of determination.

3.4. LightSpot®-FL-1 Detects and Quantifies Olaparib-induced P-gp expression Level on SUM1315 Monolayer Cultures

Thereafter, the sensitivity of LightSpot®-FL-1 fluorescent staining for the quantification of the P-gp expression level was checked, in comparison with anti-P-gp immunostaining on SUM1315 cell lines. For this study, the SUM1315 cells cultured in monolayer were treated for 3 h with increasing concentrations of Olaparib (10, 50 or 100 μM), a PARP inhibitor used for TNBC treatment. For these experiments, Olaparib was dissolved in DMSO. The final concentration of this solvent was always 0.1% in all cell-culture conditions (Figure 6). The fluorescence intensities were normalized to DMSO control values as a basal P-gp expression level. The results showed that, with anti-P-gp immunostaining, the basal P-gp expression level was $3.5 \pm 0.2 \times 10^3$ FU for the control 0.1% DMSO cells (Figure 6a,e). After 10 μM Olaparib treatment, the P-gp expression remained similar to control, with $3.6 \pm 0.2 \times 10^3$ FU (Figure 6b,e). In contrast, with 50 and 100 μM Olaparib, a significant increase in P-gp expression level was detected, with $3.9 \pm 0.2 \times 10^3$ FU and $3.9 \pm 0.1 \times 10^3$ FU, respectively ($p = 10^{-15}$ & 10^{-15}, Figure 6c–e), compared to 0.1% DMSO control cells. Very interestingly, a similar P-gp expression level evolution was detected with LightSpot®-FL-1 staining (green signal) in the same experimental conditions (Figure 6f–i). Indeed, 10 μM Olaparib-treated cells presented a similar P-gp expression level, with $17.4 \pm 4.3 \times 10^3$ FU compared to the 0.1% DMSO control presenting $16.1 \pm 5.3 \times 10^3$ FU ($p = 0.77$, Figure 6f,g,j). In contrast, after 50 and 100 μM Olaparib cell treatment, significantly increased P-gp expression levels were measured with $27.0 \pm 8.6 \times 10^3$ FU and $25.5 \pm 7.7 \times 10^3$ FU, respectively ($p = 10^{-14}$ & 10^{-11}, Figure 6h–j), compared to 0.1 % DMSO controls. These results clearly highlighted the fact that the LightSpot®-FL-1 fluorescent probe presented the same P-gp detection and quantification level efficiency as anti-P-gp immunostaining.

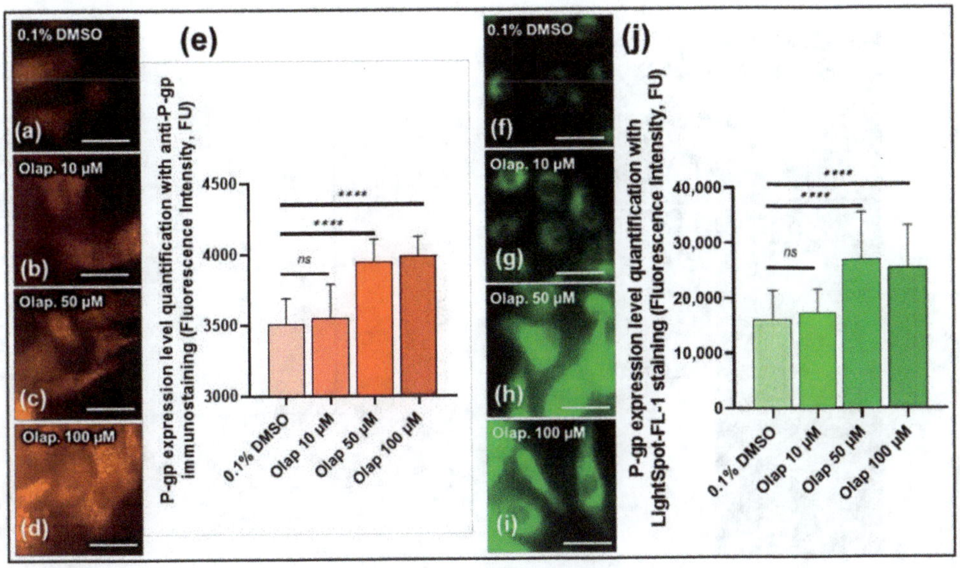

Figure 6. Comparison between anti-P-gp immunostaining and LightSpot®-FL-1 fluorescent probe staining for P-gp level expression measure on the SUM1315 cell line in monolayer culture condition after increased Olaparib concentration exposure. SUM1315 cells were treated with 10, 50 or 100 μM Olaparib for 3 h. Cells were then fixed and immunostained, combining anti-P-gp mouse antibody (F4 clone) and a goat anti-mouse secondary antibody, coupled to Alexa Fluor™ 568 (red signal) for each dose (**a–d**), and the signal was quantified using Gen5 software (BioTek®) (**e**). LightSpot®-FL-1 staining (green signal) was also utilized for the same experimental conditions (**f–i**), and quantified using Gen5 software (**j**). All pictures were acquired with the Cytation™3 MV (BioTek®, M = 4 X, scale bar = 50 μm). Significances between conditions were indicated as ns (not significant; $p > 0.05$), and **** $p < 0.0001$.

3.5. The Cell-permeant LightSpot®-FL-1 Detects and Quantifies Basal and Induced P-gp Expression in SUM1315 Spheroid Cell Mass Models

The LightSpot®-FL-1 fluorescent probe is able to penetrate into cells and cell masses. Thus, its performance for the detection and quantification of P-gp levels was also analyzed in SUM1315 models. Firstly, to develop a LightSpot®-FL-1 staining protocol with this model, SUM1315 spheroids were incubated with 1 μM LightSpot®-FL-1 fluorescent probe for 2 h. Then, four washes in D-PBS were carried out to remove the unfixed and unspecific fluorescent compound from the spheroids. At the end of LightSpot®-FL-1 incubation, the mean signal fluorescence intensity quantified in spheroids was $49.7 \pm 7.7 \times 10^3$ FU (Figure 7f). Then, green-fluorescent intensity staining decreased across each washing (Figure 7a–e). Indeed, the mean fluorescent LightSpot®-FL-1 intensity significantly decreased to $36.3 \pm 10.2 \times 10^3$ FU after 1 wash ($p = 10^{-6}$, compared to values before washes), to $21.9 \pm 11.8 \times 10^3$ FU after 2 washes ($p = 10^{-6}$, compared to values after 1 wash), to $13.4 \pm 7.2 \times 10^3$ FU after 3 washes ($p = 10^{-4}$, compared to values after 2 washes) and stabilized to $10.7 \pm 2.2 \times 10^3$ FU after 4 washes ($p = 0.1$, compared to values after 2 washes). These results suggested that, with these spheroid models, at least 3 washes are required after LightSpot®-FL-1 staining to remove the excess and unspecific fluorescent compound.

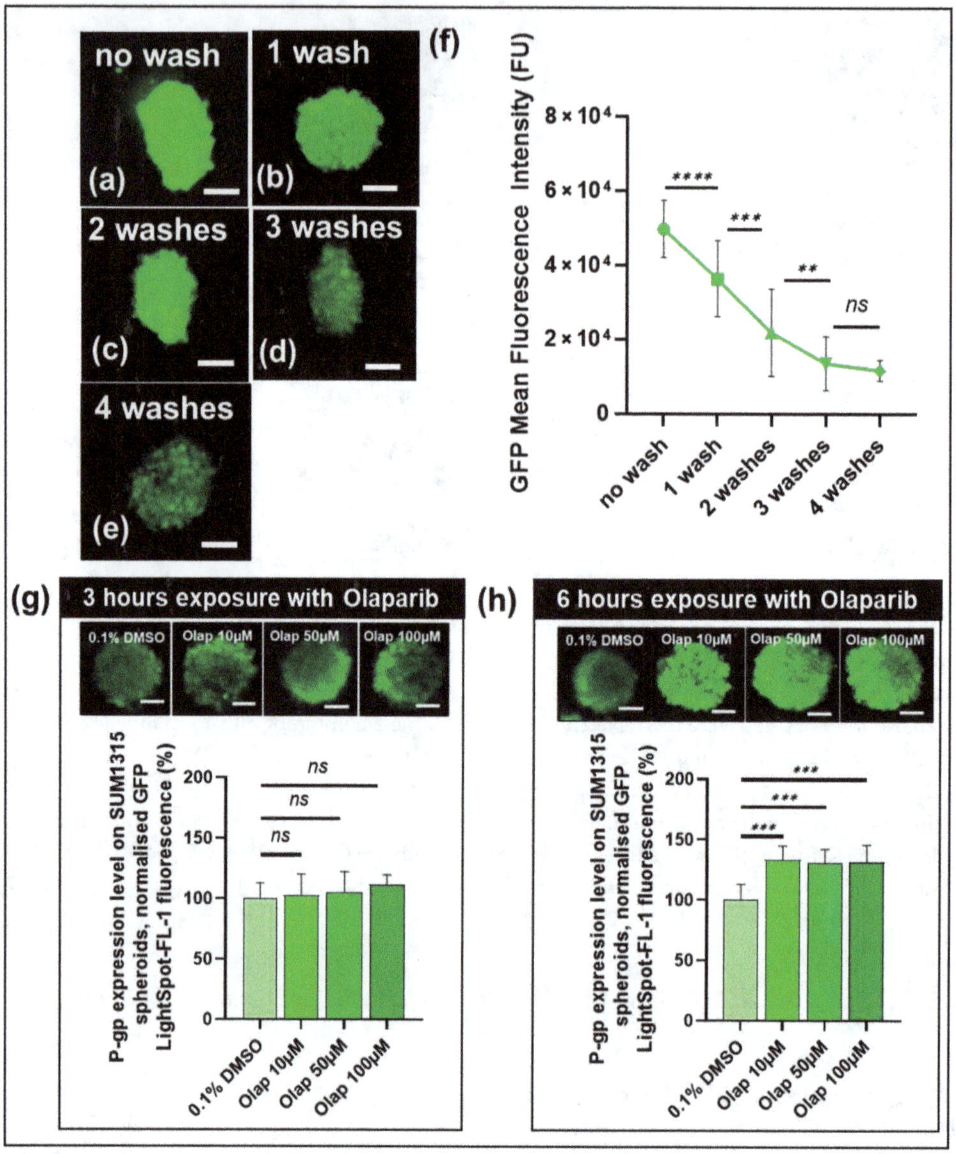

Figure 7. Development of LightSpot®-FL-1 staining on SUM1315 spheroids. SUM1315 spheroids (about 200 μm diameter) were incubated with LightSpot®-FL-1 at 1 μM and washed several times in D-PBS. Before and between each wash of 30 min, pictures of spheroids were made (**a**) for no wash, (**b**) for 1 wash, (**c**) for 2 washes, (**d**) for 3 washes, and (**e**) for 4 washes. For each wash number condition, spheroid global fluorescent intensity was quantified using Gen5 software (BioTek®) (**f**). Otherwise, SUM1315 spheroids were exposed with increasing Olaparib concentrations for 3 h (**g**) or for 6 h (**h**). After the LightSpot®-FL-1 staining, pictures were made for each dose for 3 (**g**) and 6 h (**h**) of Olaparib exposure. For each condition, spheroid global LightSpot®-FL-1 fluorescent intensity was quantified for 3 h of Olaparib-exposed spheroids (**g**) and for 6 h Olaparib-exposed spheroids (**h**). All pictures were acquired with the Cytation™3 MV (BioTek®, M = 4 X, scale bar = 50 μm). Significances between conditions were indicated as ns (not significant; $p > 0.05$), ** $p < 0.01$, *** $p < 0.001$, and **** $p < 0.0001$.

Secondly, after P-gp staining and methodology development in spheroids with LightSpot®-FL-1 tracer, experiments for P-gp level quantification were carried out with this model. As previously carried out on monolayer cultures, SUM1315 spheroids were exposed to increasing Olaparib concentrations, i.e., 10, 50 or 100 μM, for 3 h or 6 h, before being stained with a LightSpot®-FL-1 fluorescent probe. In parallel, controls with 0.1%

DMSO spheroids were conducted. For all experiments, measured fluorescent intensities were normalized by 0.1% DMSO control spheroid values. After 3 h of Olaparib exposure, no P-gp expression level difference was detected between the 0.1% DMSO control with 100.0 ± 12.7% and the other Olaparib treated spheroids, with 102.5 ± 17.5%, 105.0 ± 17.1% and 111.4 ± 8.2% for 10, 50 and 100 μM, respectively (p = 0.95, 0.62 & 0.08, Figure 7g). In contrast, after 6 h of anti-PARP exposure, an increase in P-gp level expression was detected with 133.3 ± 11.6%, 130.7 ± 11.4% and 131.4 ± 14.4% for 10, 50 and 100 μM Olaparib, respectively ($p = 10^{-10}$, 10^{-10} & 10^{-10}, Figure 7h) than 0.1% DMSO control spheroids with 100.0 ± 12.8%. These results highlighted the performance and sensitivity of the LightSpot®-FL-1 fluorescent probe to detect and quantify P-gp overexpression in SUM1315 spheroids, after their exposure to an anti-PARP-targeted therapy.

4. Discussion

The development of a tumoral multidrug resistance profile represents a real obstacle in cancer treatment, frequently leading to therapeutic failure [8]. This is a phenomenon in which tumor cells become resistant to multiple structurally and functionally different drugs during treatment [36]. This profile generally appears after initial tumoral exposure to anticancer agents, and mostly requires increasing treatment doses or adapting the treatment strategy [37]. Various molecular mechanisms are involved in multidrug resistance, including membrane efflux triggered by MDR proteins [7]. In particular, the P-gp is the most widely studied member of this family and is associated with tumoral resistance to a wide range of anticancer drugs. Indeed, its expression is often upregulated in tumors, conferring to cancer cells the ability to expulse therapeutic agents and thus limit/evade chemotherapy-mediated cell death. That is why the study of tumoral chemoresistance, established by the P-gp, is a relevant field as a way to optimize cancer treatment and limit therapeutic failure risks [20]. Indeed, the relationship between P-gp expression and treatment efficacy is widely validated for a large variety of cancer types, such as lung, bladder, ovarian, and breast cancers. This is especially of interest for aggressive and challenging tumoral subtypes, such as TNBC. This breast cancer sub-group is commonly associated with a high rate of residual disease after treatment, which increases the risk of relapse in the first 5 years after treatment [38]. One principal cause of therapeutic failure in TNBC treatment is a primary or acquired multidrug resistance profile that can include chemoresistance conferred by the P-gp [39]. Several studies have already demonstrated significant P-gp overexpression after neo-adjuvant chemotherapy that was higher for patients presenting an uncompleted pathological response [40,41]. In addition, it has been highlighted that the upregulation of P-gp expression after the neo-adjuvant chemotherapy of breast-cancer patients was associated with the metastatic spread of lymph nodes [42]. Moreover, other studies had already described the P-gp as a predictive factor of treatment outcomes [21,22]. However, this protein is very rarely used in clinics as a predictive biomarker for the prognosis of the pathology, primarily because of the lack of efficient tools allowing the detection of its presence in clinical samples.

Nowadays, two approaches allow us to evaluate the P-gp expression level at the preclinical step. Firstly, the evaluation of the P-gp involvement in xenobiotic efflux mechanisms can be indirectly studied via competitive fluorescent P-gp substrates, such as rhodamine 123, among many others [43,44]. For this approach, flow cytometry is mainly used, expressly requiring living cells in suspension. Secondly, direct P-gp quantification can be made with enzyme-linked immunosorbent assays, specific antibody immunostaining using Western blotting, immunocytochemistry or immunohistochemistry methodologies [5,45]. These approaches can be applied to cells in suspension, in monolayers, or on tissue sections, and allowed us to specifically detect and localize the P-gp. However, these approaches present difficulties regarding antibody penetration inside cells and/or cell masses and imply expensive and time-consuming experimentation. Thus, they only target extracellular-membrane P-gp, and not the intracellular part [45]. Indeed, the P-gp located on organelle membranes, such as the endoplasmic reticulum and lysosomes, also plays an important role in cellular drug resistance that must not be underestimated [46,47]. Therefore, all of these methodologies present limited interest for routine clinical applications. For this reason, the simple, direct, reliable, and cost-effective detection and quantification of P-gp in tumor cells, and more particularly in tumoral masses, represents a relevant challenge for optimizing treatment efficacy and patient care while limiting the risk of therapeutic failure.

Fluorescence microscopy, based on molecularly targeted imaging agents, may have the potential to overcome such a challenge. Indeed, it provides a way to assess protein location and expression level in biological samples, with subcellular resolution and good sensitivity. As a consequence, over the last decade, there has been a remarkable growth in the development and use of small-molecule fluorescent probes in the biological sciences, particularly in oncology for cancer detection, staging and characterization. In particular, it is well documented that this approach could complement biopsy-based histopathological diagnosis [48]. Small-molecule fluorescent probes typically consist of a target-specific ligand, conjugated through a linker to a small organic fluorophore, for detection in the biological sample. Thus, considering the construction of a P-gp-targeted fluorescent probe, we designed LightSpot®-FL-1, a peptidic P-gp inhibitor derivative conjugated to the cell-permeant, bright, and photostable BODIPY-FL fluorophore (Figure 1). This peptidic moiety derives from a series of peptidomimetic P-gp ligands, previously identified as potent and selective non-competitive inhibitors, which reversibly bind to the intracellular domain of the P-gp [49]. From there, we reasoned that such ligands were good candidates to yield an efficient P-gp fluorescent probe after conjugation with a fluorophore.

LightSpot®-FL-1 was designed to penetrate inside cells and/or cell masses to specifically label P-gp, thus allowing its direct localization and quantification. Different TNBC cell models were used to evaluate LightSpot®-FL-1 as an efficient P-gp probe: DU4475 in a suspension cell line, SW527, HCC1937, MDA-MB-231 and SUM1315 monolayer cell lines, and SUM1315 spheroids.

Firstly, the ability of LightSpot®-FL-1 to penetrate and subsist inside cells was checked by flow cytometry analysis, using TNBC SUM1315 and DU4475 cells. Of particular interest, within the first 15 min after cell exposure to the fluorescent probe, a cellular fluorescence intensity 40-fold increase for DU4475 and 5000-fold increase for SUM1315 cells was observed, followed by a stabilization of the fluorescent signal in both cell lines (Figure 2). This suggests rapid LightSpot®-FL-1 uptake and binding to its P-gp target. Then, the cell-washing step led to the successful removal of the non-specifically bound LightSpot®-FL-1 part. Indeed, after 5 min of washing, a clear decrease of cell fluorescence intensity of 30.9% for DU4475, and of 50.0% for SUM1315 cells, was detected. However, part of the fluorescent LightSpot®-FL-1 probe was clearly retained in cells, even after two hours of washing. This part corresponds to 33.3% and 13.6% of the fluorescent tracer signal measured before the washing step, for DU4475 and SUM1315 cells, respectively (Figure 2). These results indicated that the Light-Spot®-FL-1 fluorescent probe quickly penetrates and specifically persists in cells.

Thereafter, the P-gp's selective localization, detection, and quantification by LightSpot®-FL-1 staining were demonstrated by fluorescence microscopy. For this demonstration, both TNBC cell models DU4475 and SUM1315 (living or fixed) were exposed to 1 μM of the fluorescent probe for one hour, before a D-PBS wash for another hour, in order to expel excess markers out of the cells. This staining, applied to both living and fixed TNBC cells, highlighted the same membrane and cytoplasmic distribution of the LightSpot®-FL-1 compound, with an absence of cell nucleus accumulation (Figure 3). In addition, these results showed 99.5% and 94.4% fluorescent staining intensity similarities between living and fixed cell conditions, for DU4475 and SUM1315 cells, respectively (Figure 3). This demonstrated that LightSpot®-FL-1 staining can be carried out on both fresh or fixed cells, giving the same signal distribution and intensity. This property may turn out to be of particular interest for the staining of precious clinical samples. The following experiments were carried out on fixed TNBC cell models.

In order to validate P-gp-sensitive detection and quantification with the LightSpot®-FL-1 probe, the FL-1 marking was compared to anti-P-gp immunofluorescent staining using anti-P-gp F4 clone antibodies. These experiments were firstly conducted on DU4475 and SUM1315 cells and highlighted a similar staining signal and cellular distribution on both TNBC models (Figure 4). Strong colocalization between the two sets of labeling was also obtained on DU4475 cells, with a Pearson's coefficient of 92.1% and a Mander's overlap coefficient of 100.0%, which highlighted a strong spatial correlation between the two signals. Then, signal fluorescent intensities of both labeling sets were also compared for other TNBC cell lines. The correlation between the two signals for the five TNBC cell lines presented a coefficient determination R^2 of 0.99 (Figure 5). All these results demonstrated strong similarities between LightSpot®-FL-1 staining and anti-P-gp immunostaining signal localizations and intensities. These experiments allowed us to stratify several TNBC cell lines according to their P-gp level of expression, and they are consistent with the literature [35]. Thus, this innovative fluorescent probe transpires to be very efficient for the localization and quantification of P-gp on TNBC monolayer cell cultures.

In addition, the ability of the LightSpot®-FL-1 fluorescent probe to quantify the P-gp induction of expression was also checked. Indeed, our previous works had already highlighted the induction of P-gp expression in the SUM1315 cell line after exposure to 50 µM of Olaparib PARP inhibitor, using the Western blotting methodology [28]. Therefore, for these experiments, the TNBC SUM1315 cell line, cultured in monolayer, was also used as a model after their exposure to increasing Olaparib doses (10, 50 and 100 µM) over 3 h. As previously, the LightSpot®-Fl-1 staining was achieved alongside anti-P-gp immunostaining. Firstly, a non-significant increase in P-gp expression level was noted after 10 µM of Olaparib exposure, with a 2.8% and 5.7% increase for immunostaining and LightSpot®-FL-1 staining, respectively, in comparison to the DMSO control (Figure 6). In contrast, in the presence of 50 and 100 µM of Olaparib, a significant increase in P-gp level was measured with the two methodologies. Indeed, regarding the immunostaining, this increase was 11.4% for both 50 and 100 µM Olaparib concentrations, compared to the DMSO control. In contrast, for the LightSpot®-FL-1 staining, the P-gp level increased more strongly up to 55.1% after high-concentration Olaparib exposure, compared to 0.1% in the DMSO control (Figure 6). These results suggest that the LightSpot®-FL-1 seems to be more sensitive in the detection of the P-gp overexpression level, in comparison to the immunostaining method. This increased sensitivity permitted by the cell-permeant LightSpot®-FL-1 tracer might probably be due to the quantification of P-gp expressed on intracellular organelles, such as lysosomes [50].

This innovative LightSpot®-FL-1 tracer presents the ability to penetrate a cell mass. Thus, its performance for P-gp detection and quantification in cell masses was analyzed using SUM1315 spheroid models. Firstly, the P-gp staining method for SUM1315 spheroids was developed. Indeed, after 90 min of SUM1315 spheroid incubation with a 1 µM LightSpot®-FL-1 probe, homogeneous distribution of an intense green signal was detected on all spheroid areas. In order to remove unspecific tracer accumulation, spheroids were then severally washed allowing a clear drop of spheroid green-fluorescent signal of 27.0% after one wash, 66.1% after two washes, and 73.0% after 3 washes (Figure 7). Interestingly, upon this step, a stable signal persisted inside the spheroid models, with a similarity of 80.0% (no significant difference observed), despite an additional fourth washing step. Thus, these data allowed us to determine optimal conditions to directly detect and quantify the P-gp expression level inside SUM1315 spheroid models. As previously seen on monolayer cell cultures, the LightSpot®-FL-1 probe's ability to detect changes in P-gp expression level after drug exposure was assessed on SUM1315 spheroids. In these conditions, no significant increase in P-gp expression level was detected after a 3 h short-term Olaparib exposure, with 2.4%, 4.8, and 10.2% of P-gp expression variation for 10, 50, and 100 µM Olaparib doses, respectively, in comparison to DMSO controls (Figure 7). However, after a longer Olaparib exposure of 6 h, the LightSpot®-FL-1 compound allowed us to detect a significant P-gp expression level increase of 33.3%, 30.7%, and 30.7% for 10, 50, and

100 μM Olaparib, respectively, in comparison to DMSO controls (Figure 7). These results highlighted the added value of the LightSpot®-FL-1 tracer to detect and quantify drug-induced overexpression of P-gp in fixed cell masses such as spheroid models.

The present works allowed the development of the new LightSpot®-FL-1 fluorescent probe for the specific localization and quantification of the P-gp chemoresistance protein, inside in vitro preclinical TNBC models. In particular, this innovative tool turned out to be very effective for directly detecting and measuring the basal or induced expression level of the P-gp on both monolayer cultures and spheroid models. One of the added values of the LightSpot®-FL-1 is its ability to specifically detect the P-gp on fresh and also fixed cell models. This ability would be particularly interesting regarding precious biological samples and would allow the elimination of P-gp expression level modifications during experiments. Moreover, we demonstrated that this new approach is more sensitive for the detection of P-gp expression level changes than classic immunofluorescence methods. This performance may probably be due to the ability of the LightSpot®-FL-1 probe to detect not only the plasma membrane P-gp but also the intracellular P-gp expressed at the membrane organelles [46,47]. Indeed, the P-gp is expressed not only at the plasmid membrane level, but, according to the literature, it is also transiently present on intracellular organelle membranes, such as endoplasmic reticulum, Golgi apparatus and endosome/lysosome vesicles [46]. In fact, all these organelles are involved during the synthesis and traffic of the P-gp. However, the P-gp is maintained on the lysosome membrane, playing an important role in tumoral chemoresistance via lysosomal drug sequestration and degradation [50,51]. Therefore, this approach would be more complete for the detection of the global P-gp cell expression level. For this, other works are currently in progress to characterize more precisely the intracellular LightSpot®-FL-1 staining. All these characteristics make the LightSpot®-FL-1 probe very effective for the quantification and localization of the P-gp inside multicellular biological structures. In particular, this innovative tool is very promising for improving studies of the P-gp and for the clinical diagnosis of tumoral chemoresistance established by this protein. More specifically, the LightSpot®-FL-1 may help to re-introduce the tumoral P-gp expression level as a predictive biomarker of therapeutic failure or cancer relapse. This new clinical approach may turn out to be very useful as a way to improve tumor treatment that is all the most important in challenging cancer subtypes such as TNBC. In this field, our current works are focused on the development of the LightSpot®-FL-1 probe on clinical samples for the evaluation of tumoral chemoresistance.

5. Patents

These present works follow the international patent filing # PCT/EP2020/077694 from 2 October 2020, by UCA/INSERM/BIOMARQUEURS [34].

Author Contributions: Conceptualization, A.G., P.D., C.D., E.M. and M.B.; Data curation, A.G., P.D. and M.R.; Formal analysis, A.G., P.D. and M.R.; Funding acquisition, P.D. and M.B.; Investigation, A.G., P.D. and M.R.; Methodology, A.G., P.D., C.D., E.M. and M.B.; Validation, A.G., P.D., C.D., E.M. and M.B.; Writing—original draft, A.G., P.D. and M.B.; Writing—review & editing, A.G., P.D., C.D., C.A., M.D., J.G., B.V., F.P.-L., E.M. and M.B. All authors have read and agreed to the published version of the manuscript.

References

1. Juliano, R.L.; Ling, V.A. Surface Glycoprotein Modulating Drug Permeability in Chinese Hamster Ovary Cell Mutants. *Biochim. Biophys. Acta.* **1976**, *455*, 152–162. [CrossRef]
2. Holland, I.B.; Cole, S.P.C.; Kuchler, K.; Higgins, C.F. Chapter 1—Phylogenetic and Functional Classification of ABC (ATP-Binding Cassette) Systems. In *ABC Proteins: From Bacteria to Man*; Academic Press Inc., Elsevier: Amsterdam, The Netherland, 2003; pp. 3–35.
3. Bamdad, M.; Brousseau, P.; Denizeau, F. Identification of a Multidrug Resistance-like System in Tetrahymena Pyriformis: Evidence for a New Detoxication Mechanism in Freshwater Ciliates. *FEBS Lett.* **1999**, *456*, 389–393. [CrossRef]
4. Bamdad, M.; Reader, S.; Grolière, C.A.; Bohatier, J.; Denizeau, F. Uptake and Efflux of Polycyclic Aromatic Hydrocarbons by Tetrahymena Pyriformis: Evidence for a Resistance Mechanism. *Cytometry* **1997**, *28*, 170–175. [CrossRef]
5. Vache, C.; Camares, O.; Cardoso-Ferreira, M.-C.; Dastugue, B.; Creveaux, I.; Vaury, C.; Bamdad, M. A Potential Genomic Biomarker for the Detection of Polycyclic Aromatic Hydrocarbon Pollutants: Multidrug Resistance Gene 49 in Drosophila Melanogaster. *Environ. Toxicol. Chem.* **2007**, *26*, 1418–1424. [CrossRef]
6. Valton, E.; Wawrzyniak, I.; Amblard, C.; Combourieu, B.; Bayle, M.-L.; Desmolles, F.; Kwiatkowski, F.; Penault-Llorca, F.; Bamdad, M. P-Gp Expression Levels in the Erythrocytes of Brown Trout: A New Tool for Aquatic Sentinel Biomarker Development. *Biomarkers* **2017**, *22*, 566–574. [CrossRef]
7. Gottesman, M.M. Mechanisms of Cancer Drug Resistance. *Annu. Rev. Med.* **2002**, *53*, 615–627. [CrossRef] [PubMed]
8. Robey, R.W.; Pluchino, K.M.; Hall, M.D.; Fojo, A.T.; Bates, S.E.; Gottesman, M.M. Revisiting the Role of ABC Transporters in Multidrug-Resistant Cancer. *Nat. Rev. Cancer* **2018**, *18*, 452–464. [CrossRef]
9. Theodoulou, F.L.; Kerr, I.D. ABC Transporter Research: Going Strong 40 Years On. *Biochem. Soc. Trans.* **2015**, *43*, 1033–1040. [CrossRef] [PubMed]
10. Silverman, J.A. Multidrug-Resistance Transporters. *Pharm. Biotechnol.* **1999**, *12*, 353–386. [CrossRef] [PubMed]
11. Zheng, H.-C. The Molecular Mechanisms of Chemoresistance in Cancers. *Oncotarget* **2017**, *8*, 59950–59964. [CrossRef]
12. Sarkadi, B.; Homolya, L.; Szakács, G.; Váradi, A. Human Multidrug Resistance ABCB and ABCG Transporters: Participation in a Chemoimmunity Defense System. *Physiol. Rev.* **2006**, *86*, 1179–1236. [CrossRef]
13. Leonard, G.D.; Fojo, T.; Bates, S.E. The Role of ABC Transporters in Clinical Practice. *Oncologist* **2003**, *8*, 411–424. [CrossRef] [PubMed]
14. Lawlor, D.; Martin, P.; Busschots, S.; Thery, J.; O'Leary, J.J.; Hennessy, B.T.; Stordal, B. PARP Inhibitors as P-Glyoprotein Substrates. *J. Pharm. Sci.* **2014**, *103*, 1913–1920. [CrossRef]
15. Azzariti, A.; Porcelli, L.; Simone, G.M.; Quatrale, A.E.; Colabufo, N.A.; Berardi, F.; Perrone, R.; Zucchetti, M.; D'Incalci, M.; Xu, J.M.; et al. Tyrosine Kinase Inhibitors and Multidrug Resistance Proteins: Interactions and Biological Consequences. *Cancer Chemoth. Pharm.* **2010**, *65*, 335–346. [CrossRef] [PubMed]
16. Pérez-Tomás, R. Multidrug Resistance: Retrospect and Prospects in Anti-Cancer Drug Treatment. *Curr. Med. Chem.* **2006**, *13*, 1859–1876. [CrossRef]
17. Nedeljković, M.; Damjanović, A. Mechanisms of Chemotherapy Resistance in Triple-Negative Breast Cancer-How We Can Rise to the Challenge. *Cells* **2019**, *8*, 957. [CrossRef]
18. Yamada, A.; Ishikawa, T.; Ota, I.; Kimura, M.; Shimizu, D.; Tanabe, M.; Chishima, T.; Sasaki, T.; Ichikawa, Y.; Morita, S.; et al. High Expression of ATP-Binding Cassette Transporter ABCC11 in Breast Tumors Is Associated with Aggressive Subtypes and Low Disease-Free Survival. *Breast Cancer Res. Treat.* **2013**, *137*, 773–782. [CrossRef]
19. Linn, S.C.; Giaccone, G.; van Diest, P.J.; Blokhuis, W.M.D.; van der Valk, P.; van Kalken, C.K.; Kuiper, C.M.; Pinedo, H.M.; Baak, J.P.A. Prognostic Relevance of P-Glycoprotein Expression in Breast Cancer. *Ann. Oncol.* **1995**, *6*, 679–685. [CrossRef] [PubMed]
20. Robinson, K.; Tiriveedhi, V. Perplexing Role of P-Glycoprotein in Tumor Microenvironment. *Front. Oncol.* **2020**, *10*, 265. [CrossRef] [PubMed]
21. Baekelandt, M.M.; Holm, R.; Nesland, J.M.; Tropé, C.G.; Kristensen, G.B. P-Glycoprotein Expression Is a Marker for Chemotherapy Resistance and Prognosis in Advanced Ovarian Cancer. *Anticancer Res.* **2000**, *20*, 1061–1067.
22. Verrelle, P.; Frédéric, M.; Fonck, Y.; Feillel, V.; Dionet, C.; Kwiatkowski, F.; Plagne, R.; Chassagne, J. Clinical Relevance of Immunohistochemical Detection of Multidrug Resistance P-Glycoprotein in Breast Carcinoma. *J. Natl. Cancer Inst.* **1991**, *83*, 111–116. [CrossRef] [PubMed]
23. Irvin, W.J.; Carey, L.A. What Is Triple-Negative Breast Cancer? *Eur. J. Cancer* **2008**, *44*, 2799–2805. [CrossRef]
24. Prat, A.; Pineda, E.; Adamo, B.; Galván, P.; Fernández, A.; Gaba, L.; Díez, M.; Viladot, M.;

Arance, A.; Muñoz, M. Clinical Implications of the Intrinsic Molecular Subtypes of Breast Cancer. *Breast* **2015**, *24* (Suppl. 2), S26–S35. [CrossRef] [PubMed]
25. Yin, L.; Duan, J.-J.; Bian, X.-W.; Yu, S.-C. Triple-Negative Breast Cancer Molecular Subtyping and Treatment Progress. *Breast Cancer Res.* **2020**, *22*, 61. [CrossRef]
26. Liedtke, C.; Mazouni, C.; Hess, K.R.; André, F.; Tordai, A.; Mejia, J.A.; Symmans, W.F.; Gonzalez-Angulo, A.M.; Hennessy, B.; Green, M.; et al. Response to Neoadjuvant Therapy and Long-Term Survival in Patients with Triple-Negative Breast Cancer. *J. Clin. Oncol.* **2008**, *26*, 1275–1281. [CrossRef]
27. Carey, L.A.; Dees, E.C.; Sawyer, L.; Gatti, L.; Moore, D.T.; Collichio, F.; Ollila, D.W.; Sartor, C.I.; Graham, M.L.; Perou, C.M. The Triple Negative Paradox: Primary Tumor Chemosensitivity of Breast Cancer Subtypes. *Clin. Cancer. Res.* **2007**, *13*, 2329–2334. [CrossRef] [PubMed]
28. Dufour, R.; Daumar, P.; Mounetou, E.; Aubel, C.; Kwiatkowski, F.; Abrial, C.; Vatoux, C.; Penault-Llorca, F.; Bamdad, M. BCRP and P-Gp Relay Overexpression in Triple Negative Basal-like Breast Cancer Cell Line: A Prospective Role in Resistance to Olaparib. *Sci. Rep.* **2015**, *5*, 12670. [CrossRef] [PubMed]
29. Dubois, C.; Dufour, R.; Daumar, P.; Aubel, C.; Szczepaniak, C.; Blavignac, C.; Mounetou, E.; Penault-Llorca, F.; Bamdad, M. Development and Cytotoxic Response of Two Proliferative MDA-MB-231 and Non-Proliferative SUM1315 Three-Dimensional Cell Culture Models of Triple-Negative Basal-like Breast Cancer Cell Lines. *Oncotarget* **2017**, *8*, 95316–95331. [CrossRef] [PubMed]
30. Dubois, C.; Daumar, P.; Aubel, C.; Gauthier, J.; Vidalinc, B.; Mounetou, E.; Penault-Llorca, F.; Bamdad, M. The New Synthetic Serum-Free Medium OptiPASS Promotes High Proliferation and Drug Efficacy Prediction on Spheroids from MDA-MB-231 and SUM1315 Triple-Negative Breast Cancer Cell Lines. *J. Clin. Med. Res.* **2019**, *8*, 397. [CrossRef]
31. Dubois, C.; Martin, F.; Hassel, C.; Magnier, F.; Daumar, P.; Aubel, C.; Guerder, S.; Mounetou, E.; Penault-Lorca, F.; Bamdad, M. Low-Dose and Long-Term Olaparib Treatment Sensitizes MDA-MB-231 and SUM1315 Triple-Negative Breast Cancers Spheroids to Fractioned Radiotherapy. *J. Clin. Med.* **2019**, *9*, 64. [CrossRef]
32. Goisnard, A.; Dubois, C.; Daumar, P.; Aubel, C.; Depresle, M.; Gauthier, J.; Vidalinc, B.; Penault-Llorca, F.; Mounetou, E.; Bamdad, M. The New Serum-Free OptiPASS® Medium in Cold and Oxygen-Free Conditions: An Innovative Conservation Method for the Preservation of MDA-MB-231 Triple Negative Breast Cancer Spheroids. *Cancers* **2021**, *13*, 1945. [CrossRef] [PubMed]
33. Booij, T.H.; Price, L.S.; Danen, E.H.J. 3D Cell-Based Assays for Drug Screens: Challenges in Imaging, Image Analysis, and High-Content Analysis. *SLAS Discov.* **2019**, *24*, 615–627. [CrossRef]
34. Bamdad, M.; Daumar, P.; Dubois, C.; Gauthier, J.; Goisnard, A.; Mounetou, E.; Penault-Llorca, F.; Vidalinc, B. LightSpot Patent: Method for Detecting, Localising and Quantifying MDR Proteins. International Patent Application WO 2021/064191 A1, 8 April 2021.
35. Bush, T.L.; Payton, M.; Heller, S.; Chung, G.; Hanestad, K.; Rottman, J.B.; Loberg, R.; Friberg, G.; Kendall, R.L.; Saffran, D.; et al. AMG 900, a Small-Molecule Inhibitor of Aurora Kinases, Potentiates the Activity of Microtubule-Targeting Agents in Human Metastatic Breast Cancer Models. *Mol. Cancer Ther.* **2013**, *12*, 2356–2366. [CrossRef]
36. Kumar, A.; Jaitak, V. Natural Products as Multidrug Resistance Modulators in Cancer. *Eur. J. Med. Chem.* **2019**, *176*, 268–291. [CrossRef]
37. Kartal-Yandim, M.; Adan-Gokbulut, A.; Baran, Y. Molecular Mechanisms of Drug Resistance and Its Reversal in Cancer. *Crit. Rev. Biotechnol.* **2016**, *36*, 716–726. [CrossRef]
38. Dent, R.; Trudeau, M.; Pritchard, K.I.; Hanna, W.M.; Kahn, H.K.; Sawka, C.A.; Lickley, L.A.; Rawlinson, E.; Sun, P.; Narod, S.A. Triple-Negative Breast Cancer: Clinical Features and Patterns of Recurrence. *Clin. Cancer Res.* **2007**, *13*, 4429–4434. [CrossRef] [PubMed]
39. André, F.; Zielinski, C.C. Optimal Strategies for the Treatment of Metastatic Triple-Negative Breast Cancer with Currently Approved Agents. *Ann. Oncol.* **2012**, *23*, vi46–vi51. [CrossRef] [PubMed]
40. Kim, B.; Fatayer, H.; Hanby, A.M.; Horgan, K.; Perry, S.L.; Valleley, E.M.A.; Verghese, E.T.; Williams, B.J.; Thorne, J.L.; Hughes, T.A. Neoadjuvant Chemotherapy Induces Expression Levels of Breast Cancer Resistance Protein That Predict Disease-Free Survival in Breast Cancer. *PLoS ONE* **2013**, *8*, e62766. [CrossRef]
41. Zhang, Z.; Zhang, W.; Jin, Y.; Wang, H.; Gu, F.; Zhou, J.; Lao, Z.; Xu, Z.; Tang, F.; Zou, L.; et al. Evaluating the Response of Neoadjuvant Chemotherapy for Treatment of Breast Cancer: Are Tumor Biomarkers and Dynamic Contrast Enhanced MR Images Useful Predictive Tools? *J. Thorac. Dis.* **2014**, *6*, 785–794. [CrossRef]
42. Rudas, M.; Filipits, M.; Taucher, S.; Stranzl, T.; Steger, G.G.; Jakesz, R.; Pirker, R.; Pohl, G. Expression of MRP1, LRP and Pgp in Breast Carcinoma Patients Treated with Preoperative Chemotherapy. *Breast Cancer Res. Treat.* **2003**, *81*, 149–157. [CrossRef]
43. Saaby, L.; Brodin, B. A Critical View on In Vitro Analysis of P-Glycoprotein (P-Gp) Transport Kinetics. *J. Pharm. Sci.* **2017**, *106*, 2257–2264. [CrossRef]

44. Jouan, E.; Le Vée, M.; Mayati, A.; Denizot, C.; Parmentier, Y.; Fardel, O. Evaluation of P-Glycoprotein Inhibitory Potential Using a Rhodamine 123 Accumulation. *Pharmaceutics* **2016**, *8*, 12. [CrossRef] [PubMed]
45. Hamrang, Z.; Arthanari, Y.; Clarke, D.; Pluen, A. Quantitative Assessment of P-Glycoprotein Expression and Function Using Confocal Image Analysis. *Microsc. Microanal.* **2014**, *20*, 1329–1339. [CrossRef] [PubMed]
46. Fu, D.; Arias, I.M. Intracellular Trafficking of P-Glycoprotein. *Int. J. Biochem. Cell Biol.* **2012**, *44*, 461–464. [CrossRef]
47. Zhitomirsky, B.; Assaraf, Y.G. Lysosomal Sequestration of Hydrophobic Weak Base Chemotherapeutics Triggers Lysosomal Biogenesis and Lysosome-Dependent Cancer Multidrug Resistance. *Oncotarget* **2015**, *6*, 1143–1156. [CrossRef]
48. Garland, M.; Yim, J.J.; Bogyo, M. A Bright Future for Precision Medicine: Advances in Fluorescent Chemical Probe Design and Their Clinical Application. *Cell Chem. Biol.* **2016**, *23*, 122–136. [CrossRef] [PubMed]
49. Arnaud, O.; Koubeissi, A.; Ettouati, L.; Terreux, R.; Alamé, G.; Grenot, C.; Dumontet, C.; Di Pietro, A.; Paris, J.; Falson, P. Potent and Fully Noncompetitive Peptidomimetic Inhibitor of Multidrug Resistance P-Glycoprotein. *J. Med. Chem.* **2010**, *53*, 6720–6729. [CrossRef] [PubMed]
50. Yamagishi, T.; Sahni, S.; Sharp, D.M.; Arvind, A.; Jansson, P.J.; Richardson, D.R. P-Glycoprotein Mediates Drug Resistance via a Novel Mechanism Involving Lysosomal Sequestration. *J. Biol. Chem.* **2013**, *288*, 31761–31771. [CrossRef] [PubMed]
51. Hraběta, J.; Belhajová, M.; Šubrtová, H.; Merlos Rodrigo, M.A.; Heger, Z.; Eckschlager, T. Drug Sequestration in Lysosomes as One of the Mechanisms of Chemoresistance of Cancer Cells and the Possibilities of Its Inhibition. *Int. J. Mol. Sci.* **2020**, *21*, 392. [CrossRef]

6

Nitric Oxide-Releasing Drug Glyceryl Trinitrate Targets JAK2/STAT3 Signaling, Migration and Invasion of Triple-Negative Breast Cancer Cells

Sarra Bouaouiche [1,2,†], Silvia Ghione [1,2,†], Randa Sghaier [1,2], Olivier Burgy [3], Cindy Racoeur [1,2], Valentin Derangère [4], Ali Bettaieb [1,2] and Stéphanie Plenchette [1,2,*]

1 Laboratoire d'Immunologie et Immunothérapie des Cancers (LIIC), EPHE, PSL Research University, 75000 Paris, France; bouaouiche.sarra@gmail.com (S.B.); silvi.ghio50@gmail.com (S.G.); sg.randa@yahoo.fr (R.S.); Cindy.Racoeur@u-bourgogne.fr (C.R.); ali.bettaieb@u-bourgogne.fr (A.B.)
2 Laboratoire d'Immunologie et Immunothérapie des Cancers (LIIC), EA7269, Université de Bourgogne Franche-Comté, 21000 Dijon, France
3 INSERM U1231, UFR Sciences de Santé, Université de Bourgogne-Franche Comté, 21000 Dijon, France; Olivier.Burgy@u-bourgogne.fr
4 Plateforme de Transfert en Biologie du Cancer, Centre Georges-François Leclerc, 21000 Dijon, France; VDerangere@cgfl.fr
* Correspondence: stephanie.plenchette@u-bourgogne.fr or stephanie.plenchette-colas@ephe.psl.eu;

† These authors contributed equally to the work.

Abstract: Triple-negative breast cancer (TNBC) is a highly aggressive disease with invasive and metastasizing properties associated with a poor prognosis. The STAT3 signaling pathway has shown a pivotal role in cancer cell migration, invasion, metastasis and drug resistance of TNBC cells. IL-6 is a main upstream activator of the JAK2/STAT3 pathway. In the present study we examined the impact of the NO-donor glyceryl trinitrate (GTN) on the activation of the JAK2/STAT3 signaling pathway and subsequent migration, invasion and metastasis ability of TNBC cells through in vitro and in vivo experiments. We used a subtoxic dose of carboplatin and/or recombinant IL-6 to activate the JAK2/STAT3 signaling pathway and its functional outcomes. We found an inhibitory effect of GTN on the activation of the JAK2/STAT3 signaling, migration and invasion of TNBC cells. We discovered that GTN inhibits the activation of JAK2, the upstream activator of STAT3, and mediates the S-nitrosylation of JAK2. Finally, the effect of GTN (Nitronal) on lung metastasis was investigated to assess its antitumor activity in vivo.

Keywords: cancer; nitric oxide; signaling; migration; invasion; metastasis

---

1. Introduction

Triple-negative breast cancer (TNBC) is the most aggressive subtype of breast cancer among women worldwide. TNBCs represent 10–15% of all subtypes of breast cancers and are so named because of the absence of estrogen receptor (ER), progesterone receptor (PR) and no overexpression of human epidermal growth factor receptor 2 (HER2) [1]. Consequently, standard targeted therapies used for treating other subtypes of breast cancers (hormone receptor-positive or HER2-positive) are not a therapeutic option. The therapeutic care of patients afflicted with early or advanced TNBC remains chemotherapy. Although TNBC patients present higher chemosensitivity than for other subtypes of breast cancer, their prognosis remains worse [2]. In recent years, much emphasis has been put on TNBC molecular features to identify new therapeutic targets and options of treatment.

The signal transducers and activators of transcription (STAT) family encompasses key transcription factors involved in breast cancer disease. Importantly, STAT3 signaling pathways, activated through many cytokines (such as Interleukin-6 (IL-6), IL-10) and growth factors (epidermal growth factor (EGF), fibroblast growth factor (FGF), insulin-like growth factor (IGF)), promote breast cancer progression, proliferation, apoptosis, metastasis and chemoresistance [3]. It is well established that the tumor microenvironment plays a crucial role for tumor development, tumor progression and response to anticancer therapies [4,5]. A continuous dynamic cross talk between tumor cells and stroma cells accounts tremendously for tumor fate and patient prognosis. A variety of stroma cells including immune cells (from the innate and adoptive response), cancer-associated fibroblasts (CAFs) and blood vasculature mainly populate the tumor microenvironment [4,6]. Inflammatory cytokines, chemokines and growth factors are active players in the communications within the tumor microenvironment that support tumor growth, invasion, migration and initiate the metastatic cascade [7].

IL-6 is a major pro-inflammatory cytokine secreted in the tumor microenvironment from both tumor and stromal cells which influences almost all hallmarks of cancer to promote cancer growth and progression [8]. The autocrine and paracrine action of IL-6 is associated with multiple signaling pathways that support not only aggressive features of cancer cells such as invasion, migration and metastasis, but also tumor growth, survival angiogenesis, regulation of immune response and chemoresistance [9]. Tumor-associated macrophages (TAMs), cancer-associated fibroblasts (CAFs) or myeloid-derived suppressor cells (MDSCs) are major sources of IL-6 and play an important role in invasiveness and metastasis [10,11]. Various clinical studies have correlated high circulating IL-6 levels in patients with malignant tumors, as for breast cancer [12,13], prostate cancer [14], head and neck squamous cell carcinoma [15] or renal cancer [16]. Even though several studies positively correlated elevated serum IL-6 levels with a poor prognosis, further studies are required to clearly determine whether IL-6 is a cause or consequence in different types of cancer [17]. Nevertheless, in breast cancer, elevated systemic IL-6 seems to reflect poor prognosis, advanced disease and distant metastasis [13]. The classical and alternative IL-6 signaling pathways activate JAKs with subsequent activation of the signal transducer and activator of transcription-3 (STAT3), a key transcription factor inducing numerous effector genes involved in cancer promotion and malignancy [18–20]. IL-6/STAT3 activity is also often associated with metastatic processes including epithelial-mesenchymal transition (EMT), degradation of extracellular matrix and cell migration [20]. Typically, IL-6 exerts its effect through two functional receptor complexes composed of a transmembrane form IL-6 receptor alpha (mIL-6 Rα) or a soluble form (sIL-6 R) that provides IL-6 binding specificity and interaction with the signal-transducing chains (gp130). JAK1 and JAK2 are critical tyrosine kinases that trigger the phosphorylation and activation of STAT3 on tyrosine 705 (Tyr 705) and subsequent dimer formation that initiates its translocation into the nucleus [19]. The IL-6/JAK2/STAT3 axis represents an important therapeutic target [18]. IL-6 also mediates its effect through the activation of other oncogenic signaling pathways including PI3K/AKT and MAPK/ERK pathways [8]. Thus, neutralizing either IL-6 or related signaling pathways represent an attractive therapeutic target in cancer. However, anti-IL-6 therapies have mainly demonstrated no benefit in several types of cancer [21]. Hence, new anticancer strategies targeting the IL-6 signaling axis are needed. Here, we considered a nitric oxide (NO)-based strategy to prevent the IL-6/JAK2/STAT3 axis. NO is an important signaling molecule now understood to play a dual role in cancer as a positive or negative regulator of multiple signaling pathways [22]. Some phase II clinical trials in advanced non-small cell lung cancer and prostate cancer patients reveal that the use of glyceryl trinitrate (GTN) may have beneficial effects in combination with chemotherapy (vinorelbine and cisplatin) and/or radiotherapy [23,24]. Interestingly, cisplatin can increase IL-6 cytokine production and then cellular migration and proliferation in non-small cell lung cancer cells [25]. However, further phase III trials in advanced non-small cell lung cancer patients treated with platinum-based doublet as first-line therapy (carboplatin/gemcitabine or carboplatin/paclitaxel) with GTN did not present clinical benefit [26]. Better knowledge is required to define how GTN should be utilized in cancer therapy.

In the present study we investigated the effect of carboplatin in promoting IL-6-mediated TNBC cell migration. We then examined the ability of GTN, a NO-releasing drug, to counteract the IL-6/JAK2/STAT3 axis migration, invasion and metastasis of TNBC cells.

2. Results

2.1. *Effect of Carboplatin on the Production of IL-6 in TNBC Cells*

Firstly, we investigated the effect of carboplatin on the expression of the pro-inflammatory cytokine IL-6 in TNBC cells from mouse (4T1 cells) and human (MDA-MB-231) origin. The 4T1 cells and MDA-MB-231 cells were exposed to a subtoxic concentration of carboplatin for 6 h (Supplementary Figure S1). We found that carboplatin induces an increase in IL-6 at the mRNA level in TNBC cells. A significant augmentation of the level of IL-6 mRNA was found in 4T1 cells after 6 h of treatment with carboplatin (Figure 1A). Similarly, we found that carboplatin induces the expression of IL-6 in MDA-MB-231 cells after 6 h of treatment (Figure 1B). Exposure of RAW 264.7 cells to a subtoxic concentration of carboplatin showed no significant changes in IL-6 mRNA levels, neither after 48 h of treatment (Figure 1C), nor at 6 h and 24 h (data not shown).

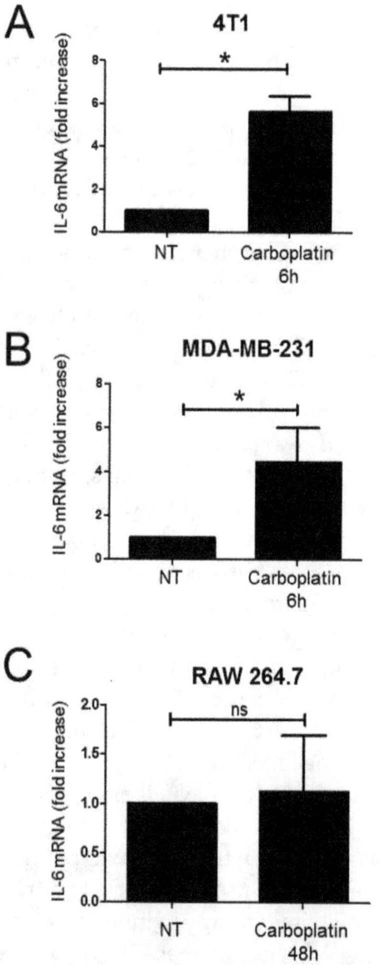

Figure 1. Carboplatin increases IL-6 production in TNBC cells. (**A**) 4T1 cells, (**B**) MDA-MB-231 cells and (**C**) RAW 264.7 cells were treated with carboplatin (10 μM, 750 nM and 10 μM, respectively) at the indicated time and IL-6 mRNA levels were determined by RT-qPCR. Data are shown as fold increase with mean +/− SD of three independent experiments performed in duplicate. *p* values were determined using a one-tailed Mann–Whitney test. Statistically significant differences are indicated: * $p < 0.05$; ns: not significant.

2.2. *GTN Inhibits JAK2/STAT3 Signaling Pathway*

The JAK2/STAT3 signaling pathway can be activated by IL-6. By immunoblotting analyses, we confirmed that the JAK2/STAT3 signaling pathway, in 4T1 and MDA-MB-231 cells, is activated as attested by the phosphorylation of JAK2 (Tyr1007/1008) and STAT3 (Tyr705), either by carboplatin or recombinant IL-6 treatment (Figure 2A–D). We investigated the effect of the NO donor GTN on the JAK2/STAT3 signaling pathway activation following carboplatin or recombinant IL-6 treatment. GTN induces the release of NO as attested by the increase in nitrite (NO_2^-) levels. This effect is not modified upon carboplatin exposure (Supplementary Figure S2). GTN induces a modest cytotoxic effect against 4T1 and MDA-MB-231 cells after 48 h, but not after 24 h exposure (Supplementary Figure S3). In agreement, GTN has no significant impact on early apoptosis in TNBC cells (4T1 and MDA-MB-231) after 24 h and 48 h of treatment. It induces only a low amount of early/late apoptosis in MDA-MB-231 cells after 48 h treatment (Supplementary Figure S4). GTN treatment in combination with either carboplatin or IL-6 significantly decreased p-JAK2 and subsequent p-STAT3 in TNBC cells (Figure 2A–D). To confirm the capacity of carboplatin to activate the JAK2/STAT3 signaling pathway through IL-6, we treated 4T1 cells with carboplatin with or without an IL-6 neutralizing antibody. Immunoblot analysis revealed that elevated levels of p-STAT3 and p-JAK2 stimulated by carboplatin can be blocked by the IL-6 neutralizing antibody and confirm the role of carboplatin in mediating IL-6 production and JAK2/STAT3 activation (Figure 2E).

These results suggest that GTN can inhibit the activation of the JAK2/STAT3 signaling pathway. We further explored the effect of NO on the phosphorylation state of JAK2. We therefore employed the erythroleukemic cell line HEL 92.1.7, characterized by the single point mutation JAK2-V617F, a gain-of-function mutant form of JAK2, versus the erythroleukemic cell line K562 that contains the non-mutated form of JAK2. As expected, a high level of basal expression of p-JAK2 was observed in the HEL 92.1.7 cell line as compared to K562 cells. Treatment of HEL 92.1.7 cells with GTN results in a significant decrease in p-JAK2 and subsequent diminution of p-STAT3 (Figure 2F).

Taken together, these results indicated that NO can counteract the JAK2/STAT3 pathway via the inhibition of p-JAK2.

2.3. *NO Promotes JAK2 S-Nitrosylation*

A myriad of signaling pathways regulated by NO occur through protein post-translational modification by S-nitrosylation. We investigated whether NO donors could promote the S-nitrosylation of JAK2 that may inhibit its kinase activity and downstream activation of the signaling pathway. To examine whether JAK2 can be S-nitrosylated, MDA-MB-231 and 4T1 cells were treated with GTN, with or without carboplatin, or another NO donor (S-nitrosocysteine (SNOC)) and then subjected to biotin-switch assay. We identified JAK2 as a target of NO. Interestingly, GTN alone only slightly induces the S-nitrosylation of JAK2, as seen only in MDA-MB-231 cells (Figure 3A). Interestingly, in both MDA-MB-231 and 4T1 cell lines, the combination therapy GTN/carboplatin markedly induced the S-nitrosylation of JAK2 (Figure 3A,B). In addition, SNOC (massive and rapid delivery of NO) induced the S-nitrosylation of JAK2 in both cell lines.

This result suggested that S-nitrosylation may be a regulatory mechanism for JAK2 activity.

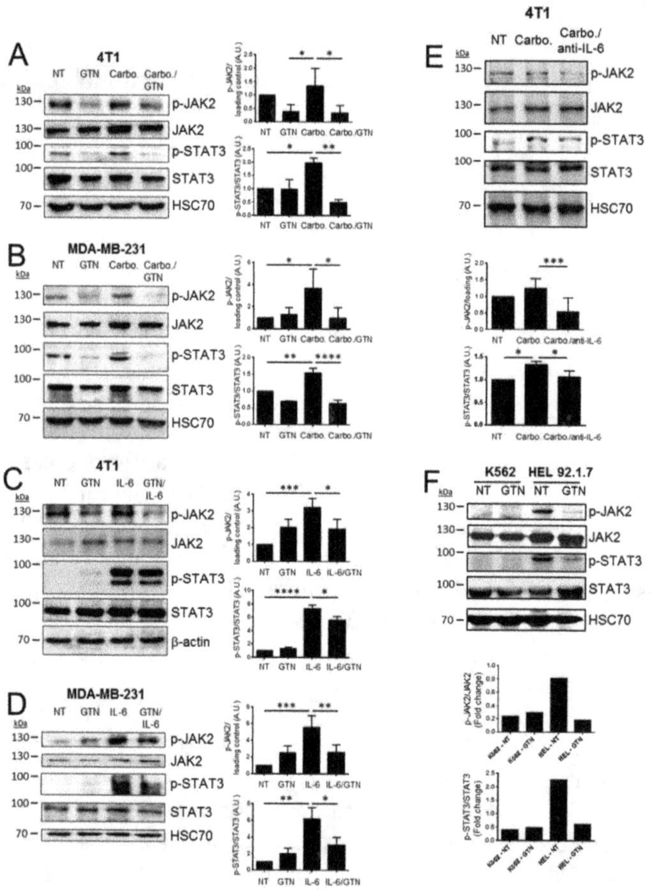

Figure 2. GTN inhibits IL-6-mediated JAK2/STAT3 signaling in TNBC cells. (**A**) 4 T1 cells and (**B**) MDA-MB-231 cells were treated with glyceryl trinitrate (GTN, 250 μM) and/or carboplatin (10 μM for 4T1 cells, 750 nM for MDA-MB-231 cells) or left untreated (non-treated, NT) for 48 h. (**C**) 4T1 cells and (**D**) MDA-MB-231 cells were treated with GTN (250 μM), recombinant murine or human IL-6 (rec-IL-6, 10 ng/mL), rec-IL-6/GTN or left untreated (non-treated, NT) for 6 h and 24 h respectively. (**E**) 4T1 cells were treated with carboplatin in presence or absence of neutralizing IL-6 antibody (anti-IL-6), or left untreated (non-treated, NT). (**F**) K562 and HEL 92.1.7 were treated with GTN 250 μM for 48 h. (**A–F**) The levels of phosphorylated JAK2 (p-JAK2), total JAK2, phosphorylated STAT3 (p-STAT3) and total STAT3 were analyzed by Western blot. HSC70 or β-actin was used as a loading control in all Western blots performed. The blots presented are representative of at least three independent experiments. (**A–E**) The histograms present quantification using densitometric analyses of at least three independent experiments: mean ratio p-JAK2/loading control (p-JAK2 normalized to the loading control either HSC70 or β-actin due to non-specific increase in JAK2 basal levels in 4T1 cells in response to treatment) and mean ratio p-STAT3/STAT3. (**F**) The histograms present quantification of one representative experiment (from three independent experiments). Statistically significant differences were determined using a one-way ANOVA test (with a Fisher's LSD test). * $p < 0.05$; ** $p < 0.01$; *** $p < 0.0001$; **** $p < 0.00001$. (**E**) Statistical analysis for ratio p-STAT3/STAT3: * $p < 0.1$.

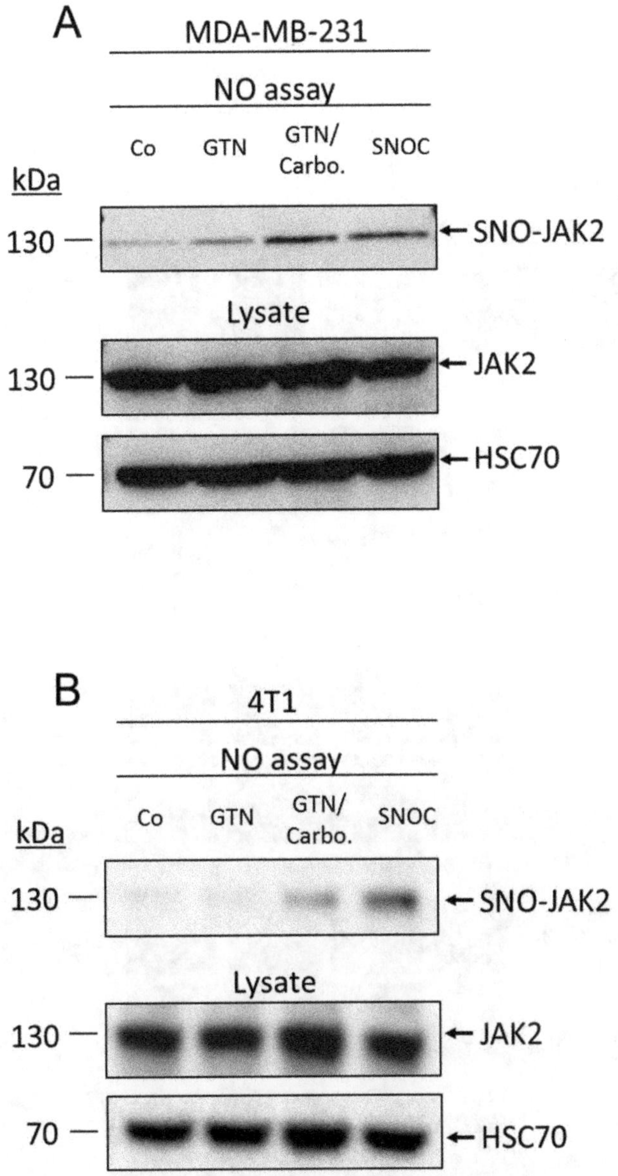

Figure 3. GTN promotes JAK2 S-nitrosylation. (**A**) MDA-MB-231 cells or (**B**) 4T1 cells were treated with carboplatin (750 nM and 10 μM, respectively) and/or GTN (250 μM) for 24 h, and S-nitrosocysteine (SNOC 1 mM) for 15 min. S-nitrosylation of JAK2 was demonstrated by using the biotin switch assay method. Total lysates were immunoblotted with JAK2 and HSC70 as a loading control.

2.4. Effect of GTN on IL-6-Mediated Wound Healing in TNBC Cells

IL-6 plays an important role as a migration factor in vitro and in vivo. Wound healing assays were performed with recombinant IL-6 added to TNBC cells. To completely preclude any stimulation of cell proliferation by IL-6, we performed an MTS assay. We demonstrated that IL-6, upon 24 h of treatment, induced no modification in the rate of proliferation of TNBC cells (Figure 4A,B). We found that recombinant IL-6 increases the wound healing ability of both 4T1 and MDA-MB-231 cells (Figure 4C,D). We explored the effect of GTN on the ability of IL-6 to stimulate wound healing in TNBC cells. The wound healing activity of TNBC cells remains unchanged following treatment with GTN alone in comparison with non-treated (NT) control cells. However, combined treatment of IL-6 with GTN inhibits the wound healing activity of both 4T1 and MDA-MB-231 cells (Figure 4C,D). To confirm the role of NO in the inhibition of the wound healing by the NO donor GTN, cells stimulated with IL-6 along with GTN were treated in presence or absence of the NO scavenger cPTIO. We showed that in presence of cPTIO, the inhibitory effect of GTN on IL-6-mediated wound healing is abrogated in both 4T1 and MDA-MB-231 cells (Figure 4E,F).

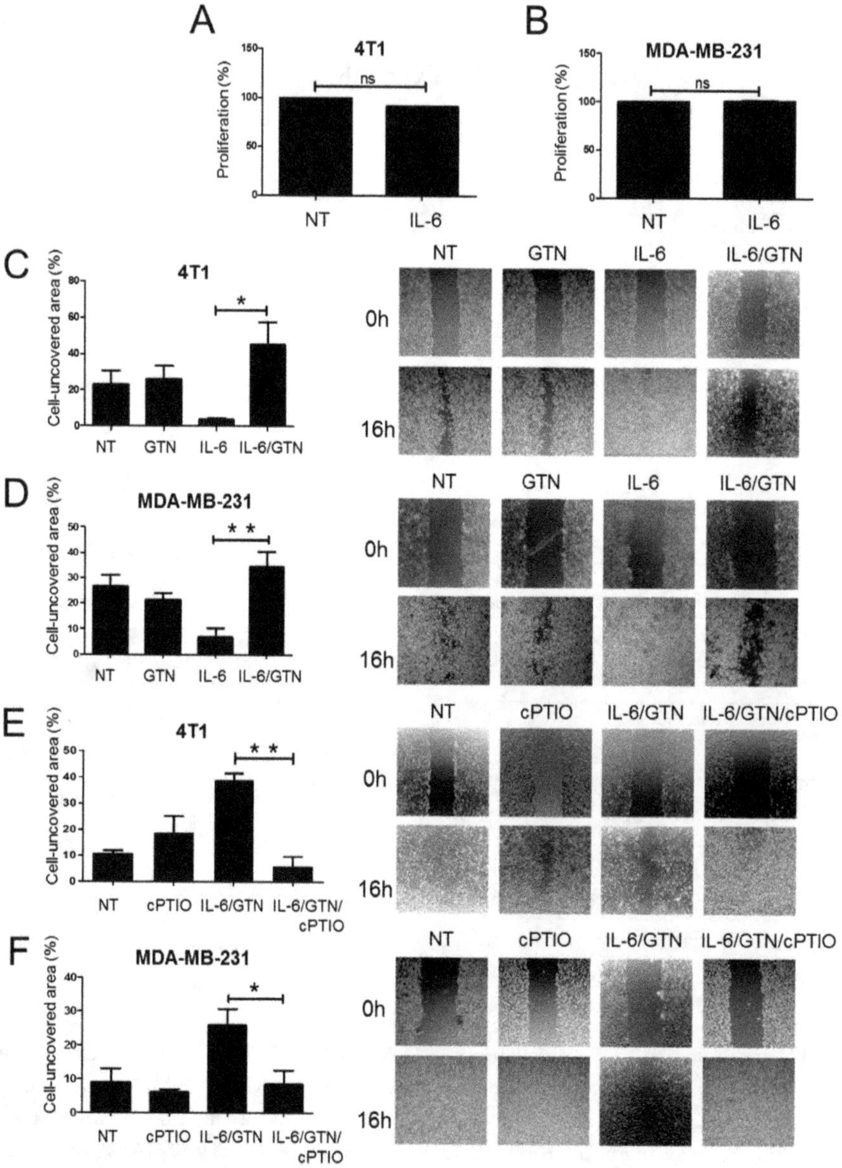

Figure 4. GTN prevents recombinant IL-6-induced wound healing in TNBC cells. (**A**) 4T1 and (**B**) MDA-MB-231 cells were treated with murine or human recombinant IL-6 (10 ng/mL), respectively, for 24 h and MTS proliferation assay analysis was performed. Results indicate means +/− SD of three independent experiments. (**C–F**) The in vitro wound healing assays. (**C**) 4T1 and (**D**) MDA-MB-231 cells were treated for 16 h with GTN (250 μM), and/or recombinant IL-6 (10 ng/mL) or left untreated (NT). Data are shown as percentage of cell-covered area. (**E**) 4T1 and (**F**) MDA-MB-231 cells were treated for 16 h with IL-6/GTN, and/or cPTIO (50 μM) or left untreated (NT). Results are expressed as mean +/− SEM of three independent experiments. Images are representative of three independent experiments. Statistically significant differences were determined using a one-way ANOVA test. * $p < 0.05$; ** $p < 0.01$; ns: not significant.

Altogether, these data suggested that GTN can counteract the IL-6 responsiveness of TNBC for wound healing migration in a NO-dependent manner.

2.5. *In Vitro Effects of GTN on Migration and Invasion of TNBC Cells*

To further address cell migration, we explored the impact of GTN on TNBC cells using the transwell cell migration assay. The 4T1 cells were seeded in the upper compartment and conditioned medium from carboplatin-treated 4T1 cells was incubated in the lower compartment. To figure out whether IL-6 secreted from carboplatin-treated cells could promote 4T1 cell migration, an IL-6 neutralizing antibody was added to the conditioned medium in the lower compartment. We found significant effect of the IL-6 neutralizing antibody on carboplatin-mediated 4T1 migration activity. Moreover, the addition of GTN into the conditioned medium significantly abrogated carboplatin-mediated 4T1 migration activity (Figure 5A). We then performed a co-culture experiment using the transwell migration system. The 4T1 cells were seeded in the upper compartment while co-cultured 4T1 and RAW 264.7 cells (ratio 3:1) were seeded in the lower compartment and stimulated with the indicated treatment. The percentage of 4T1 cells migrating is more important in the presence of co-cultured 4T1/RAW 264.7 cells compared to 4T1 cells alone (data not shown). Carboplatin treatment slightly increases 4T1 cell migration. The addition of an IL-6 neutralizing antibody along with carboplatin treatment significantly affected 4T1 cell migration, and even more following GTN treatment (Figure 5B). The transwell cell invasion assays were performed with conditioned media from carboplatin-treated 4T1 cells, then treated without or with an IL-6-neutralizing antibody (lower chamber) or GTN (upper-chamber). We observed a significant increase in 4T1 cell invasion in the presence of conditioned media from carboplatin-treated 4T1 cells. Cell invasion in response to GTN was significantly reduced. In the presence of the IL-6-neutralizing antibody, there seemed to be a trend that approximated but did not reach statistical significance (Figure 5C). We investigated the role of GTN on the EMT process. The EMT was stimulated by TGF-β1 in 4T1 cells attested by the upregulation of mesenchymal markers [27]. We found that TGF-β1-induced EMT in 4T1 cells increased the level of expression of the mesenchymal markers MMP9, Vimentin, Snail and Twist, and to a further extent upon carboplatin exposure. However, in response to GTN, the level of the mesenchymal markers was reduced (Figure 5D).

Altogether, these results indicate that GTN may have a broader impact on 4T1 cell invasion than the IL-6-neutralizing antibody.

2.6. *In Vivo Effect of GTN in a Syngeneic Model of Murine Metastatic TNBC*

The anti-metastatic effect of GTN was undertaken in vivo using a syngeneic model of murine TNBC with 4T1 cells which metastasize to the lungs. Mice were injected with 4T1 cells, and after seven days, mice were treated twice a week with Nitronal (glyceryl trinitrate) infusion solution or saline (NaCl). After a month, we analyzed the lung tissue for the presence of metastases by hematoxylin-eosin staining of formalin-fixed paraffin-embedded lung sections from five untreated and five Nitronal-treated mice (Figure 6A). The areas of tumor lesions (% of lung sections) were evaluated for each mouse in both the control and treated groups. Compared to control mice, Nitronal-treated mice showed a decrease in the area of tumor lesions (%). The one-sided p-value from the Mann–Whitney test is 0.086 (statistical significance considering a 90% confidence interval ($p < 0.1$)) (Figure 6B).

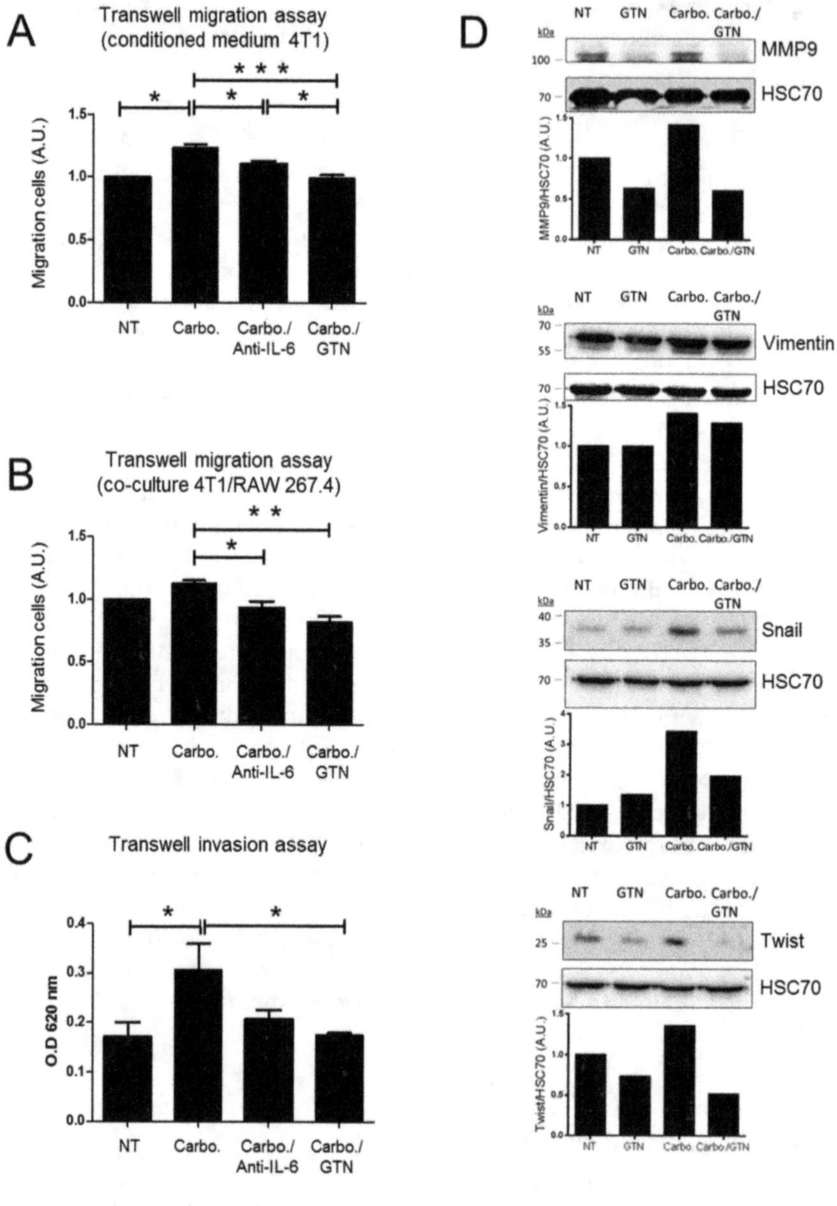

Figure 5. GTN prevents carboplatin-induced 4T1 cell migration and invasion in transwell systems. (**A**) Transwell migration assays were performed using 4T1 cells (upper chamber) incubated with conditioned media from 4T1 cells previously treated or not with carboplatin (10 μM) for 48 h (lower chamber). IL-6 neutralizing antibody (100 ng/mL) or GTN (250 μM) were added for an additional 16 h of treatment. (**B**) Transwell migration assays were performed using 4T1 cells (upper chamber) incubated with 4T1/RAW 267.4 co-culture (ratio 3:1) (lower chamber) treated with carboplatin (10 μM) alone or with either IL-6 neutralizing antibody (100 ng/mL) or GTN (250 μM) for 16 h of treatment. (**A**,**B**) The migration of control 4T1 cells is set at 1 arbitrary unit (A.U.) and the cancer cell migration following the indicated treatment is compared to control cells. (**C**) Transwell invasion assays were carried out using 4T1 cells (upper chamber) incubated with conditioned media from 4T1 cells previously treated or not with carboplatin (10 μM) for 48 h (lower chamber). GTN (250 μM) or IL-6 neutralizing antibody (100 ng/mL) was added within the conditioned media (lower chamber) for 16 h. Migrating and invading cells were stained with crystal violet and quantified by measuring the optical density (OD) at 620 nm. Results are means +/− SEM of three independent experiments. (**D**) Western blot analysis of MMP9, Snail, Vimentin and Twist in 4T1 cells treated with TGF-β1 (10 ng/mL) for 24 h, and then treated with GTN (250 μM) carboplatin (10 μM), carboplatin/GTN for 24 h. Densitometric analysis of proteins relative to HSC70 levels (one experiment representative of three independent experiments). Statistically significant differences were determined using a one-way ANOVA test. * $p < 0.05$; ** $p < 0.01$; *** $p < 0.0001$.

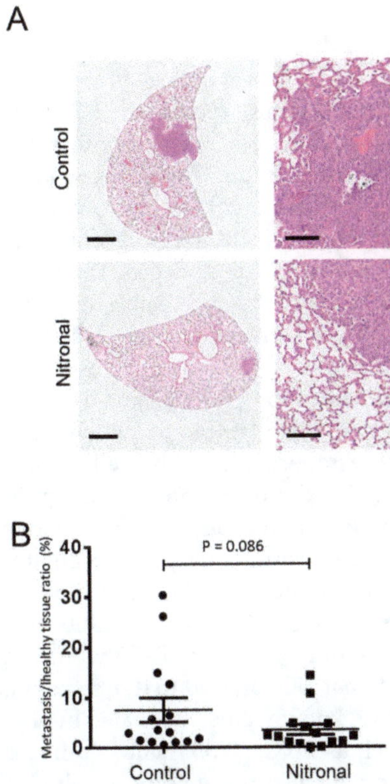

Figure 6. In vivo effect of Nitronal on lung metastases of 4T1 TNBC cells. (**A**) Representative immunohistochemistry images of lung sections from control or treated mice bearing 4T1 tumors. Lung metastases are visualized by hematoxylin-eosin staining of formalin-fixed paraffin-embedded sections. (**B**) Metastatic areas per lung sections for each animal were quantified as described in material and methods. Graph shows mean +/− SEM of 15 mice per group. Scale bar (left panel, 1 mm; right panel, 100 μm). Statistically significant differences were determined using a t-test with 90% confidence level and *, $p < 0.1$, considered statistically significant.

3. Discussion

TNBC is an aggressive disease with a high rate of metastasis, poor prognosis and few therapeutic options. One current therapeutic strategy for TNBC targets DNA repair complexes (by means of platinum derivatives and taxanes). Cisplatin- or carboplatin-containing regimens (cisplatin/gemcitabine, carboplatin/paclitaxel, carboplatin/gemcitabine) are recommended for first-line and second-line therapy [28]. A platinum-based regimen including carboplatin is recommended for patients with TNBC to increase pathologic complete response [29]. However, chemoresistance to platinum derivatives arose in various types of solid cancers. In this study we show that carboplatin enhances IL-6 expression and secretion by TNBC cells to activate the JAK2/STAT3 signaling pathway and cell migration. In TNBCs and many other human cancers, IL-6 is recognized as a major cytokine produced by multiple cell types within the tumor microenvironment, and which has important roles in tumor development and progression. IL-6 is involved in various oncogenic activities (cell proliferation, cell survival, migration, invasiveness and resistance towards anticancer therapy), therefore making IL-6 signaling cascades in breast cancer a target of choice.

Therapeutic strategies of IL-6 signaling blockade have been developed for several inflammatory diseases [21,30]. However, up to now, IL-6-based therapies have demonstrated no clinical efficacy in breast cancers and also in other various types of cancer patients [30,31]. More recently, a phase II clinical trial evaluating a selective JAK1/2 inhibitor in patients with metastatic triple-negative breast cancer (tumors demonstrating p-STAT3 expression) also demonstrated limited clinical efficacy [32]. A better understanding of IL-6/IL-6 R regulation and signaling needs to be taken into account to improve IL-6-based therapies in breast cancers.

NO-releasing drugs have gained growing interest as anti-cancer agents offering new treatment options for targeting various signaling pathways simultaneously [22,33]. NO is a free radical and highly reactive molecule that exerts a dual role in cancer, either pro-tumoral or anti-tumoral [22]. Protein post-translation modification by S-nitrosylation display decisive roles in regulating several signaling pathways involved in growth, cell survival or invasion. In this study we report that GTN inhibits TNBC cell migration and invasion in vitro, most likely via the IL-6/JAK2/STAT3 axis. We demonstrate that GTN prevents carboplatin-induced IL-6 to activate the JAK2-STAT3 pathway. We also report for the first time that GTN promoted the S-nitrosylation of JAK2 which may be associated with the inhibition of phosphorylation and activation of JAK2 and STAT3. The S-nitrosylation of JAK2 had never been reported so far; however, JAK2 nitration (Tyr1007 and Tyr1008) was described to prevent its activity [34]. Strikingly, data from the biotin switch assay demonstrates that the level of S-nitrosylated JAK2 is more important in TNBC cells treated with GTN along with carboplatin, than with GTN alone. The S-nitrosylation of JAK2 most likely directly regulate its kinase activity. Our finding is in agreement with a previous report that provided evidence for a cysteine-based redox-sensitive switch that regulates JAK2 catalytic activity [35]. Furthermore, it has been demonstrated that another NO donor, S-nitrosoglutathione (GSNO), selectively S-nitrosylates STAT3 at Cys259 and inhibits its accessibility to JAK2 [36,37]. Further studies would determine whether STAT3 would be targeted in this context. Altogether, these results suggest that NO can lead to IL-6 signaling blockade. Although p53 is a downstream target of STAT3, known to be attenuated by IL-6 via the JAK/STAT3 pathway in various cell types such as LNCap (p53 wild-type) and 22Rv1 (one wild-type copy of p53 and one mutated copy of p53) prostate cancer cells [38], we did not find any changes in p53 level upon IL-6 exposure on MDA-MB-231 cells (data not shown).

Conversely, high expression of iNOS in TNBC correlates with tumor aggressiveness (progression and metastasis), chemoresistance and poor outcome [39]. The role of iNOS inhibitors on TNBC aggressiveness has been studied. Importantly, preclinical studies using the pan-NOS inhibitor L-NMMA has demonstrated efficacy in decreasing tumorigenicity of TNBC, reducing tumor growth and lung metastasis [40]. Furthermore, the use of L-NMMA in combination with docetaxel has demonstrated enhanced chemotherapy response in TNBC PDX models and represents an interesting therapeutic approach [41].

Nevertheless, the dual nature of NO in cancer, pro- or anti-tumorigenic, is still a subject of intense debate. NO action and cellular outcomes largely rely on the role of many factors in the tumor microenvironment, particularly for TNBC, a subtype of breast cancer characterized by a profound intratumoral heterogeneity.

A growing number of studies provide evidence that coordinated cytokine expression is critical for the growth and malignancy of TNBCs.

Together, IL-6 and CCL5 are key enhancers of TNBC tumor growth and metastasis [42]. Indeed, within the tumor microenvironment, IL-6 secreted by TNBC cells upregulates CCL5 expression in lymphatic endothelial cells by activating the IL-6 receptor, STAT3, which subsequently enhances transcription of the *CCL5* gene. Importantly, the simultaneous blockade of CCR5 and IL-6 receptor signaling firmly inhibits TNBC tumor growth and prevents TNBC metastasis [42].

In TNBC, the tandem expression of IL-6 and IL-8 is also critical for growth and resistance to apoptosis [43]. Importantly, several reports suggest that both IL-6 and IL-8 play a critical role in the aggressiveness of breast cancer and of other types of cancer [44]. Recently, a study demonstrated that a synergistic IL-6 and IL-8 signaling pathway is required to influence cancer cell motility and metastases. Mechanistically, the pathway likely occurs through the downstream signaling of WASF3 and Arp2/3 and subsequent regulation of actin cytoskeleton dynamics [45]. Simultaneous inhibition of IL-6 and IL-8 receptors decreases the expression of WASF3 and Arp2/3, and reduces metastasis in mice [45]. In accordance with this finding, previous clinical studies had shown that the elevated serum concentrations of IL-6 and IL-8 of breast cancer patients correlate with the stage of the disease, the recurrence, and are indicators of poor prognosis [46–48]. However, the prognostic role of IL-6 and IL-8 association in breast cancer may differ according to breast cancer subtype. Indeed, high levels of IL-6 and IL-8 are associated with breast cancer recurrence only among patients with HER2 tumors [12].

In our current study we found that carboplatin enhances the expression of IL-8 at the mRNA level (data not shown). However, further studies are needed to determine whether GTN could block both IL-6 and IL-8 signaling to prevent cell migration and invasion. In support to this, our in vivo studies indicate a decrease in metastatic lesions upon the NO-donor GTN. Various clinical trials to evaluate the effectiveness of GTN in a combined regimen (chemotherapy and/or radiotherapy) has been conducted [23,24,26,49–51]. Although some clinical benefit were observed for non-small cell lung cancer (NSCLC) patients (GTN combined with vinorelbine and cisplatin) and prostate cancer patients (GTN after surgery or radiotherapy) in phase II clinical trials [23,24], additional data are required to define how GTN should be utilized in cancer therapy. Although we cannot extrapolate to humans the concentration of GTN used for our in vitro and in vivo findings, we provide here a new rationale to overcome chemotherapy-induced IL-6 production that should be considered for future GTN-based clinical trials.

In conclusion, we demonstrated that GTN can act upstream of STAT3 activation within the JAK2-STAT3 signaling. Our study provides evidence to consider the potential efficacy of IL-6 blockade in TNBC by the NO-donor GTN.

4. Materials and Methods

4.1. Cancer Cell Lines

Human MDA-MB-231 and murine 4T1 TNBC cell lines and murine macrophage-like cell line RAW 264.7 were obtained from ATCC. All cell lines were cultured in RPMI 1640 supplemented with 10% of fetal bovine serum (FBS) (37 °C, 5% CO_2), and were tested and certified as mycoplasma-free before use.

4.2. Drug, Reagents and Recombinant Proteins

The NO-releasing drug glyceryl trinitrate (GTN) was purchased from Merk (Lyon, France). Nitronal (GTN) infusion solution, 1 mg/mL (Pohl-Boskamp, Hohenlockstedt, Germany) was used for in vivo experiments. S-nitrosocysteine (SNOC), was prepared as described previously [52]. Carboplatin was obtained from the Centre Georges François Leclerc (CGFL) pharmacy. S-methylmethane thiosulfonate (MMTS), and carboxyP-TIO (cPTIO) were purchased from Sigma-Aldrich and biotin-HPDP from Perbio Science (Brebières, France). Recombinant murine and human IL-6 were purchased from Peprotech (Neuilly sur Seine, France) and TGF-β1 from R&D systems (Bio-Techne, Lille, France).

4.3. Quantitative Real-Time Polymerase Chain Reaction (RT-qPCR)

Total RNA was extracted from cells using Trizol (Invitrogen, Thermo Fischer Scientific, Illkirch-Graffenstaden, France). Using M-MLV reverse transcriptase, random primers and RNAse inhibitor, 500 ng of RNA were reverse transcribed into cDNA according manufacturer's protocol (Promega, Charbonnières-les-Bains, France). cDNA was quantified by real-time PCR with Sybr Green PCR Master mix (Invitrogen) on a 7500 fast Real-Time PCR System (Life technologies, Thermo Fischer Scientific, Illkirch-Graffenstaden, France). mRNA abundance was calculated according to the change-in-cycling-threshold (ΔCt) method and data represented relatively to reference gene mRNA (β-actin). Primers: hIL-6 for: ACCCCCAGGAGAAGATTCCA; hIL-6 rev: GGGTCAGGGGTGGTTATTGC; hActβ for: AGAGCTACGAGCTGCCTGAC; hActβ rev: AGCACTGTGTTGGCGTACAG; mIL-6 for: AGCCAGAGTCCTTCAGAGAGAT; mIL-6 rev: GAGAGCATTGGAAATTGGGGT; mActβ for: TTCTTTGCAGCTCCTTCGTT; mActβ rev: ATGGAGGGGAATACAGCCCC.

4.4. Griess Assay

The Griess assay quantifies the conversion of NO to nitrite (NO_2^-). Cells were seeded in 96-well plates in complete RPMI medium (200 µL/well). After 24 h and 48 h of treatment, NO_2^- level was quantified by incubating 100 µL of culture supernatant with 100 µL of Griess' reactives (solutions A and B at 1:1 ratio). Solution A composition: N-1-(Napthyl)ethylenediamine hypochlorite. Solution B composition: p-aminobenzene-sulfonamide/H_3 PO_4 5%. After 15 min incubation, absorbance was read at 550 nm (corrected at 690 nm).

4.5. Proliferation Assay (MTS)

Cells were seeded in 96-well plates in complete RPMI medium (200 µL/well). After 48 h of treatment, cell proliferation was evaluated by adding MTS ((3-(4,5-dimethyl-2-yl)-5-(3-carboxymethoxythenyl)-2-(4-sulfophenyl)-2H-tetrazolium) (Promega). Absorbance was read after 2 h at 490 nm.

4.6. Apoptosis Quantification

Cells were seeded in 6-well plates in complete RPMI medium (2 mL/well). After 24 h and 48 h of treatment, apoptosis was evaluated by flow cytometry using AnnexinV-FITC/7-AAD staining (BD Biosciences, Le Pont de Claix, France). The percentage of apoptotic cells were evaluated.

4.7. Wound Healing Assay

MDA-MB-231 and 4T1 cells were seeded into 6-well tissue culture plate at a density that, after growth overnight, allowed cells to reach approximately 80% confluence as a monolayer. A straight scratch was made on the monolayer using a 200 µL pipette tip. Then, the cells were washed gently with PBS three times and further cultured with RPMI complete medium. Representative pictures were taken, to measure gap width at 0 h and after 16 h of incubation. Four pictures per experimental condition and time point were used to measure gap width using ImageJ software (Rockville, MD, USA)

4.8. Transwell Migration and Invasion Assays

Migration and invasion assays were performed using transwell systems (24-well inserts without or with Matrigel, respectively, 8 µm pore size; Corning). Briefly, 4T1 cells were seeded onto the top chamber in RPM1 complete medium. The bottom chamber was filled with RPMI complete medium (10% FBS) in the presence or absence of the indicated treatment. After 16 h, cells were removed gently from the top side of the transwell using a cotton-tipped swab. Each insert was fixed with methanol, stained with crystal violet and solubilized with 37% acetic acid. Then, optical density at 620 nm was measured.

4.9. Biotin Switch Assay (BSA)

The BSA was performed as described previously [53]. Briefly, 50×10^6 of cells were treated with GTN or SNOC at the indicated concentration and for the indicated time. Cells were harvested, washed three times in phosphate-buffered saline (PBS) and lysed in non denaturating nitrosothiol, SNO lysis buffer (50 mM Tris-HCl, pH 7.4, 300 mM NaCl, 5 mM ethylenediaminetetraacetic (EDTA), 0.1 mM neocuproine, 1% Triton X-100) supplemented with 1 X protease inhibitors cocktail. All protein samples were normalized to 0.5 mg/mL in 10 mL of lysis buffer and free thiols were blocked by four volumes of blocking buffer (HENS buffer: 250 mM Hepes, pH 7.7, 1 mM EDTA, 0.1 mM neocuproine, 1% sodium dodecyl sulfate; containing 20 mM methyl methanethiosulfonate (MMTS)) at 50 °C for 20 min. After removing excess MMTS and washing proteins extracts twice by acetone precipitation, protein pellets were re-suspended in 1 mL of HENS buffer containing 1 mM ascorbate and 1 mM biotin-HPDP. Proteins were then recovered by two precipitations with acetone. Total biotinylated proteins were purified by precipitation on neutravidin beads and eluted with 2X blue Laemmli buffer (10 min, 95 °C) for further analysis by Western blotting.

4.10. Animal and Ethics Statement

Seven-week-old female Balb/c mice (total number of animals used $n = 15$) were purchased from the animal care facility at the University of Burgundy (France). The mice were acclimatized to the conventional housing system for 7 days before the period of study. All animals were observed by the animal care staff on a daily basis. Behavioral observations during the experiment were monitored by the research staff. Mice were housed at 22 +/− 2 °C in a 12 h light/dark cycle. For ethical reasons, when the volume of the primary tumor reached ~1500 mm^3, mice are sacrificed. During the period of this study, no mice were excluded. The experiments were approved by the local Ethics Committee "Comité d'éthique de l'expérimentation animale Grand Campus Dijon" (C2 EA Grand Campus Dijon no 105) protocol code 23450.

4.11. In Vivo Syngeneic Mouse Model of Breast Metastasis Formation

Mice (one cage of 10 mice in a first experiment and one cage of 20 mice in a second experiment) were subcutaneously inoculated in the right flank with mycoplasma-free 4T1 cells (1 × 10^4 cells in 100 μL) under anesthesia by continuous inhalation of 4% isoflurane gas. After 1 week, mice were randomly assigned to two groups ($n = 5$ per cage in the first experiment and $n = 10$ in the second experiment), control group (0.9% NaCl) or treated group (Nitronal® 1 mg/mL, Pohl Boskamp, Hohenlockstedt, Germany). No sample size calculation was done. S.G., O.B., C.R. and S.P. were aware of the group allocation at the different stages of the experiment. Both groups were injected subcutaneously twice a week with (100 μL of either Nitronal or 0.9% NaCl). All mice received 9 injections in total (either Nitronal or 0.9% NaCl), over a time period of 29 days. After, all the mice were sacrificed and lung tissues were excised, inflated and fixed in formalin for histology analysis [54].

4.12. Histology and Metastases Assessment

Several sections of lungs were paraffin-embedded and stained by hematoxylin and eosin (H&E) (Histology facility CellimaP, University of Burgundy). Metastatic areas per total lung section areas were quantified using QuPath software (Version: 0.2.3, University of Edinburgh [55]). The result is reported as the percentage (%) of metastatic area to total lung area per lung section.

4.13. Western Blotting

Whole-cell lysates were prepared by lysing the cells in lysis buffer (150 mM NaCl, 150 mM Tris HCl, pH 7.4, 1% SDS and 1 mM sodium orthovanadate, supplemented with 1 X protease inhibitor cocktail). Viscosity of protein extract was reduced by sonication or reduced by several passages through a 26-gauge needle. Protein concentrations were measured using the Bio-Rad DC protein assay kit (Marnes-la-Coquette, France). Thirty or fifty micrograms of protein were incubated in loading buffer (125 mM Tris-HCl, pH 6.8, 10% β-mercaptoethanol, 4.6% SDS, 20% glycerol and 0.003% bromophenol blue) for 5 min at 95 °C. Proteins were separated by sodium dodecyl sulfate–polyacrylamide gel electrophoresis (SDS-PAGE) and transferred to nitrocellulose membrane (Bio-Rad). Membranes were blocked in Tris-buffered saline (TBS) containing 8% BSA at room temperature for one hour, and incubated with primary antibody diluted in TBS 0.1% Tween-20 with 2% BSA overnight at 4 °C. Membranes were washed three times in TBS 0.1% Tween-20 and further incubated with corresponding secondary antibody for one hour at room temperature. After 3 washes in TBS 0.1% Tween-20, proteins were revealed using the enhanced chemiluminescence detection kit and ChemiDoc imager (Bio-Rad).

4.14. Antibodies

The antibodies used in this study included the following: anti-IL-6 neutralizing antibody (R&D systems), rabbit anti-JAK2, rabbit anti-phospho (Tyr1007-10008)-JAK2, rabbit anti-STAT3, rabbit anti-phospho (Tyr705)-STAT3, rabbit anti-Vimentin, rabbit anti-Snail (Cell Signaling); mouse anti-Twist, mouse anti-MMP9, goat anti-β-actin, mouse anti-HSC70 (Santa Cruz); peroxidase affinipure anti-mouse IgG and peroxidase affinipure anti-rabbit IgG (Jackson ImmunoResearch).

4.15. Statistical Analysis

Statistical analyses were performed using GraphPad Prism software (version 6.01, www.graphpad.com, 21 September 2012). Significant differences were evaluated using the one-way ANOVA test or the one-tailed Mann–Whitney test used for comparing data (means +/− SEM) from in vitro experiments. For in vivo analysis, the one-tailed Mann–Whitney non-parametrical test was used to compare the control group versus the treated group (means with SEM) with 90% confidence level. $p < 0.1$ was considered statistically significant.

Author Contributions: Conceptualization, S.P.; Formal analysis, S.B., S.G., R.S., O.B., C.R., V.D., A.B. and S.P.; Funding acquisition, S.P.; Investigation, S.B., S.G., R.S., O.B., C.R. and S.P.; Methodology, S.B., S.G., R.S., O.B., C.R., V.D. and S.P.; Project administration, S.P.; Software, V.D.; Supervision, S.P.; Validation, S.B., S.G., R.S., O.B. and C.R.; Visualization, S.B., S.G., R.S. and S.P.; Writing—original draft, S.B., S.G. and S.P.; Writing—review & editing, S.B., S.G., R.S., O.B., C.R., V.D., A.B. and S.P. All authors have read and agreed to the published version of the manuscript.

References

1. Bianchini, G.; Balko, J.M.; Mayer, I.A.; Sanders, M.E.; Gianni, L. Triple-negative breast cancer: Challenges and opportunities of a heterogeneous disease. *Nat. Rev. Clin. Oncol.* **2016**, *13*, 674–690. [CrossRef]
2. Di Leo, A.; Curigliano, G.; Diéras, V.; Malorni, L.; Sotiriou, C.; Swanton, C.; Thompson, A.; Tutt, A.; Piccart, M. New approaches for improving outcomes in breast cancer in Europe. *Breast* **2015**, *24*, 321–330. [CrossRef]
3. Ma, J.H.; Qin, L.; Li, X. Role of STAT3 signaling pathway in breast cancer. *Cell Commun. Signal.* **2020**, *18*, 33. [CrossRef]
4. Qiu, S.Q.; Waaijer, S.J.H.; Zwager, M.C.; de Vries, E.G.E.; van der Vegt, B.; Schröder, C.P. Tumor-associated macrophages in breast cancer: Innocent bystander or important player? *Cancer Treat. Rev.* **2018**, *70*, 178–189. [CrossRef]
5. Martins, D.; Schmitt, F. Microenvironment in breast tumorigenesis: Friend or foe? *Histol. Histopathol.* **2018**, 18021. [CrossRef]
6. Barbazán, J.; Matic Vignjevic, D. Cancer associated fibroblasts: Is the force the path to the dark side? *Curr. Opin. Cell Biol.* **2018**, *56*, 71–79. [CrossRef]
7. Yaacoub, K.; Pedeux, R.; Tarte, K.; Guillaudeux, T. Role of the tumor microenvironment in regulating apoptosis and cancer progression. *Cancer Lett.* **2016**, *378*, 150–159. [CrossRef]
8. Heinrich, P.C.; Behrmann, I.; Haan, S.; Hermanns, H.M.; Müller-Newen, G.; Schaper, F. Principles of interleukin (IL)-6-type cytokine signalling and its regulation. *Biochem. J.* **2003**, *374*, 1–20. [CrossRef]
9. Grivennikov, S.; Karin, M. Autocrine IL-6 signaling: A key event in tumorigenesis? *Cancer Cell* **2008**, *13*, 7–9. [CrossRef]
10. Landskron, G.; De la Fuente, M.; Thuwajit, P.; Thuwajit, C.; Hermoso, M.A. Chronic inflammation and cytokines in the tumor microenvironment. *J. Immunol. Res.* **2014**, *2014*, 149185. [CrossRef]
11. Hou, L.; Xie, S.; Li, G.; Xiong, B.; Gao, Y.; Zhao, X.; Hu, J.; Deng, S.; Jiang, J. IL-6 Triggers the Migration and Invasion of Oestrogen Receptor-Negative Breast Cancer Cells via Regulation of Hippo Pathways. *Basic Clin. Pharmacol. Toxicol.* **2018**, *123*, 549–557. [CrossRef] [PubMed]
12. Cho, Y.A.; Sung, M.K.; Yeon, J.Y.; Ro, J.; Kim, J. Prognostic role of interleukin-6, interleukin-8, and leptin levels according to breast cancer subtype. *Cancer Res. Treat.* **2013**, *45*, 210–219. [CrossRef] [PubMed]
13. Dethlefsen, C.; Højfeldt, G.; Hojman, P. The role of intratumoral and systemic IL-6 in breast cancer. *Breast Cancer Res. Treat.* **2013**, *138*, 657–664. [CrossRef] [PubMed]
14. Nakashima, J.; Tachibana, M.; Horiguchi, Y.; Oya, M.; Ohigashi, T.; Asakura, H.; Murai, M. Serum interleukin 6 as a prognostic factor in patients with prostate cancer. *Clin. Cancer Res.* **2000**, *6*, 2702–2706.

15. Nakashima, J. Prognostic significance of interleukin-6 in patients with prostate cancer. *Nihon Rinsho* **2002**, *60*, 165–169.
16. Gudbrandsdottir, G.; Aarstad, H.H.; Bostad, L.; Hjelle, K.M.; Aarstad, H.J.; Bruserud, Ø.; Tvedt, T.H.A.; Beisland, C. Serum levels of the IL-6 family of cytokines predict prognosis in renal cell carcinoma (RCC). *Cancer Immunol. Immunother.* **2021**, *70*, 19–30. [CrossRef]
17. Lippitz, B.E.; Harris, R.A. Cytokine patterns in cancer patients: A review of the correlation between interleukin 6 and prognosis. *Oncoimmunology* **2016**, *5*, e1093722. [CrossRef]
18. Bournazou, E.; Bromberg, J. Targeting the tumor microenvironment: JAK-STAT3 signaling. *JAKSTAT* **2013**, *2*, e23828. [CrossRef]
19. Yu, H.; Lee, H.; Herrmann, A.; Buettner, R.; Jove, R. Revisiting STAT3 signalling in cancer: New and unexpected biological functions. *Nat. Rev. Cancer* **2014**, *14*, 736–746. [CrossRef]
20. Yu, H.; Pardoll, D.; Jove, R. STATs in cancer inflammation and immunity: A leading role for STAT3. *Nat. Rev. Cancer* **2009**, *9*, 798–809. [CrossRef]
21. Rossi, J.F.; Lu, Z.Y.; Jourdan, M.; Klein, B. Interleukin-6 as a therapeutic target. *Clin. Cancer Res.* **2015**, *21*, 1248–1257. [CrossRef]
22. Plenchette, S.; Romagny, S.; Laurens, V.; Bettaieb, A. NO and cancer: Itinerary of a double agent. *Med. Sci. (Paris)* **2016**, *32*, 625–633. [CrossRef]
23. Yasuda, H.; Yamaya, M.; Nakayama, K.; Sasaki, T.; Ebihara, S.; Kanda, A.; Asada, M.; Inoue, D.; Suzuki, T.; Okazaki, T.; et al. Randomized phase II trial comparing nitroglycerin plus vinorelbine and cisplatin with vinorelbine and cisplatin alone in previously untreated stage IIIB/IV non-small-cell lung cancer. *J. Clin. Oncol.* **2006**, *24*, 688–694. [CrossRef]
24. Siemens, D.R.; Heaton, J.P.; Adams, M.A.; Kawakami, J.; Graham, C.H. Phase II study of nitric oxide donor for men with increasing prostate-specific antigen level after surgery or radiotherapy for prostate cancer. *Urology* **2009**, *74*, 878–883. [CrossRef]
25. Kiss, E.; Abdelwahab, E.H.M.M.; Steib, A.; Papp, E.; Torok, Z.; Jakab, L.; Smuk, G.; Sarosi, V.; Pongracz, J.E. Cisplatin treatment induced interleukin 6 and 8 production alters lung adenocarcinoma cell migration in an oncogenic mutation dependent manner. *Respir Res* **2020**, *21*, 120. [CrossRef]
26. Davidson, A.; Veillard, A.S.; Tognela, A.; Chan, M.M.; Hughes, B.G.; Boyer, M.; Briscoe, K.; Begbie, S.; Abdi, E.; Crombie, C.; et al. A phase III randomized trial of adding topical nitroglycerin to first-line chemotherapy for advanced nonsmall-cell lung cancer: The Australasian lung cancer trials group NITRO trial. *Ann. Oncol.* **2015**, *26*, 2280–2286. [CrossRef]
27. Hao, Y.; Baker, D.; Ten Dijke, P. TGF-β-Mediated Epithelial-Mesenchymal Transition and Cancer Metastasis. *Int. J. Mol. Sci.* **2019**, *20*, 2767. [CrossRef]
28. Wahba, H.A.; El-Hadaad, H.A. Current approaches in treatment of triple-negative breast cancer. *Cancer Biol. Med.* **2015**, *12*, 106–116. [CrossRef]
29. Korde, L.A.; Somerfield, M.R.; Carey, L.A.; Crews, J.R.; Denduluri, N.; Hwang, E.S.; Khan, S.A.; Loibl, S.; Morris, E.A.; Perez, A.; et al. Neoadjuvant Chemotherapy, Endocrine Therapy, and Targeted Therapy for Breast Cancer: ASCO Guideline. *J. Clin. Oncol.* **2021**, JCO2003399. [CrossRef]
30. Heo, T.H.; Wahler, J.; Suh, N. Potential therapeutic implications of IL-6/IL-6R/gp130-targeting agents in breast cancer. *Oncotarget* **2016**, *7*, 15460–15473. [CrossRef]
31. Kang, S.; Tanaka, T.; Narazaki, M.; Kishimoto, T. Targeting Interleukin-6 Signaling in Clinic. *Immunity* **2019**, *50*, 1007–1023. [CrossRef]
32. Stover, D.G.; Gil Del Alcazar, C.R.; Brock, J.; Guo, H.; Overmoyer, B.; Balko, J.; Xu, Q.; Bardia, A.; Tolaney, S.M.; Gelman, R.; et al. Phase II study of ruxolitinib, a selective JAK1/2 inhibitor, in patients with metastatic triple-negative breast cancer. *NPJ Breast Cancer* **2018**, *4*, 10. [CrossRef] [PubMed]
33. Plenchette, S.; Romagny, S.; Laurens, V.; Bettaieb, A. S-Nitrosylation in TNF superfamily signaling pathway: Implication in cancer. *Redox Biol.* **2015**, *6*, 507–515. [CrossRef]
34. Elsasser, T.H.; Kahl, S.; Li, C.J.; Sartin, J.L.; Garrett, W.M.; Rodrigo, J. Caveolae nitration of Janus kinase-2 at the 1007Y-1008Y site: Coordinating inflammatory response and metabolic hormone readjustment within the somatotropic axis. *Endocrinology* **2007**, *148*, 3803–3813. [CrossRef]
35. Smith, J.K.; Patil, C.N.; Patlolla, S.; Gunter, B.W.; Booz, G.W.; Duhé, R.J. Identification of a redox-sensitive switch within the JAK2 catalytic domain. *Free Radic. Biol. Med.* **2012**, *52*, 1101–1110. [CrossRef]
36. Singh, I.; Kim, J.; Singh, A.K.; Sharma, A.K.; Won, J.S. STAT3 Regulation By S-Nitrosylation: Implication In Cancer. *Redox Biol.* **2015**, *5*, 416–417. [CrossRef]
37. Kim, J.; Won, J.S.; Singh, A.K.; Sharma, A.K.; Singh, I. STAT3 regulation by S-nitrosylation:

Implication for inflammatory disease. *Antioxid. Redox Signal.* **2014**, *20*, 2514–2527. [CrossRef]
38. Cheteh, E.H.; Sarne, V.; Ceder, S.; Bianchi, J.; Augsten, M.; Rundqvist, H.; Egevad, L.; Östman, A.; Wiman, K.G. Interleukin-6 derived from cancer-associated fibroblasts attenuates the p53 response to doxorubicin in prostate cancer cells. *Cell Death Discov.* **2020**, *6*, 42. [CrossRef]
39. Walsh, E.M.; Keane, M.M.; Wink, D.A.; Callagy, G.; Glynn, S.A. Review of Triple Negative Breast Cancer and the Impact of Inducible Nitric Oxide Synthase on Tumor Biology and Patient Outcomes. *Crit Rev. Oncog.* **2016**, *21*, 333–351. [CrossRef]
40. Granados-Principal, S.; Liu, Y.; Guevara, M.L.; Blanco, E.; Choi, D.S.; Qian, W.; Patel, T.; Rodriguez, A.A.; Cusimano, J.; Weiss, H.L.; et al. Inhibition of iNOS as a novel effective targeted therapy against triple-negative breast cancer. *Breast Cancer Res.* **2015**, *17*, 25. [CrossRef]
41. Dávila-González, D.; Choi, D.S.; Rosato, R.R.; Granados-Principal, S.M.; Kuhn, J.G.; Li, W.F.; Qian, W.; Chen, W.; Kozielski, A.J.; Wong, H.; et al. Pharmacological Inhibition of NOS Activates ASK1/JNK Pathway Augmenting Docetaxel-Mediated Apoptosis in Triple-Negative Breast Cancer. *Clin. Cancer Res.* **2018**, *24*, 1152–1162. [CrossRef]
42. Jin, K.; Pandey, N.B.; Popel, A.S. Simultaneous blockade of IL-6 and CCL5 signaling for synergistic inhibition of triple-negative breast cancer growth and metastasis. *Breast Cancer Res.* **2018**, *20*, 54. [CrossRef]
43. Hartman, Z.C.; Poage, G.M.; den Hollander, P.; Tsimelzon, A.; Hill, J.; Panupinthu, N.; Zhang, Y.; Mazumdar, A.; Hilsenbeck, S.G.; Mills, G.B.; et al. Growth of triple-negative breast cancer cells relies upon coordinate autocrine expression of the proinflammatory cytokines IL-6 and IL-8. *Cancer Res.* **2013**, *73*, 3470–3480. [CrossRef]
44. Chavey, C.; Bibeau, F.; Gourgou-Bourgade, S.; Burlinchon, S.; Boissière, F.; Laune, D.; Roques, S.; Lazennec, G. Oestrogen receptor negative breast cancers exhibit high cytokine content. *Breast Cancer Res.* **2007**, *9*, R15. [CrossRef]
45. Jayatilaka, H.; Tyle, P.; Chen, J.J.; Kwak, M.; Ju, J.; Kim, H.J.; Lee, J.S.H.; Wu, P.H.; Gilkes, D.M.; Fan, R.; et al. Synergistic IL-6 and IL-8 paracrine signalling pathway infers a strategy to inhibit tumour cell migration. *Nat. Commun.* **2017**, *8*, 15584. [CrossRef]
46. Salgado, R.; Junius, S.; Benoy, I.; Van Dam, P.; Vermeulen, P.; Van Marck, E.; Huget, P.; Dirix, L.Y. Circulating interleukin-6 predicts survival in patients with metastatic breast cancer. *Int. J. Cancer* **2003**, *103*, 642–646. [CrossRef]

7

Thrombospondin-1 Silencing Improves Lymphocyte Infiltration in Tumors and Response to Anti-PD-1 in Triple-Negative Breast Cancer

Elie Marcheteau [1,2,3], Thomas Farge [1,3], Michaël Pérès [1], Guillaume Labrousse [1,3], Julie Tenet [1,3], Stéphanie Delmas [2], Maud Chusseau [2], Raphaëlle Duprez-Paumier [4], Camille Franchet [4], Florence Dalenc [4], Caroline Imbert [1], Justine Noujarède [1,3], Céline Colacios [1,3], Hervé Prats [1,3], Florence Cabon [1,2,3,†] and Bruno Ségui [1,3,5,*,†]

1 Centre de Recherches en Cancérologie de Toulouse, INSERM UMR1037, CNRS UMR5071, 2 Avenue Hubert Curien, CEDEX 1, 31047 Toulouse, France; emarcheteau@neovirtech.com (E.M.); thomas.farge@inserm.fr (T.F.); m.peres@chru-nancy.fr (M.P.); guillaume.labrousse@inserm.fr (G.L.); julie.tenet@univ-tlse.fr (J.T.); caroline.imbert@inserm.fr (C.I.); justine.noujarede@bric.ku.dk (J.N.); celine.colacios@inserm.fr (C.C.); herve.prats@inserm.fr (H.P.); florence.cabon@inserm.fr (F.C.)

2 SeleXel, 1 Place Pierre Potier, BP 50624, CEDEX 1, 31106 Toulouse, France; stephanie.delmas@evotec.com (S.D.); maud.chusseau@imavita.com (M.C.)

3 Université Toulouse III—Paul Sabatier, 118 Rte de Narbonne, 31062 Toulouse, France

4 Institut Claudius Regaud, Institut Universitaire du Cancer de Toulouse-Oncopole, 1 Av. Irène Joliot-Curie, 31100 Toulouse, France; Duprez-Paumier.raphaelle@iuct-oncopole.fr (R.D.-P.); franchet.camille@iuct-oncopole.fr (C.F.); dalenc.florence@iuct-oncopole.fr (F.D.)

5 Equipe Labellisée par la Fondation ARC—Association Pour la Recherche sur le Cancer, 94803 Villejuif, France

* Correspondence: bruno.segui@inserm.fr;

† These authors contributed equally: Florence Cabon and Bruno Ségui.

Simple Summary: Triple-negative breast cancer (TNBC) is associated with a poor prognosis, and the development of better therapeutic strategies is required. Herein, we investigated the role of the anti-angiogenic thrombospondin-1 (TSP1) in TNBC. TSP1 expression in tumor biopsies from TNBC patients was associated with a bad prognosis and a weak content of tumor-infiltrating lymphocytes (TILs). In the 4T1 mouse TNBC model, TSP1 knockdown reduced TGF-β activation and enhanced the content of TILs. Moreover, TSP1 knockdown decreased lung metastasis in syngeneic Balb/c immunocompetent mice but not in immunodeficient nude mice. Finally, TSP1 knockdown enhanced anti-PD-1 immunotherapy efficacy. Thus, targeting TSP1 may be considered as a putative therapeutic strategy in TNBC in combination with immunotherapy.

Abstract: Triple-negative breast cancer (TNBC) is notoriously aggressive with a high metastatic potential, and targeted therapies are lacking. Using transcriptomic and histologic analysis of TNBC samples, we found that a high expression of thrombospondin-1 (TSP1), a potent endogenous inhibitor of angiogenesis and an activator of latent transforming growth factor beta (TGF-β), is associated with (i) gene signatures of epithelial–mesenchymal transition and TGF-β signaling, (ii) metastasis and (iii) a reduced survival in TNBC patients. In contrast, in tumors expressing low levels of TSP1, gene signatures of interferon gamma (IFN-γ) signaling and lymphocyte activation were enriched. In TNBC biopsies, TSP1 expression inversely correlated with the CD8+ tumor-infiltrating lymphocytes (TILs) content. In the 4T1 metastatic mouse model of TNBC, TSP1 silencing did not affect primary tumor development but, strikingly, impaired metastasis in immunocompetent but not in immunodeficient nude mice. Moreover, TSP1 knockdown increased tumor vascularization and T lymphocyte infiltration and decreased TGF-β activation in immunocompetent mice. Noteworthy was the finding that TSP1 knockdown increased CD8+ TILs and their programmed cell death 1 (PD-1) expression and sensitized 4T1 tumors to anti-PD-1 therapy. TSP1 inhibition might thus represent an innovative targeted approach to impair TGF-β activation and breast cancer cell metastasis and improve lymphocyte infiltration in tumors, and immunotherapy efficacy in TNBC.

Keywords: THBS1; TSP1; angiogenesis; metastasis; immunotherapy; tumor-infiltrating lymphocytes

1. Introduction

Triple-negative breast cancer (TNBC) remains associated with a poor prognosis, and the development of better therapeutics represents a major unmet clinical need. In metastatic settings, chemotherapy still represents the mainstay of treatment. Advances in genomics and molecular profiling have helped better define subtypes of TNBC with distinct biologic drivers to guide the therapeutic development of targeted therapies, including vascular endothelial growth factor A (VEGF-A), a major pro-angiogenic growth factor [1], immune checkpoint inhibitors for programmed cell death ligand 1 (PD-L1)-positive TNBC [2] and poly (ADP-ribose) polymerase (PARP) inhibitors for breast cancer 1/2 (BRCA1/2) mutant TNBC [3,4]. Whereas a PARP inhibitor has recently been shown to improve the prognosis of BRCA1/2 mutant TNBC [5], the usefulness of checkpoint inhibitors of the PD-1/PD-L1 axis needs to be better defined.

Thrombospondin-1 (TSP1) is a major endogenous anti-angiogenic protein secreted by various cell types, including cancer cells [6]. TSP1 is frequently repressed in the early stages of tumor development, contributing to an increased tumor angiogenesis [7]. Intriguingly, TSP1 is overexpressed in advanced stages of many tumor types such as prostate, pancreas, glioblastoma, breast and gallbladder cancers and melanoma [8–10]. Moreover, whereas TSP1 is expressed at very low levels in the normal breast, a high TSP1 level is associated with a bad prognosis in breast cancer [11]. Accordingly, TSP1 levels are higher in the plasma of metastatic patients as compared to non-metastatic patients [12–14]. TSP1 has pleiotropic functions and is considered as a major activator of transforming growth factor beta (TGF-β), a potent immunosuppressive and pro-metastatic cytokine [15–17]. As a matter of fact, it has been shown that TSP1 modulates the immune response and metastasis of cancer cells [9,18]. To the best of our knowledge, whether TSP1-dependent metastasis relies on its capacity to modulate the immune response remains to be established.

Herein, we investigated the impact of TSP1 expression in tumor biopsies from TNBC patients on immune responses and prognosis. In the 4T1 mouse TNBC model, we next analyzed the consequence of TSP1 knockdown on TGF-β activation, immune response and metastasis, in syngeneic Balb/c immunocompetent mice and in immunodeficient nude mice. Finally, we evaluated the impact of TSP1 knockdown on anti-PD-1 immunotherapy efficacy.

2. Materials and Methods

2.1. In Silico Analyses

Kaplan–Meier plots were generated with Kaplan–Meier Plotter, an online public database combining 35 independent transcriptomic studies, totaling 5143 breast tumor samples (www.kmplot.com (accessed on 1 April 2019) [19]). This database was used to determine the relevance of TSP1 mRNA expression to the overall survival (OS). Patients' clinical data were collected and implemented in the online tool, allowing specific analysis in TNBC patients. The hazard ratio (HR) and 95% confidence intervals, as well as log rank *p*, were calculated and displayed on the webpage.

The TCGA-BRCA [20] (The Cancer Genome Atlas Research Network, Breast cancer) RNA-seq database was downloaded from TCGA servers with patients' clinical data to perform transcriptomic analysis on TNBC only samples ($n = 122$). Patients were then classified as a function of their TSP1 (*THBS1*, ENSG00000137801) mRNA expression to segregate low and high TSP1 patients according to the median. We performed gene set enrichment analysis (GSEA) on these two groups using the GSEA v2.0 tool, developed from a joint project of UC San Diego (La Jolla, CA, USA) and Broad Institute (Cambridge, MA, USA) [19,21] and curated gene signatures available on their website. Normalized enrichment scores (NESs), *p*-values and false discovery rates were added to the figures as displayed by the GSEA result file.

2.2. Patients

A total of 12 patients with primary breast cancer (TNBC) were included in this study between July 2015 and February 2018. Patients who received neoadjuvant chemotherapy were excluded. Clinical characteristics of patients and tumor pathological features were obtained from their medical reports and followed the standard procedures adopted by the Claudius Regaud Institute.

2.3. Immunohistochemistry

IHC analysis of patient samples was performed on formalin-fixed, paraffin-embedded sections of the initial tumor biopsies with the indicated antibodies. The percentage of stained tumor cells was assessed for each biomarker. Antibodies against CD8 (clone SP57, Roche diagnostic, Meylan, France) and TSP1 (clone MA5-11330, Thermo Scientific, Villebon sur Yvette, France) were used. Alternatively, the proportion of TILs was determined as previously recommended [22].

2.4. Cell Lines and Transduction

4T1, a 6-thioguanine-resistant cell line selected from the 410.4 tumor without mutagen treatment, was obtained from ATCC and tested to be mycoplasma-free. Cells were maintained in Dulbecco's modified Eagle's medium (DMEM) with high glucose supplemented with 10% FBS.

Lentiviral vector pLKO.1 expressing the non-target shRNA (SHC002) or shRNA construct targeting TSP1 exon 5 (TRCN0000039696) was purchased from Sigma-Aldrich (Saint-Quentin-Fallavier, France). Plasmids were transfected into cells in culture using the TransIT-X2 Dynamic Delivery System (MIRUS BIO). Lentiviral vector pTRIP (Dharmacon, Illkirch, France) expressing Luciferase Firefly was produced in HEK293FT cells by the tri-transfection method using calcium phosphate. Lentiviral particles were harvested 72 h after transfection. For lentiviral transduction, 5×10^4 cells were seeded onto a 12-well plate and incubated for 6 h with lentivirus in OPTI-MEM.

2.5. Animal Model

Six-week-old female BALB/cOlaHsd mice were purchased from Envigo (Gannat, France). Experiments respected institutional guidelines and were approved by the Institutional Animal Care and Research Advisory Committee (CEEA-122). To assess tumor growth, 0.1 million cells expressing luciferase were injected into the Balb/c female mammary fat pad. Tumor growth was monitored twice a week using a caliper.

2.6. Quantification of Lung Metastasis

Evaluation of the metastatic load was performed by quantification of luciferase mRNAs in lungs by RT-qPCR and normalized Cyclophilin-A. Primers' sequences were as follows:

- Luciferase forward primer: 5′TCTAAAACGGATTACCAGGGATTT;
- Luciferase reverse primer: 5′ACCGGGAGGTAGATGAGATGTG;
- Cyclophilin A forward primer: 5′GTCAACCCCACCGTGTTCTT;
- Cyclophilin A reverse primer: 5′CTGCTGTCTTTGGGACCTTGT.

2.7. Immunotherapy in Mice

A neutralizing anti-mouse PD-1 antibody was administered i.p. at 0.2 mg on days 4, 6, 9 and 11 after tumor graft. Anti-PD-1 antibody (clone RMP1-14) and isotype control antibodies (clone 2A3) were purchased from BioXcell (Supplied by Euromedex, Souffelweyersheim, France).

2.8. Flow Cytometry

On day 11, mice were sacrificed, and tumors were collected and digested with Mouse Tumor Dissociation kit and GentleMacs (Miltenyi, Paris, France). Cells were counted and incubated with anti-CD16/32 blocking antibodies prior to incubation. Cells were stained with LIVE/DEAD reactive dye (Invitrogen, Villebon sur Yvette, France), and cell surface staining was performed on tumor-infiltrating and draining lymph node cells using anti-CD45 (clone 30-F11), anti-Thy-1 (clone 30-H12), anti-CD4 (clone GK1.5), anti-CD8 (clone 53–6.7) or anti-PD-1 (clone J43) antibody. Intracellular staining of Foxp3 (anti-mouse Foxp3 clone FJK-16s) and Ki67 (anti-mouse Ki67 clone B56) was performed with fix perm solution (eBioscience, Villebon sur Yvette, France). Cells were analyzed with a BD LSR Fortessa X-20 (BD Biosciences, Le Pont-de-Claix, France), followed by Flow-jo software analysis.

2.9. Statistical Analysis

Statistical significance of difference between groups was evaluated using the GraphPad Prism software (Ritme, Paris, France). Results are expressed as mean $\pm$ SEM or range, as appropriate. The Mann–Whitney test was used to compare two groups. Comparison between tumor growth curves was performed using a two-way ANOVA test. Significance was assumed at $p < 0.05$.

3. Results

3.1. TSP1 Expression Is Associated with a Poor Prognosis in TNBC Patients and a Low CD8+ T Cell Infiltration in Tumors

We first evaluated the correlation between TSP1 expression and prognosis in tumor samples of patients affected with breast cancer. Analysis of transcriptomic data combined from 35 independent studies (www.kmplot.com (accessed on 1 April 2019) [19]) showed that the TSP1 mRNA level, encoded by the *THBS1* gene, was significantly associated with a reduced survival in breast cancers, including ER-/PR-/HER2-TNBC (Figure 1A). Of note, the hazard ratio (HR) was higher in TNBC (HR = 1.85) as compared to all breast cancers (HR = 1.19), indicating that high TSP1 levels may contribute to tumor aggressiveness in TNBC patients mainly. To obtain insight into the putative mechanisms associated with TSP1 expression and cancer progression, we evaluated gene expression pathways by Gene Set Enrichment Analysis (GSEA) of 122 tumor samples from the TCGA TNBC cohort. The "Epithelial Mesenchymal Transition" and "Hallmarks of the TGF-β signaling" pathways were significantly enriched in tumors expressing high TSP1 levels (Figure 1B and Supplementary Figure S1A,B), whereas low expression of TSP1 was associated with the "Lymphocyte activation" and "Hallmarks of the interferon gamma response" pathways (Figure 1C and Supplementary Figure S1C,D). Accordingly, expression of genes encoding IFNγ, CD8α and CD8β was significantly increased in tumor samples with a low TSP1 expression (Figure 1D). We next analyzed TSP1 expression and TILs in primary tumor samples from TNBC patients in a prospective cohort by immunohistochemistry. We found an inverse correlation between TSP1 expression and T cell tumor infiltration, including CD8+ TILs (Figure 2A,B).

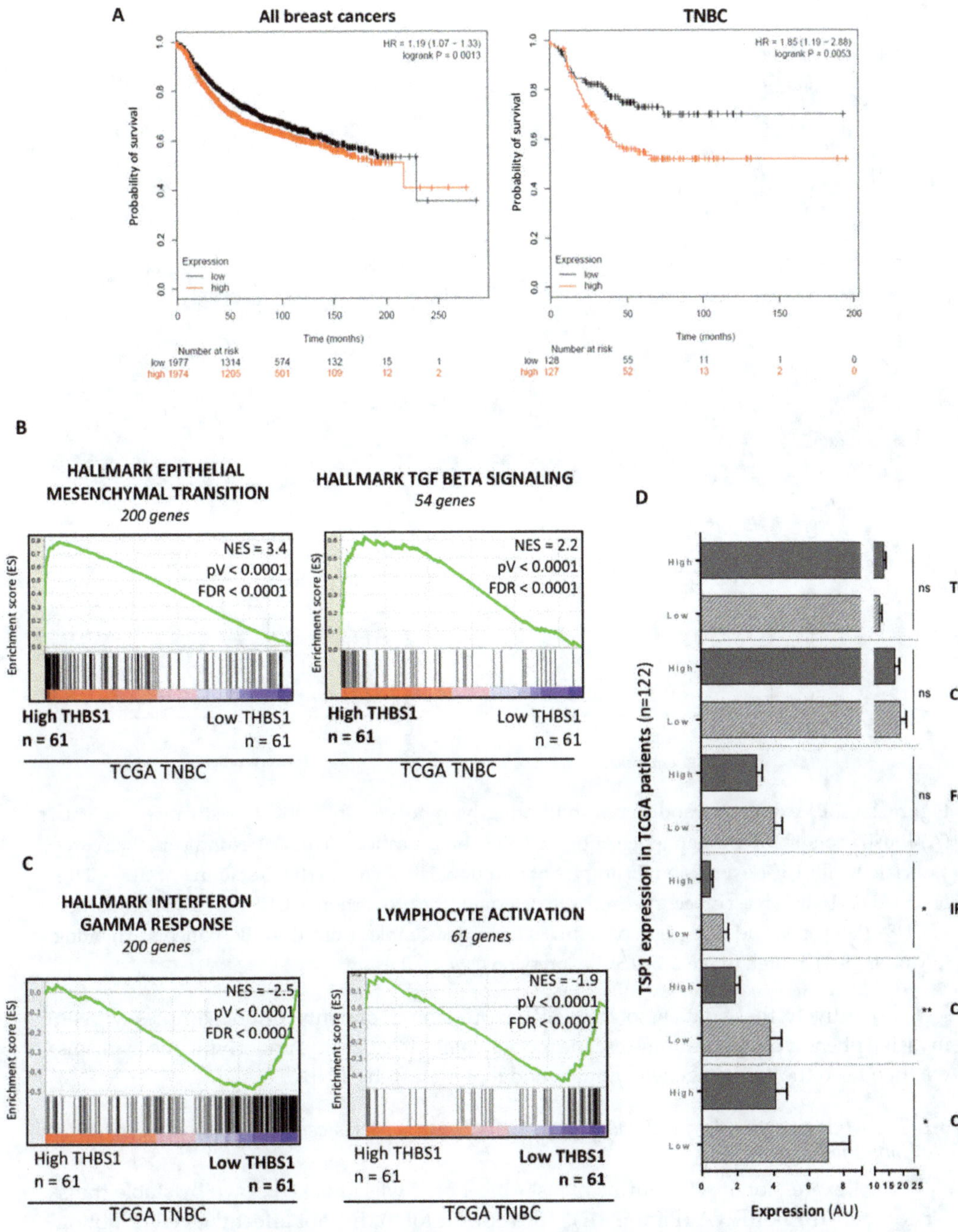

Figure 1. Impact of TSP1 expression on prognostic value in breast cancer. Schemes follow the same formatting. (**A**) Kaplan–Meier relapse-free survival analysis relating to TSP1 mRNA levels in 3951 breast cancer patients (left panel) and the same analysis in a cohort of 253 TNBC patients (right panel). Hazard ratios (HRs), 95% confidence intervals and log rank *p*-values are indicated in the graphs. (**B**,**C**) Gene Set Enrichment Analysis of gene signatures was performed from transcriptomes of the human TNBC TCGA database. Kolmogorov–Smirnov statistical test was performed. (**D**) mRNA expression in low and high TSP1 mRNA-expressing tumor samples from the human TNBC TCGA database. Mann–Whitney statistical test was performed. *, $p < 0.05$; **, $p < 0.01$; ns, not significant. Abbreviations: AU, Arbitrary Units; CD4, cluster of differentiation 4; CD8a, cluster of differentiation 8a; CD8b, cluster of differentiation 8b; FDR, false discovery rate; Foxp3, forkhead box protein P3; HR, Hazard Ratio; IFNγ, interferon γ; NES: normalized enrichment score; TGFβ, transforming growth factor β; TNBC, triple-negative breast cancer; TCGA, the cancer genome atlas; TSP1, Thrombospondin-1.

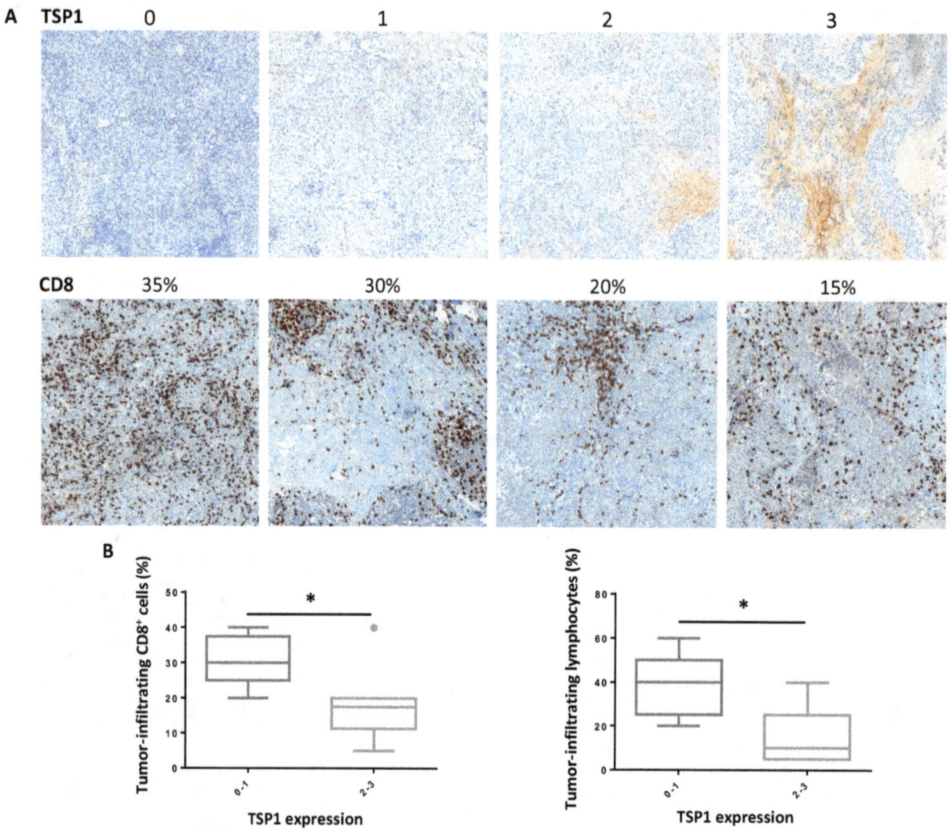

Figure 2. TSP1 expression and tumor-infiltrating lymphocytes in TNBC breast cancer patients. (**A**) Illustration of TSP1 immunodetection in TNBC breast cancer. The values indicate the scores associated with TSP1 expression. Examples of immunohistochemical (IHC) staining of CD8+ TILs obtained on TNBC breast cancer specimens to determine the proportion of CD8+ TILs. (**B**) Proportion of CD8+ (left panel) and total (right panel) TILs on tumor samples from 12 TNBC patients exhibiting low (score 0–1) or high (score 2–3) TSP1 expression (*: $p < 0.05$).

Collectively, these data associate TSP1 expression in patients' tumor samples with an invasive phenotype and immune escape mechanisms. To study the underlying mechanisms, we then used the 4T1 syngeneic mouse model of metastatic TNBC.

3.2. *TSP1 Inhibition in Murine Breast Cancer Cells Thwarts Metastasis in Immunocompetent but Not Immunodeficient Mice*

TSP1 expression in 4T1 murine breast cancer cells was knocked down by stable transfection of a TSP1-shRNA (Figure 3A). TSP1 knockdown did not affect the cell doubling time in vitro (Figure 3B). In vivo, the tumor take-rate and growth of the 4T1 control (4T1 shCTL) and TSP1 knocked-down (4T1 shTSP1) cells orthotopically implanted in the mammary fat pad were not significantly different in syngeneic immunocompetent Balb/c mice (Figure 3C). However, TSP1 knockdown in 4T1 cells reduced their lung metastatic diffusion in immunocompetent mice (Figure 3D). Under our experimental conditions, six out of nine wild-type mice (66%) grafted with 4T1 shCTL cells showed metastatic nodules on the lungs compared to two out of nine wild-type mice (22%) injected with 4T1 shTSP1 cells (Figure 3D). To quantify the total metastatic load, we measured the luciferase mRNA level by RT-qPCR (Figure 3E). The metastatic lung dissemination of 4T1shT cells was significantly reduced as compared to 4T1 shCTL cells (Figure 3E). To assess the involvement of the adaptive immune response in the modulation of tumor progression, we performed the same experiments in nude mice, which lack T cells. The primary tumor growth (Figure 3C) as well as lung metastases (Figure 3D,E) was enhanced in nude mice, as compared to immunocompetent mice. Strikingly, TSP1 knockdown did not compromise 4T1 lung metastasis in nude mice.

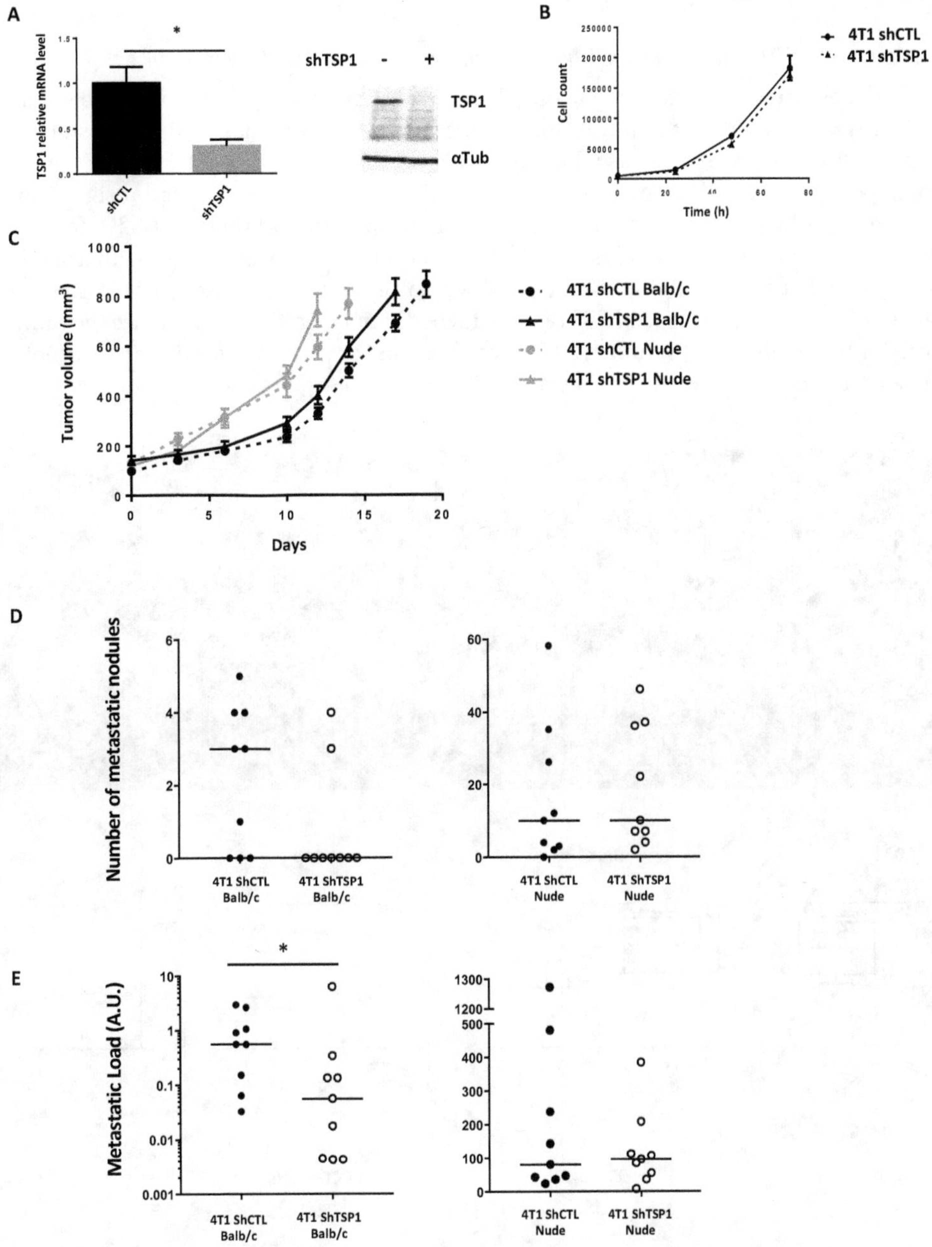

Figure 3. Impact of TSP1 expression in 4T1 mouse breast cancer model. (**A**) TSP1 mRNA (left panel) and protein (right panel) expression in 4T1 shCTL and 4T1 shTSP1 was evaluated by RT-qPCR and Western blot, respectively. Left panel, data are means ± SEM of $n = 3$ independent experiments. (**B**) In vitro cell proliferation of 4T1 shCTL and 4T1 shTSP1, data are means ± SEM of triplicate determination of one representative experiment of three independent experiments. (**C**) Growth of 4T1 shCTL and 4T1 shTSP1 orthotopic tumors over time in Balb-c mice (black) and nude mice (gray). (**D**,**E**) Lungs were collected from 9 mice of each group (left panels: wild-type mice; right panels: nude mice) when primary tumors reached 1000 mm^3. Visible lung metastatic nodules on the lung surface were counted (**D**). Alternatively, RNA was extracted from lungs, and metastatic load in lungs was quantified by measurement of luciferase mRNA level normalized to cyclophilin A (**E**). Bars indicate the medians (*: $p < 0.05$).

Collectively, these data demonstrate that, whereas TSP-1 is not mandatory for 4T1 primary tumor growth, it contributes to lung metastasis. Since TSP1 knockdown had no effect in nude mice, we hypothesized that TSP1 impairs T cell-dependent immune responses, facilitating 4T1 lung metastasis.

3.3. Impacts of TSP1 Knockdown on Tumor Vascularization and T Cell Infiltration

The most striking feature regarding TSP1 inhibition in 4T1 tumors was the significant increase in the density of intratumoral blood vessels, as evaluated by CD31 staining (Figure 4A,B). This increased vascularization, observed at day 11 on IHC cuts of tumors, appeared to be, at least partly, functional since the same samples showed a significant decrease in CAIX-positive hypoxic zones in 4T1 shTSP1 tumors (Figure 4A,B). In good agreement with our in silico analyses, TSP1 knockdown was also associated with a significant decrease in active TGF-β in tumors, and with a significant increase in CD8α staining (Figure 4A,B). As a matter of fact, TSP1 knockdown did not significantly enhance the tumor density of high endothelial venules (HEV), which are major gateways for lymphocyte entry in breast tumors (Supplementary Figure S2) [23].

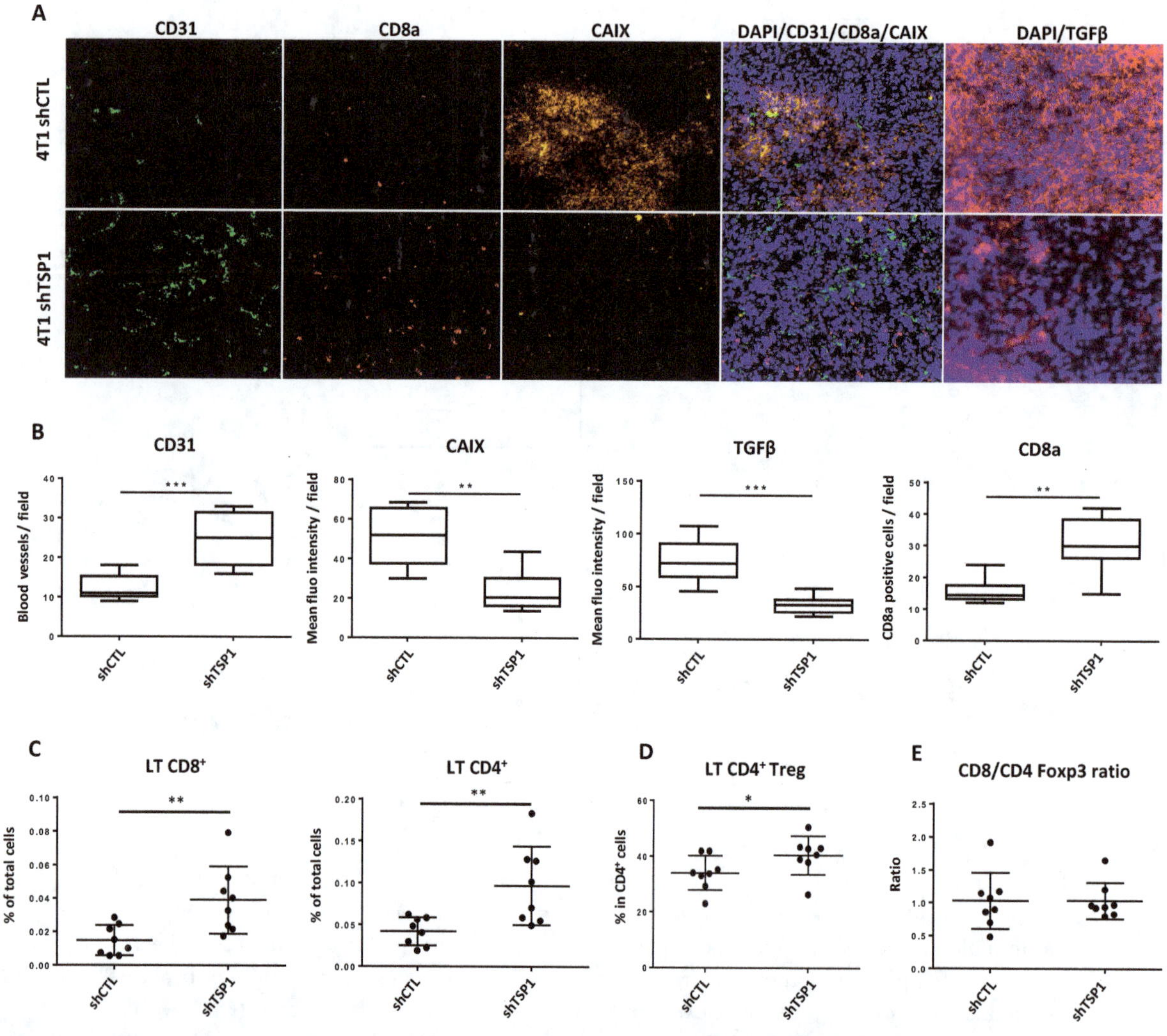

Figure 4. Impact of TSP1 expression on tumor microenvironment in 4T1 mouse breast cancer model. (**A**) Immunodetection of CD31, CD8α, CA-IX and active TGF-β in 4T1 shCTL and 4T1 shTSP1 tumors 11 days after cell injection in Balb/c mice. (**B**) Quantification in 4T1 shCTL and 4T1 shTSP1 tumors of blood vessels, CD8+ TILs, CA-IX and active TGF-β-positive area. Data obtained in 8 mice are represented as Tukey boxes. (**C–E**) Alternatively, tumors were collected at day 11 and dissociated, and the tumor cell content was analyzed by using flow cytometry (n = 8 mice per group). Bars are means ± SEM (*: $p < 0.05$; **: $p < 0.01$; ***: $p < 0.001$).

To further investigate the consequences of TSP1 knockdown on the immune response, we performed flow cytometry analyses of lymphocytes in the tumor bed (Figure 4C–E), and tumor-draining lymph nodes (Supplementary Figure S3B). These experiments confirmed the significant increase in the proportion of CD8+ T cells among the total cells in TSP1 knockdown tumors and showed similar trends for CD4+ T cells and regulatory T cells (Figure 4D). Of note, the CD8/CD4 and CD8/CD4 Foxp3 ratios remained unchanged (Figure 4E and Supplementary Figure S3A), likely reflecting a non-selective increase in lymphocyte tumor infiltration upon TSP1 knockdown. The augmentation of TILs in shTSP1 tumors was not associated with significant changes in the proliferation of T cells, as evaluated by KI67 staining (Supplementary Figure S3A). Whereas TSP1 knockdown in 4T1 cells did not alter the T cell content in tumor-draining lymph nodes, it significantly increased the CD8+ T cell/Treg ratio (Supplementary Figure S3B). The latter observation indicates that the effects of TSP1 knockdown in tumor cells on the immune response are unlikely restricted to the primary tumors, enhancing the immune response in tumor-draining lymph nodes.

Collectively, these data show that TSP1 knockdown increases functional tumor angiogenesis and lymphocyte tumor infiltration.

3.4. TSP1 Knockdown Enhances Anti-PD-1 Therapy Efficacy in Mice

Only a small proportion of patients affected with TNBC exhibit objective clinical responses upon targeting PD-1 or PD-L1 with blocking monoclonal antibodies [24,25]. Tumor vascular normalization has been shown to enhance the efficacy of anti-PD-1 therapy in mice [26]. We thus sought to evaluate a potential role of TSP1 in anti-PD-1 therapy. As immunotherapy-induced anti-tumor immune responses depend on the expression of PD-1 and its ligands (i.e., PD-L1/2) [27], we first analyzed the expression of the *PDCD1* (encoding PD-1), *PDCD1LG1* (encoding PD-L1) and *PDCD1LG2* (encoding PD-L2) genes in TNBC tumor samples expressing TSP1 at low or high levels from the TCGA database. High TSP1 expression was associated with a significant reduction in PD-1 levels. Whereas the expression of PD-L2 was similar in both groups, PD-L1 expression was slightly, yet not significantly, reduced in TNBC tumor samples exhibiting high levels of TSP-1 (Figure 5A).

We next analyzed the expression of PD-1 on CD8+ TILs from 4T1 shCTL and shTSP1 tumors in mice (Figure 5B). Whereas the proportion of PD-1+ cells among CD8+ TILs was similar in both groups (Figure 5C), the proportion of PD-1+ CD8+ TILs among total cells significantly increased upon TSP1 knockdown (Figure 5D), likely reflecting the increase in CD8+ T cell infiltration in 4T1 shTSP1 tumors (as shown in Figure 4). Moreover, PD-1 expression was significantly augmented on CD8+ TILs, as evaluated by the increase in the mean fluorescence intensity (Figure 5E). Thus, TSP1 knockdown was associated with a PD-1 expression increase at the cell surface of CD8+ TILs from 4T1 tumors in mice. Finally, we investigated the impact of TSP1 knockdown on anti-PD-1 therapy in immunocompetent mice (Figure 5F and Supplementary Figure S4). We found that the anti-PD-1 therapy efficacy towards 4T1 tumors was significantly enhanced by TSP1 knockdown under our experimental conditions (Figure 5F).

Collectively, the data indicate that silencing TSP1 is associated with an upregulation of PD-1 on CD8+ TILs and enhances the efficacy of anti-PD-1 therapy in TNBC.

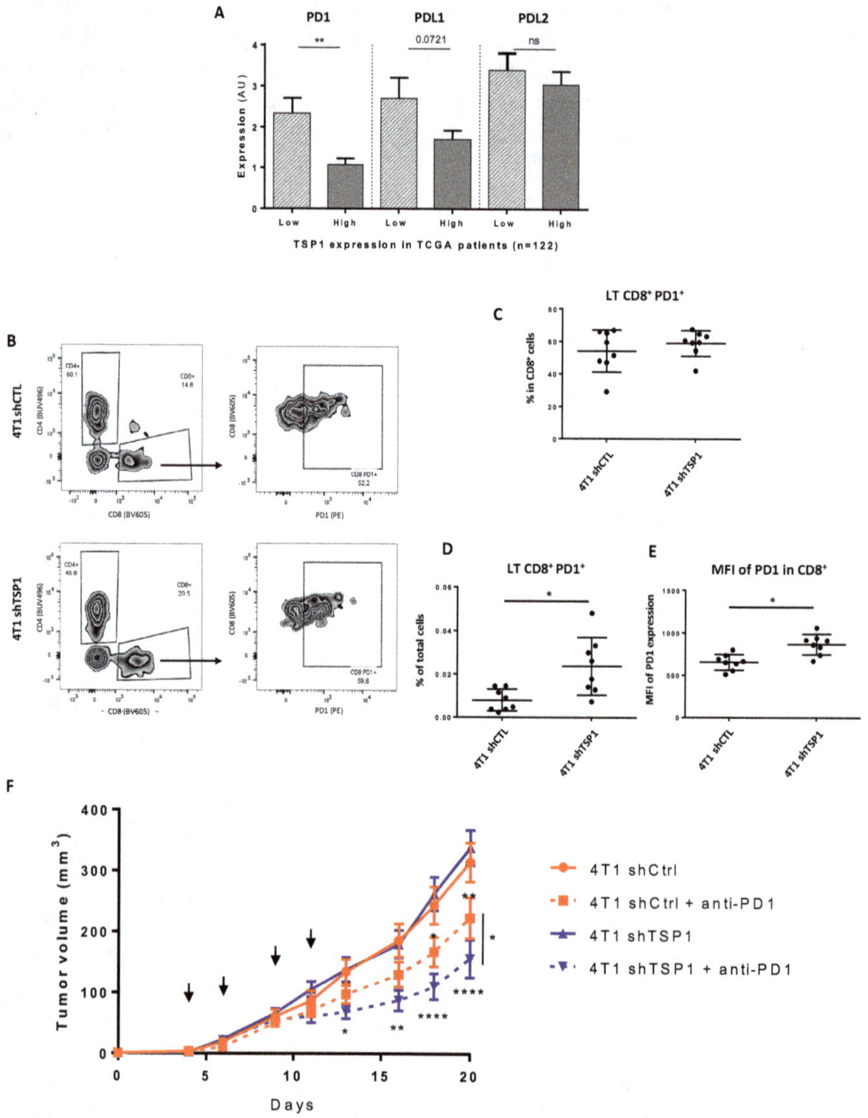

Figure 5. Impact of TSP1 expression on PD-1 expression and anti-PD-1 treatment in 4T1 mouse breast cancer model. (**A**) Analysis of PD-1, PD-L1 and PD-L2 expression in TCGA patients was performed depending on the median expression of TSP1 (**: $p < 0.01$). (**B–E**) At day 11, PD-1 expression on CD8+ TILs was quantified by flow cytometry on 4T1 shCTL and 4T1 shTSP1 tumors from Balb-c mice (*: $p < 0.05$) (**B**). Proportion of PD-1+ cells among CD8+ TILs (**C**) or total cells (**D**). Mean fluorescence intensity (MFI) of PD-1 expression on CD8+ TILs (**E**). (**F**): 1×10^5 4T1 shCTL or 4T1 shTSP1 breast carcinoma cells were orthotopically injected into the mammary fat pad of WT Balb/c mice. Mice received four injections of anti-PD-1 antibodies at days 4, 6, 9 and 11 (black arrows) at 10 mg/kg. Alternatively, mice were injected with isotype control. Tumor volumes were determined with a caliper at the indicated days. Data are means ± SEM obtained from 8 mice per group from one experiment. A two-way ANOVA with the Tukey multiple comparison test was used, and differences were statistically significant (*: $p < 0.05$; **: $p < 0.01$; ****: $p < 0.0001$).

4. Discussion

Tumor angiogenesis plays a critical role in cancer progression and resistance to therapies. Normalization of tumor vessels is an interesting strategy for cancer treatment [28,29]. We provide evidence that TSP1, produced by breast cancer cells, not only impairs functional tumor angiogenesis but also likely contributes to immune escape mechanisms, leading to metastasis and resistance to anti-PD-1 therapy in TNBC.

Our analyses of public human breast cancer databases strongly indicate that a high expression of the TSP1 mRNA is associated with a bad prognosis in TNBC. The TSP1 mRNA level was significantly associated with a reduced survival in breast cancers, as depicted in Figure 1A. One should note, however, that in all breast cancers, the HR is rather low (HR = 1.19 (1.07–1.33)) between patients exhibiting high and low levels of TSP1 mRNA. In sharp contrast, the HR (HR = 1.85 (1.19–2.88)) was greater in TNBC, indicating that a high TSP1 mRNA expression level in tumor samples can be considered as an independent bad prognosis biomarker in TNBC, but not in all breast cancers. In agreement with this observation, a sustained expression of TSP1 is also associated with the most aggressive stages of renal, prostate and pancreatic cancers [9,30]. The dosage of TSP1 in plasma shows that a high level is associated with a ganglionic infringement in breast cancer [31]. In 2015, the team of Campone also associated TSP1 with the metastatic relapse of TNBC and proposed its use as a marker of bad prognosis [10]. Thus, with regard to our own results, and those from the literature, the expression of TSP1 is correlated with tumor aggressiveness in numerous cancers, including TNBC.

Whereas our pilot study based on IHC analyses is limited due to the low number of cases (i.e., 12 patients with TNBC), the inverse correlation between anti-cancer immune response and TSP1 expression is further documented by our in silico analyses on 253 TNBC patients. In TNBC, we were also able to highlight that the strong expression of TSP1 was associated with a gene signature of epithelial–mesenchymal transition (EMT) and TGF-β signaling, a potent inductor of EMT. In addition, gene signatures of lymphocyte activation and IFN-γ response were both enriched in TNBC specimens expressing low TSP1 levels. On biopsies of patient tumors, we observed that CD8+ T cell infiltration was statistically increased in tumors expressing low TSP1 levels. The set of our data suggests that TSP1 not only contributes to the activation of TGF-β and the EMT process but also to immune escape. TGF-β signaling, as evaluated by a TGF-β-dependent gene signature, is enriched in tumor samples exhibiting high TSP1 mRNA levels (see Figure 1B). However, TGF-β mRNA levels are similar in tumor samples exhibiting high or low TSP1 expression levels (see Figure 1D). Those data further reinforce the notion that TSP1 acts at the protein rather than at the mRNA level, in order to activate the latent forms of TGF-β.

Considering the functional interaction between TSP1 and CD47, we cannot rule out the idea that it contributes to stimulating tumor progression, by impairing tumor vasculature normalization and/or the immune response. Indeed, TSP1 drives human and mouse endothelial cell senescence in a CD47-dependent manner [32]. CD47 is also expressed on various cancer cell types, including breast cancer cells, and behaves as a "don't eat me signal" [33]. Thus, its interaction with TSP1 could prevent tumor cell phagocytosis by antigen-presenting cells, thereby limiting the priming of the immune response towards tumor cells.

To clarify the role of TSP1 in vivo, we selected the 4T1 cell line, which is a TNBC mouse model with a strong metastatic potential. We did not observe any impact on the growth of the primary tumors by knocking down TSP1 in the tumor cells. However, TSP1 knockdown triggered a significant increase in the tumor blood vessel density. These vessels were also more functional since we noticed a significant decrease in hypoxia. It is thus interesting to note that the vascular normalization and better oxygenation of tumors do not inevitably lead to an increase in the primary tumor size in this 4T1 model. We quantified lung metastases, and we show that TSP1 inhibition by shRNA entails a significant reduction in the number of animals presenting this type of metastatic dissemination. Thus, we provide evidence that TSP1 expressed by 4T1 cells is pro-metastatic, as observed in other tumor types [9,12,34–37]. Noteworthy, we show that the anti-metastatic effect of TSP1 silencing in syngeneic mice is abolished in immunodeficient mice (i.e., nude mice), which strongly suggests that the TSP1 pro-metastatic effect in our preclinical TNBC model depends on its capacity to inhibit the adaptive immune response.

Our transcriptomic data analysis in human TNBC samples suggests that TSP1 plays an important role in the inhibition of lymphocyte-dependent immune responses, driving the tumor progression and aggressive phenotype of this type of cancer. On TNBC biopsies, we noticed a negative correlation between TSP1 protein expression and total TILs, as evaluated by morphological criteria [22], including CD8+ TILs. These TILs are associated with a good prognosis in breast cancers, including in TNBC, and a better response to chemotherapies compared with poorly infiltrated tumors [30,31,38].

To estimate the role of TSP1 on the immune response, we studied lymphocyte infiltration in primary tumors that developed in immunocompetent mice transplanted with 4T1 shCTL or 4T1 shTSP1 cells. We noticed a significant increase in the infiltration of CD8+, CD4+ and Foxp3+ T cells when TSP1 was knocked down. It should be noted that the CD8+/CD4+ T cells and CD8+ T cell/Treg ratios remained constant. We therefore highlight, for the first time, that the inhibition of TSP1 expression enhanced tumor infiltration by various T lymphocyte subpopulations, including not only CD8+ and CD4+ T cells but also Tregs. These results are in line with studies showing that high tumor infiltration with both CD8+ T cells and Tregs can be associated with a good prognosis in breast cancers [38–40]. Of note, considering that Foxp3 can be upregulated in conventional T cells upon activation in humans [41], unlike in mice, the infiltration of Tregs in human samples based on the sole analysis of Foxp3 expression may conduct to misinterpretation.

Furthermore, we noticed an increase in the expression of PD-1 on CD8+ T cells in 4T1shTSP1 tumors. This increase, observed at day 11, probably reflects a better activation state, rather than an exhausted phenomenon of lymphocytes. Indeed, the CD8+ TILs were KI67+, indicating their proliferative capacity. TSP1 inhibition allows rendering 4T1 tumors significantly more sensitive to anti-PD-1 treatment. This effect could be connected to the increase in tumor vascularization, allowing a better intratumoral diffusion of anti-PD-1. In addition, the increase in target cells in tumors (i.e., CD8+ PD-1+ TILs) constitutes a predictive element of the response to anti-PD-1 [42].

5. Conclusions

This proof-of-concept study indicates that targeting TSP1 may represent a good strategy in TNBC to facilitate the anti-tumor immune response. Moreover, TSP1 could be considered as a bad prognosis biomarker in patients affected with TNBC and as a therapeutic target in combination with anti-PD-1 blocking antibody.

Author Contributions: Conceptualization, H.P., F.C. and B.S.; funding acquisition, H.P., F.C. and B.S.; investigation, E.M., T.F., R.D.-P. and C.F.; methodology, E.M., T.F., M.P., G.L., J.T., S.D., M.C., C.I., J.N. and C.C.; project administration, H.P., F.C. and B.S.; resources, M.P., F.D. and C.C.; supervision, H.P., F.C. and B.S.; writing—original draft, E.M., F.C. and B.S.; writing—review and editing, E.M., J.T., C.F., F.D., C.C., H.P., F.C. and B.S. All authors have read and agreed to the published version of the manuscript.

References

1. Miles, D.W.; Dieras, V.; Cortes, J.; Duenne, A.A.; Yi, J.; O'Shaughnessy, J. First-line bevacizumab in combination with chemotherapy for HER2-negative metastatic breast cancer: Pooled and subgroup analyses of data from 2447 patients. *Ann. Oncol.* **2013**, *24*, 2773–2780. [CrossRef] [PubMed]
2. Kwapisz, D. Pembrolizumab and atezolizumab in triple-negative breast cancer. *Cancer Immunol. Immunother.* **2021**, *70*, 607–617. [CrossRef] [PubMed]
3. Robson, M.; Im, S.A.; Senkus, E.; Xu, B.; Domchek, S.M.; Masuda, N.; Delaloge, S.; Li, W.; Tung, N.; Armstrong, A.; et al. Olaparib for Metastatic Breast Cancer in Patients with a Germline BRCA Mutation. *N. Engl. J. Med.* **2017**, *377*, 523–533. [CrossRef]
4. Litton, J.K.; Rugo, H.S.; Ettl, J.; Hurvitz, S.A.; Goncalves, A.; Lee, K.H.; Fehrenbacher, L.; Yerushalmi, R.; Mina, L.A.; Martin, M.; et al. Talazoparib in Patients with Advanced Breast Cancer and a Germline BRCA Mutation. *N. Engl. J. Med.* **2018**, *379*, 753–763. [CrossRef]
5. Tutt, A.N.J.; Garber, J.E.; Kaufman, B.; Viale, G.; Fumagalli, D.; Rastogi, P.; Gelber, R.D.; de Azambuja, E.; Fielding, A.; Balmana, J.; et al. Adjuvant Olaparib for Patients with BRCA1- or BRCA2-Mutated Breast Cancer. *N. Engl. J. Med.* **2021**, *384*, 2394–2405. [CrossRef] [PubMed]
6. Clezardin, P.; Frappart, L.; Clerget, M.; Pechoux, C.; Delmas, P.D. Expression of thrombospondin (TSP1) and its receptors (CD36 and CD51) in normal, hyperplastic, and neoplastic human breast. *Cancer Res.* **1993**, *53*, 1421–1430.

7. Sid, B.; Sartelet, H.; Bellon, G.; El Btaouri, H.; Rath, G.; Delorme, N.; Haye, B.; Martiny, L. Thrombospondin 1: A multifunctional protein implicated in the regulation of tumor growth. *Crit. Rev. Oncol. Hematol.* **2004**, *49*, 245–258. [CrossRef]
8. Daubon, T.; Léon, C.; Clarke, K.; Andrique, L.; Salabert, L.; Darbo, E.; Pineau, R.; Guérit, S.; Maitre, M.; Dedieu, S.; et al. Deciphering the complex role of thrombospondin-1 in glioblastoma development. *Nat. Commun.* **2019**, *10*, 1146. [CrossRef] [PubMed]
9. Firlej, V.; Mathieu, J.R.; Gilbert, C.; Lemonnier, L.; Nakhle, J.; Gallou-Kabani, C.; Guarmit, B.; Morin, A.; Prevarskaya, N.; Delongchamps, N.B.; et al. Thrombospondin-1 triggers cell migration and development of advanced prostate tumors. *Cancer Res.* **2011**, *71*, 7649–7658. [CrossRef]
10. Campone, M.; Valo, I.; Jézéquel, P.; Moreau, M.; Boissard, A.; Campion, L.; Loussouarn, D.; Verriele, V.; Coqueret, O.; Guette, C. Prediction of Recurrence and Survival for Triple-Negative Breast Cancer (TNBC) by a Protein Signature in Tissue Samples. *Mol. Cell Proteom.* **2015**, *14*, 2936–2946. [CrossRef]
11. Fontana, A.; Filleur, S.; Guglielmi, J.; Frappart, L.; Bruno-Bossio, G.; Boissier, S.; Cabon, F.; Clézardin, P. Human breast tumors override the antiangiogenic effect of stromal thrombospondin-1 in vivo. *Int. J. Cancer* **2005**, *116*, 686–691. [CrossRef] [PubMed]
12. Yee, K.O.; Connolly, C.M.; Duquette, M.; Kazerounian, S.; Washington, R.; Lawler, J. The effect of thrombospondin-1 on breast cancer metastasis. *Breast Cancer Res. Treat.* **2009**, *114*, 85–96. [CrossRef] [PubMed]
13. Jiménez, B.; Volpert, O.V.; Crawford, S.E.; Febbraio, M.; Silverstein, R.L.; Bouck, N. Signals leading to apoptosis-dependent inhibition of neovascularization by thrombospondin-1. *Nat. Med.* **2000**, *6*, 41–48. [CrossRef]
14. Stenina-Adognravi, O. Invoking the power of thrombospondins: Regulation of thrombospondins expression. *Matrix Biol.* **2014**, *37*, 69–82. [CrossRef]
15. Seoane, J.; Gomis, R.R. TGF-β Family Signaling in Tumor Suppression and Cancer Progression. *Cold Spring Harb. Perspect. Biol.* **2017**, *9*. [CrossRef] [PubMed]
16. Drabsch, Y.; ten Dijke, P. TGF-β signalling and its role in cancer progression and metastasis. *Cancer Metastasis Rev.* **2012**, *31*, 553–568. [CrossRef] [PubMed]
17. Crawford, S.E.; Stellmach, V.; Murphy-Ullrich, J.E.; Ribeiro, S.M.; Lawler, J.; Hynes, R.O.; Boivin, G.P.; Bouck, N. Thrombospondin- 1 is a major activator of TGF-beta1 in vivo. *Cell* **1998**, *93*, 1159–1170. [CrossRef]
18. Miller, T.W.; Kaur, S.; Ivins-O'Keefe, K.; Roberts, D.D. Thrombospondin-1 is a CD47-dependent endogenous inhibitor of hydrogen sulfide signaling in T cell activation. *Matrix Biol.* **2013**, *32*, 316–324. [CrossRef]
19. Gyorffy, B.; Lanczky, A.; Eklund, A.C.; Denkert, C.; Budczies, J.; Li, Q.; Szallasi, Z. An online survival analysis tool to rapidly assess the effect of 22,277 genes on breast cancer prognosis using microarray data of 1809 patients. *Breast Cancer Res. Treat.* **2010**, *123*, 725–731. [CrossRef]
20. Koboldt, D.C.; Fulton, R.S.; McLellan, M.D.; Schmidt, H.; Kalicki-Veizer, J.; McMichael, J.F.; Fulton, L.L.; Dooling, D.J.; Ding, L.; Mardis, E.R.; et al. Comprehensive molecular portraits of human breast tumours. *Nature* **2012**, *490*, 61–70. [CrossRef]
21. Subramanian, A.; Tamayo, P.; Mootha, V.K.; Mukherjee, S.; Ebert, B.L.; Gillette, M.A.; Paulovich, A.; Pomeroy, S.L.; Golub, T.R.; Lander, E.S.; et al. Gene set enrichment analysis: A knowledge-based approach for interpreting genome-wide expression profiles. *Proc. Natl. Acad. Sci. USA* **2005**, *102*, 15545–15550. [CrossRef]
22. Salgado, R.; Denkert, C.; Demaria, S.; Sirtaine, N.; Klauschen, F.; Pruneri, G.; Wienert, S.; Van den Eynden, G.; Baehner, F.L.; Penault-Llorca, F.; et al. The evaluation of tumor-infiltrating lymphocytes (TILs) in breast cancer: Recommendations by an International TILs Working Group 2014. *Ann. Oncol.* **2015**, *26*, 259–271. [CrossRef]
23. Martinet, L.; Garrido, I.; Filleron, T.; Le Guellec, S.; Bellard, E.; Fournie, J.J.; Rochaix, P.; Girard, J.P. Human solid tumors contain high endothelial venules: Association with T- and B-lymphocyte infiltration and favorable prognosis in breast cancer. *Cancer Res.* **2011**, *71*, 5678–5687. [CrossRef] [PubMed]
24. Adams, S.; Schmid, P.; Rugo, H.S.; Winer, E.P.; Loirat, D.; Awada, A.; Cescon, D.W.; Iwata, H.; Campone, M.; Nanda, R.; et al. Pembrolizumab Monotherapy for Previously Treated Metastatic Triple-Negative Breast Cancer: Cohort A of the Phase 2 KEYNOTE-086 Study. *Ann. Oncol.* **2019**, *30*, 397–404. [CrossRef] [PubMed]
25. Adams, S.; Loi, S.; Toppmeyer, D.; Cescon, D.W.; De Laurentiis, M.; Nanda, R.; Winer, E.P.; Mukai, H.; Tamura, K.; Armstrong, A.; et al. Pembrolizumab Monotherapy for Previously Untreated, PD-L1-Positive, Metastatic Triple-Negative Breast Cancer: Cohort B of the Phase 2 KEYNOTE-086 Study. *Ann. Oncol.* **2019**, *30*, 405–411. [CrossRef] [PubMed]
26. Cartier, A.; Leigh, T.; Liu, C.H.; Hla, T. Endothelial sphingosine 1-phosphate receptors promote vascular normalization and antitumor therapy. *Proc. Natl. Acad. Sci. USA* **2020**, *117*, 3157–3166. [CrossRef]

27. Dong, Y.; Sun, Q.; Zhang, X. PD-1 and its ligands are important immune checkpoints in cancer. *Oncotarget* **2017**, *8*, 2171–2186. [CrossRef]
28. Folkman, J. Angiogenesis. *Annu. Rev. Med.* **2006**, *57*, 1–18. [CrossRef]
29. Folkman, J. Antiangiogenesis in cancer therapy—Endostatin and its mechanisms of action. *Exp. Cell Res.* **2006**, *312*, 594–607. [CrossRef]
30. Miyashita, M.; Sasano, H.; Tamaki, K.; Hirakawa, H.; Takahashi, Y.; Nakagawa, S.; Watanabe, G.; Tada, H.; Suzuki, A.; Ohuchi, N.; et al. Prognostic significance of tumor-infiltrating CD8+ and FOXP3+ lymphocytes in residual tumors and alterations in these parameters after neoadjuvant chemotherapy in triple-negative breast cancer: A retrospective multicenter study. *Breast Cancer Res.* **2015**, *17*, 124. [CrossRef] [PubMed]
31. Byrne, G.J.; Hayden, K.E.; McDowell, G.; Lang, H.; Kirwan, C.C.; Tetlow, L.; Kumar, S.; Bundred, N.J. Angiogenic characteristics of circulating and tumoural thrombospondin-1 in breast cancer. *Int. J. Oncol.* **2007**, *31*, 1127–1132. [CrossRef]
32. Meijles, D.N.; Sahoo, S.; Al Ghouleh, I.; Amaral, J.H.; Bienes-Martinez, R.; Knupp, H.E.; Attaran, S.; Sembrat, J.C.; Nouraie, S.M.; Rojas, M.M.; et al. The matricellular protein TSP1 promotes human and mouse endothelial cell senescence through CD47 and Nox1. *Sci. Signal.* **2017**, *10*. [CrossRef] [PubMed]
33. Willingham, S.B.; Volkmer, J.P.; Gentles, A.J.; Sahoo, D.; Dalerba, P.; Mitra, S.S.; Wang, J.; Contreras-Trujillo, H.; Martin, R.; Cohen, J.D.; et al. The CD47-signal regulatory protein alpha (SIRPa) interaction is a therapeutic target for human solid tumors. *Proc. Natl. Acad. Sci. USA* **2012**, *109*, 6662–6667. [CrossRef]
34. Hu, C.; Wen, J.; Gong, L.; Chen, X.; Wang, J.; Hu, F.; Zhou, Q.; Liang, J.; Wei, L.; Shen, Y.; et al. Thrombospondin-1 promotes cell migration, invasion and lung metastasis of osteosarcoma through FAK dependent pathway. *Oncotarget* **2017**, *8*, 75881–75892. [CrossRef] [PubMed]
35. Jayachandran, A.; Anaka, M.; Prithviraj, P.; Hudson, C.; McKeown, S.J.; Lo, P.H.; Vella, L.J.; Goding, C.R.; Cebon, J.; Behren, Thrombospondin 1 promotes an aggressive phenotype through epithelial-to-mesenchymal transition in human melanoma. *Oncotarget* **2014**, *5*, 5782–5797. [CrossRef] [PubMed]
36. McElroy, M.K.; Kaushal, S.; Tran Cao, H.S.; Moossa, A.R.; Talamini, M.A.; Hoffman, R.M.; Bouvet, M. Upregulation of thrombospondin-1 and angiogenesis in an aggressive human pancreatic cancer cell line selected for high metastasis. *Mol. Cancer* **2009**, *8*, 1779–1786. [CrossRef]
37. Nucera, C.; Porrello, A.; Antonello, Z.A.; Mekel, M.; Nehs, M.A.; Giordano, T.J.; Gerald, D.; Benjamin, L.E.; Priolo, C.; Puxeddu, E.; et al. B-Raf(V600E) and thrombospondin-1 promote thyroid cancer progression. *Proc. Natl. Acad. Sci. USA* **2010**, *107*, 10649–10654. [CrossRef]
38. Yeong, J.; Thike, A.A.; Lim, J.C.; Lee, B.; Li, H.; Wong, S.C.; Hue, S.S.; Tan, P.H.; Iqbal, J. Higher densities of Foxp3(+) regulatory T cells are associated with better prognosis in triple-negative breast cancer. *Breast Cancer Res. Treat.* **2017**, *163*, 21–35. [CrossRef]
39. Ladoire, S.; Arnould, L.; Mignot, G.; Coudert, B.; Rébé, C.; Chalmin, F.; Vincent, J.; Bruchard, M.; Chauffert, B.; Martin, F.; et al. Presence of Foxp3 expression in tumor cells predicts better survival in HER2-overexpressing breast cancer patients treated with neoadjuvant chemotherapy. *Breast Cancer Res. Treat.* **2011**, *125*, 65–72. [CrossRef] [PubMed]
40. Fridman, W.H.; Pagès, F.; Sautès-Fridman, C.; Galon, J. The immune contexture in human tumours: Impact on clinical outcome. *Nat. Rev. Cancer* **2012**, *12*, 298–306. [CrossRef] [PubMed]
41. Morgan, M.E.; van Bilsen, J.H.; Bakker, A.M.; Heemskerk, B.; Schilham, M.W.; Hartgers, F.C.; Elferink, B.G.; van der Zanden, L.; de Vries, R.R.; Huizinga, T.W.; et al. Expression of FOXP3 mRNA is not confined to CD4+CD25+ T regulatory cells in humans. *Hum. Immunol.* **2005**, *66*, 13–20. [CrossRef] [PubMed]
42. Tumeh, P.C.; Harview, C.L.; Yearley, J.H.; Shintaku, I.P.; Taylor, E.J.; Robert, L.; Chmielowski, B.; Spasic, M.; Henry, G.; Ciobanu, V.; et al. PD-1 blockade induces responses by inhibiting adaptive immune resistance. *Nature* **2014**, *515*, 568–571. [CrossRef] [PubMed]

8

High Drug Resistance in Feline Mammary Carcinoma Cell Line (FMCm) and Comparison with Human Breast Cancer Cell Line (MCF-7)

Ana Salomé Correia [1,2], Rita Matos [2,3,4], Fátima Gärtner [3,4], Irina Amorim [2,3,4] and Nuno Vale [1,5,*]

1 OncoPharma Research Group, Center for Health Technology and Services Research (CINTESIS), Rua Dr. Plácido da Costa, 4200-450 Porto, Portugal; anncorr07@gmail.com
2 Department of Molecular Pathology and Immunology, Institute of Biomedical Sciences Abel Salazar (ICBAS), University of Porto, Rua de Jorge Viterbo Ferreira 228, 4050-313 Porto, Portugal; ritam@ipatimup.pt (R.M.); iamorim@ipatimup.pt (I.A.)
3 Institute of Molecular Pathology and Immunology of the University of Porto (IPATIMUP), Rua Júlio Amaral de Carvalho 45, 4200-135 Porto, Portugal; fgartner@ipatimup.pt
4 i3S, Instituto de Investigação e Inovação em Saúde da Universidade do Porto, Rua Alfredo Allen 208, 4200-135 Porto, Portugal
5 Department of Community Medicine, Health Information and Decision (MEDCIDS), Faculty of Medicine, University of Porto, Al. Prof. Hernâni Monteiro, 4200-319 Porto, Portugal
* Correspondence: nunovale@med.up.pt;

Simple Summary: The repurposing and combination of drugs are important therapeutic strategies in cancer therapy, being important for combating drug resistance and improving therapeutical regimens. This paper outlines the use of candidate drugs that are to be repurposed, and combines clinically approved drugs in breast cancer, aiming to understand the response of feline mammary carcinoma cells to this therapeutic approach, previously applied in human breast cancer cells. By using cell viability assays, we revealed that feline mammary carcinoma cells were highly resistant to these tested approaches, contrasting with human breast cancer cells.

Abstract: Drug repurposing and drug combination are important therapeutic approaches in cancer therapy. Drug repurposing aims to give new indications to drugs, rather than the original indication, whereas drug combination presupposes that the effect that is obtained should be more beneficial than the effect obtained by the individual drugs. Previously, drug repurposing and the combination of different drugs was evaluated in our research group against human breast cancer cells (MCF-7 cells). Our results demonstrated that the response obtained through the combination of drugs, when compared with the single drugs, led to more synergic responses. Therefore, using potential drugs for repurposing, combined with a reference drug in breast cancer (5-Fluorouracil), was the major aim of this project, but for the first time using the feline mammary carcinoma cell line, FMCm. Surprisingly, the feline neoplastic cells demonstrated considerable resistance to the drugs tested in isolation, and the combination was not effective, which contrasted with the obtained MCF-7 cells' response.

Keywords: FMCm cells; MCF-7 cells; drug combination; drug resistance

---

1. Introduction

In female cats, mammary cancer is the third most common neoplasia. 85–90% of these pathologies present a malignant phenotype, having extremely high mortality rates and a mean survival time of about one year [1,2]. Besides local recurrence, metastatic disease is also commonly observed, mainly involving regional lymph nodes, lungs, pleura, and liver [3]. The most common therapeutic approach is surgery, which can be used alone or, depending on the status of the disease, in combination with chemotherapeutic agents. Combination chemotherapy using doxorubicin and cyclophosphamide, or carboplatin is the more common chemotherapeutic regimen [4]. Additionally, emerging studies suggest that histone deacetylases inhibitors and microtubules inhibitors are potential candidates for the treatment of feline mammary carcinoma, inducing cell death [5]. Previously, the FMCm cell line (Feline Mammary Carcinoma) was demonstrated to be highly tumorigenic and metastatic, leading to the observation of both primary and metastatic lesions, particularly in animals that have the expression of all the complex of cadherin-catenin [6]. Recently, our research group reported a new model of the drug combination, using classical and repurposed drugs. This combination model proved to be very effective, because the repurposed drug displayed a better profile than the drug currently used in therapy, and the effect of both generated even more satisfactory results when tested in the MCF-7 cell line [7]. Drug repurposing is an approach that aims to give new indications for already approved drugs. This methodology has the advantage of allowing lower inherent costs and shorter periods of time until the final approval of the drug, because details about side effects and other parameters such as pharmacokinetics and interactions between drugs are already investigated [8]. The investigation of drugs approved for indications that do not include cancer can most likely offer beneficial treatment options for oncologic patients [9]. Some examples are presented in Table 1. Regarding drug combination, studies point out that this approach has several benefits, such as a better overall efficacy, decreased toxicity levels and the possibility to circumvent drug resistance [10]. Thus, drug combination is increasingly used in clinical practice, highlighting oncological therapy [11]. In fact, when combined, two drugs can produce different therapeutic effects, being pharmacodynamically synergistic (when the effect of the combination is greater than the individual drugs), additive (the effect of the combination is equal to the single drugs), or antagonistic (the effect of the combination is lesser than the single drugs) [12]. Thus, if two drugs are synergic, it is possible to minimize adverse effects and improve overall efficacy. In the context of cancer, a lot of clinical trials are testing combinations that include several therapeutic modalities such as chemotherapeutic drugs, hormonal therapies, and molecularly targeted therapies [13]. However, despite a growing number of studies, the selection of treatment regimens for breast cancer remains a complex procedure. We therefore intended to study the degree of resistance of FMCm cells to most of the drugs previously used in our MCF-7 model (Table 1).

Table 1. Repurposed drugs used in this project, as well as their major clinical indication, pharmacodynamics, and mechanism of action [14]. Some examples of studies in breast cancer with these drugs are also presented.

Drug	Indication	Pharmacodynamics	Mechanism of Action	Examples of Evidence in Breast Cancer
Verapamil	Angina Cardiac arrhythmias Cardiomyopathies Hypertension	Blocks calcium channels.	Inhibits calcium channels of L-type by binding to a specific area of their alpha-1 subunit.	Verapamil is a P-Glycoprotein inhibitor and leads to enhanced sensitivity levels of breast cancer cells to other drugs, such as paclitaxel [15].
Aspirin	Pain Fever Inflammation Reduction of risk of myocardial infarction	Destabilizes the production of prostaglandins by targeting cyclooxygenase (COX)-1 and -2.	By binding COX enzymes, disrupts the conversion of arachidonic acid to thromboxane A2.	In MCF-7 cells, aspirin in combination with tamoxifen led to cell cycle arrest (in G0/G1 phase of cell cycle), decreasing the levels of cyclinD1 [16].
Losartan	Hypertension Reduction of the risk of stroke	Blocks Angiotensin II receptor.	Impedes angiotensin II binding to the receptor AT1 (Angiotensin Receptor Type I) in tissues like the adrenal gland.	By targeting AT1, this drug inhibits breast cancer cells proliferation and the progression of the cancer to an invasive phenotype [17].
Chloroquine	Infections of *P. vivax*, *P. malariae*, *P. ovale*, and *P. falciparum*. Off label for rheumatic diseases	Inhibits heme polymerase.	Inhibits heme polymerase, disrupting the conversion of heme to hemazoin, process that kills the parasite.	By blocking KCNH1 channels, this drug decreases migration of MDA-MB-231 breast cancer cells [18].
Cimetidine	Acid-reflux disorders Peptic ulcer disease Heartburn Acid indigestion	Antagonizes Histamine H2-receptor.	Binds to an H2-receptor in gastric cells, blocking histamine effects.	In breast cancer cells, Cimetidine can decrease cell adhesion, presenting antimetastatic effects [19].

Table 1. *Cont.*

Itraconazole	Fungal infections, such as aspergillosis and onychomycosis	Inhibits the fungal enzyme cytochrome P450 14α-demethylase.	Interacts with 14-α demethylase, necessary to convert lanosterol to ergosterol and maintain fungal viability.	Itraconazole inhibits the Hedgehog pathway, leading to elevated levels of cell death [20].
Isoniazid	Mycobacterial infections, such as *M. tuberculosis*	Inhibits the production of bacterial mycolic acids.	In, *M. tuberculosis*, inhibits InhA (enoyl reductase).	Few studies in breast cancer. However, being an inhibitor of monoamine oxidase A, it may improve outcomes in prostate cancer, where elevated levels of this enzyme correlate with aggressiveness [21].
Pravastatin	Hyperlipidemia, Prevention of some coronary events	Decreases the plasmatic concentration of low-density lipoprotein (LDL) cholesterol.	Inhibits HMG-CoA reductase, reducing cholesterol levels.	Statins promote cell cycle arrest and increased reactive oxygen species (ROS) production, enhancing oxidative stress [22].
Tacrine	Alzheimer's Disease	Enhances cholinergic function.	Inhibits cholinesterase enzymes, leading to prolonged action of acetylcholine.	The conjugation of this drug with model amphipathic peptide (MAP) (leads to high toxicity levels to MCF-7 cells [23].

The major aim of this project was to investigate, in FMCm cells, the response to potentially repurposed drugs combined with a clinically used drug (5-Fluorouracil) for mammary cancer therapy. The big goal is that the combination of both drugs presents beneficial effects when compared to the isolated effect of each drug. Additionally, we aimed to discern the effects triggered in these two breast cancer cell lines: feline and human. The experimental work that is described was carried out in FMCm cells (Figure 1). This cell line is characterized as a feline mammary adenocarcinoma cell line, originating from a regional lymph node metastatic lesion of a 12-years-old Japanese female cat diagnosed with a stage III primary mammary adenocarcinoma with great metastatic potential [24], being adherent, anchorage-dependent, and growing as a monolayer (Figure 1).

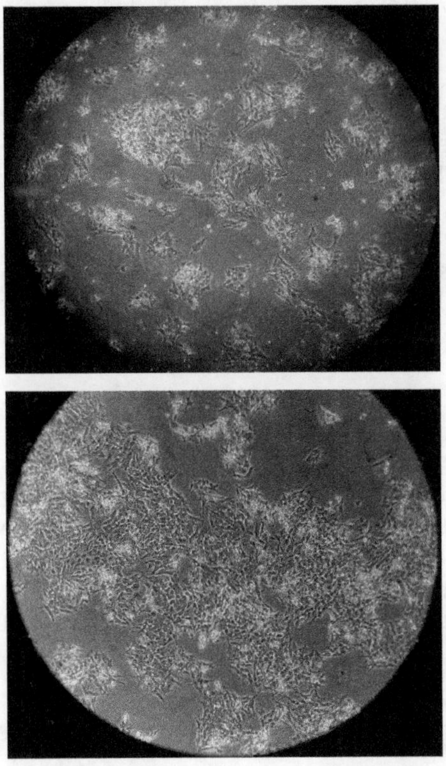

Figure 1. FMCm cells (**A**) with a confluency of 70%, 48 h, and (**B**) with a confluency of 80%, 72 h. All images were obtained through the optical microscope Lionheart^{TM} FX Automated (20×).

2. Materials and Methods

2.1. Materials

Dulbecco's Modified Eagle's Medium (DMEM), RPMI 1640 Medium, DMEM/F-12, Fetal Bovine Serum (FBS), and Penicillin-Streptomycin mixture were obtained from Milipore Sigma (Merck KGaA, Darmstadt, Germany). Human Insulin was purchased from NovoNordisk (Bagsværd, Denmark); Thiazolyl Blue Tetrazolium Bromide (MTT; cat. no. M5655), 5-Fluorouracil (5-FU; cat.no F6627), Verapamil hydrochloride (cat. no. V4629), 2-Acetoxybenzoic acid (Aspirin; cat. no. A2093), Losartan potassium (cat. no. 61188), Chloroquine diphosphate salt (cat. no. C6628), Cimetidine (cat. no. C4522), Itraconazole (cat. no. I6657), 9-Amino-1,2,3,4-tetrahydroacridine hydrochloride hydrate (Tacrine hydrochloride; cat. no. A79922) and Isonicotinic acid hydrazide (Isoniazid; cat. no. I3377) were purchased from Sigma-Aldrich (Merck KGaA, Darmstadt, Germany). Pravastatin (cat. no. 0010342) was purchased from Cayman Chemical Company (Ann Arbor, MI, USA).

2.2. Cell Culture and Treatments

Regarding the cell culture, FMCm (Passage 2; IPATIMUP, Porto, Portugal), MCF-7 (Passage 5; American Type Culture Collection, Manassas, VA, USA) and MCF-10A (Passage 7; American Type Culture Collection) were cultivated in RPMI 1640, DMEM and DMEM/F-12, respectively (10% FBS, 1% of a solution of penicillin/streptomycin (1000 U/mL; 10 mg/mL)). Additionally, DMEM/F-12 was supplemented with 2 μg/mL of human insulin, 20 ng/mL of epidermal growth factor and 1 μM hydrocortisone, as previously described [7]. All cells were incubated at 37 °C (with 5% CO_2). Experiments were executed with cells in a 70–80% confluence. Before each experiment, cells were trypsinized (0.25% trypsin-EDTA), centrifuged (1100 rpm, 5 min), and seeded at an optimal density of 3×10^4 cells/mL in 96-well plates, attaching for 24 h. For the treatment of MCF-7 and MCF-10A, all the drugs were applied in a concentration of 50 μM, as previously described [7]. For FMCm cells, all the compounds under study were dissolved in Dimethylsulfoxide (DMSO) and applied to the cells at final concentrations of 50 μM (dissolved in culture media). Controls were composed of DMSO 0.1% *v/v*.

2.3. Cell Viability Assays

The values of cellular viability after 72 h of treatment were determined by performing an MTT (3-(4,5-dimethylthiazol-2-yl) -2,5-diphenyltetrazolium bromide) tetrazolium reduction assay. To evaluate the viability of the cells after drug exposure, an MTT assay was performed. Cells were seeded in 96-well plates (37 °C for 24 h). Then, the treatments were added to the cells for a total time of 72 h. After that, the cell medium was removed and 100 μL of MTT solution (0.5 mg/mL in PBS) was added to each plate well. Then, the cells were incubated at 37 °C for 3 h, protected from light. Finally, 100 μL/well of DMSO was added after MTT solution removal. Absorbance readings (570 nm) were then carried out (Sinergy HT, BioTek Instruments, Winooski, VT, USA).

2.4. Statistical Analysis

The results are presented as the mean ± standard error of the mean (SEM). Differences between controls and cells subjected to treatment were analyzed by using a one-way ANOVA and by Dunnett's test. Differences between the combination of drugs and the more efficacious drug of the combination were analyzed by a Student's t-test. Statistical significance was considered when $p < 0.05$. All the tests were performed with SigmaPlot 12.0 (San Jose, CA, USA), except the Student's t-test, which was performed with GraphPad Prism 7 (San Diego, CA, USA).

3. Results and Discussion

5-FU was chosen as the reference anti-neoplastic drug for this project, highlighting a strong profile for this drug to be used in combination therapeutic regimens in breast cancer therapy, having the potential to increase its efficacy and safety profile. Briefly, this drug, as well as its metabolites, leads to damage in RNA and DNA [25]. Based on literature research about drugs with the potential to be repurposed, as well as the interests of the research group, six and nine drugs were tested in FMCm and MCF-7 cell lines in combination with 5-FU, respectively, to make a screening of drugs to be combined with 5-FU. Each drug was used in a concentration of 50 μM, acting for 72 h. The use of a breast cell line (MCF-10A, nontumoral) compared to a breast cancer cell line (MCF-7) led us to understand that the use of the concentration of 50 μM allowed us to distinguish responses between tumoral and nontumoral cells, even with the more effective drugs (Figure 2) [7]. Thus, this is an effective concentration for cancer cells, with very few effects in normal breast cells, justifying the use of this concentration for further work. The results were obtained by a MTT viability assay (Figures 3 and 4).

In MCF-7 cells, our results revealed that the drug with more efficacy regarding cell viability reduction was chloroquine (6.5 ± 0.4% of cellular viability), being more effective than single and combined drugs. The combinations of 5-FU with losartan, aspirin, cimetidine, pravastatin, tacrine, and isoniazid were not effective. However, two combinations of drugs were effective: 5-FU in combination with verapamil and itraconazole, a potential synergistic drug combination. The exposure of MCF-7 cells to 5-FU combined with these drugs led to a reduction in cellular viability (versus the more effective drug of the precise combination) of 23% for verapamil and 17% for itraconazole, respectively. Values of cell viability of approximately 12% and 25% were, indeed, obtained with the combinations of 5-FU/verapamil and 5-FU/itraconazole, respectively. Determined in our group, the obtained IC_{50} values for the more effective isolated drugs (5-FU, verapamil, itraconazole and chloroquine) are confirmed by the values presented in Table 2. The other drugs presented an IC_{50} value of more than 100 μM, highlighting the fact that they were not effective in these experimental conditions.

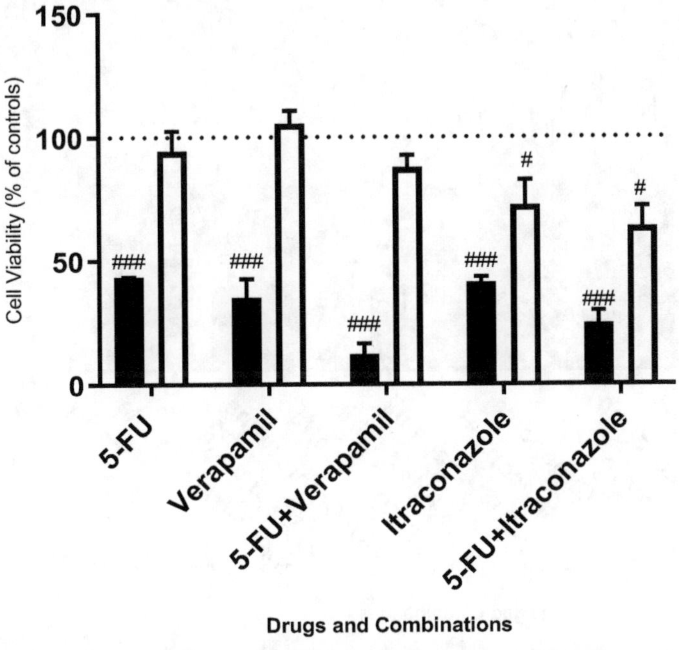

Figure 2. Cell viability values of 5-FU, verapamil, itraconazole and the combination of 5-FU with verapamil and itraconazole in MCF-7 cells (black bars) and MCF-10A cells (white bars), 72 h. All the compounds were added to cells in sextuplicates. The results (mean ± SEM) are presented as a percentage of the control (100%) of four independent experiments. ### $p < 0.001$ and # $p < 0.05$ vs. controls, Adapted from [7].

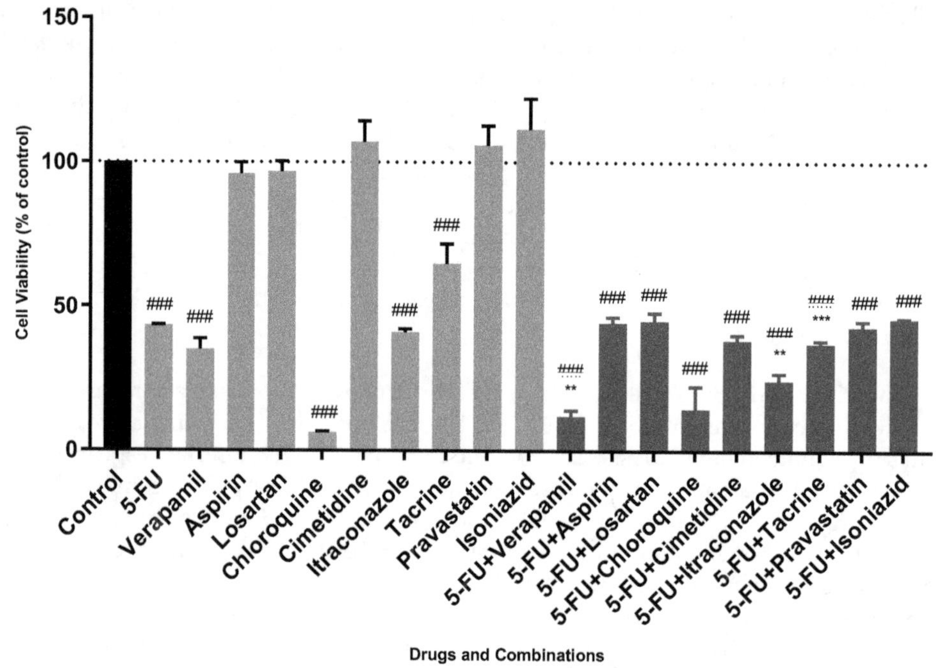

Figure 3. Cell viability values of single drugs and drug combinations in MCF-7 cells. All the compounds were added to cells in sextuplicates. The results (mean ± SEM) are presented as a percentage of the control (100%) of four independent experiments. ### $p < 0.001$ vs. control; ** $p < 0.01$ and *** $p < 0.001$ vs. the more effective drug of the combination. Reproduced from [7].

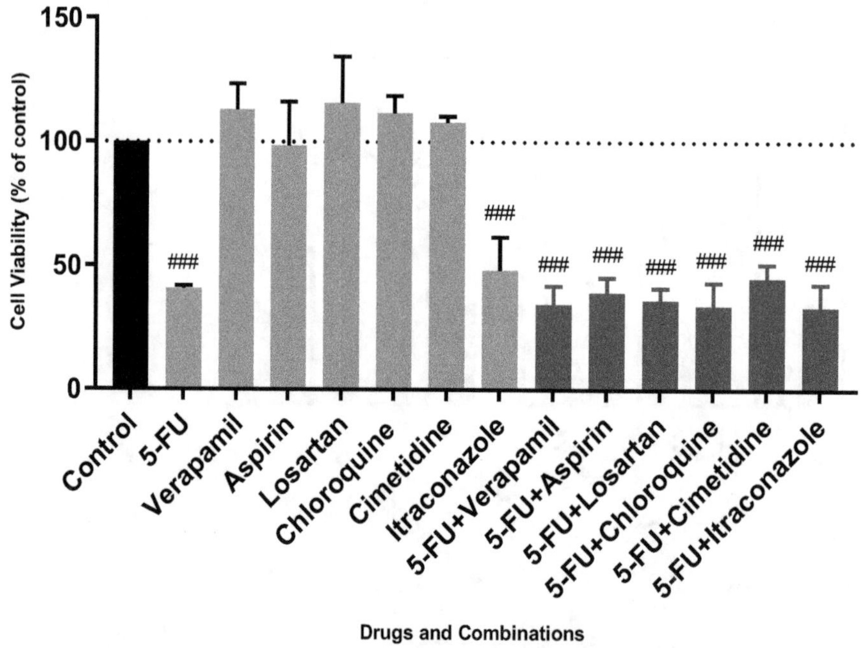

Figure 4. Cell viability values of single drugs and drug combinations in FMCm cells. All the compounds were added to cells in sextuplicates. The results (mean ± SEM) are presented as a percentage of the control (100%) of four independent experiments. ### $p < 0.001$ vs. control.

Table 2. IC_{50} values of 5-FU, verapamil, itraconazole and chloroquine in MCF-7 cells.

Drug	IC_{50} (μM)
5-FU	11.8 ± 1.8
Verapamil	29.5 ± 4.5
Itraconazole	2.1 ± 0.6
Chloroquine	16.0 ± 2.3

Regarding FMCm cells, it is possible to realize that none of the tested drug combinations efficiently reduced cell viability when compared with the single drugs. The lower cell viability value reached with drug combinations was obtained with 5-FU combined with chloroquine (33.9 ± 5.4%), which was not shown to be advantageous relative to the most effective drug of that combination (5-FU) with values of 40.6 ± 1.1%. Clearly, the drug combinations produce an effect almost equal to that of 5-FU alone, showing that the effects of the combination on cell viability are only due to the action of 5-FU and not from the combination of both drugs. In general, feline mammary carcinomas have high mortality rates, being associated with a poor prognosis. Studies in nude mice, with the FMCm cell line, demonstrated that these cells were very aggressive and had a high metastatic and tumorigenic potential [1,3,26]. An interesting finding is that, in these studies, metastasis expressed P- and E-cadherin [4] (Table 3), potentially linked with the resistance of the cells observed in our project. Indeed, the overexpression of P-cadherin in tumors that express E-cadherin is correlated with more aggressive behaviors and a worse tumor prognosis in comparison with carcinomas that express only one type of these molecules [6,27,28]. It is important to consider that the mechanism of action of the tested drugs is unknown in the oncology field. Thus, they can interact differently in FMCm cells from how they interact in MCF-7 cells, which has indeed been demonstrated in this project. For example, in the MCF-7 cells, the drug combinations 5-FU+Verapimil and 5-FU+Itraconazole appeared to show synergism, which was not observed in FMCm cells. In addition to what was mentioned above, verapamil and itraconazole may act in specific pathways when combined with 5-FU in human cells. Knowing that verapamil and itraconazole act, respectively, in inhibiting calcium channels and inhibiting the 14α-demethylase enzyme, it is expected that these factors are more related to human breast cancer and not to feline breast cancer. Another interesting example that can be observed in this study is the fact that chloroquine is effective in human breast cancer, in contrast to feline breast cancer. These data may reveal that the molecular pathways by which chloroquine acts in breast cancer are overexpressed in human cells and not in feline cells. For example, it is known that chloroquine, in cancer, seems to be related to signaling pathways such as the inhibition of the secretion of transforming growth factor β, inducing cellular apoptosis [29]. With this study, a strong possibility is that this cellular pathway is not as relevant in feline breast cancer. Thus, it is easy to understand that studies on other signaling pathways of feline breast cancer, which differs from humans, are needed. Nevertheless, 5-FU was effective in feline cells. Typically, this drug enters the cell and is intracellularly converted into fluorodeoxyuridine monophosphat, fluorodeoxyuridine triphosphate, and fluorouridine triphosphate. These metabolites inhibit thymidylate synthase and disrupt DNA and RNA synthesis [30,31]. In sum, in addition to all the aggressiveness underlying the FMCm cell line, molecular pathways different from those observed in human breast cancer need to be explored in more detail. Drug repurposing and combination, as observed in this study, are interesting techniques in this segment, providing new insights into possible molecular pathways present in this type of cancer, such as differences between breast cancer in humans and felines.

Table 3. Brief description of the P- and E-cadherin molecules.

Molecule	Description
P-cadherin	Cell-to-cell adhesion glycoprotein. Overexpression is connected to tumor-enhancing effects in breast cancer and other types of cancer, such as ovarian [32].
E-cadherin	Mediates cell adhesion and junction formations, being a part of the adherents junctions. In a general way, loss/decrease of its expression is linked with tumor progression and metastatic lesions [33].

4. Conclusions

In Feline Mammary Carcinoma cells, our results demonstrated that no combination of drugs had any advantage over the respective individual drugs, contrasting with the human breast cancer MCF-7 cells. This may most likely be due to the characteristics of this cell line, which is particularly aggressive and highly tumorigenic and metastatic. Indeed, the obtained results with chloroquine were very revealing of the resistance of FMCm cells, contrasting with the high loss of cellular viability observed with this drug in MCF-7 cells. In fact, this drug was very active in MCF-7, in agreement with the literature [34], but inactive in FMCm cells, and for the first time this evidence was reported in this project. In sum, the feline neoplastic cells showed considerable resistance to the drugs and drug combinations tested in this study when compared with MCF-7 cells, suggesting that molecular pathways involved in breast cancer differ highly between feline and human cancers, being important to explore this difference in more detail. As observed in this study, drug repurposing and drug combination are interesting approaches to provide new insights about differences in feline and human breast cancer, opening doors to more detailed studies focusing on molecular pathways and pharmacodynamics.

Author Contributions: Formal analysis, N.V.; Funding acquisition, F.G.; I.A. and N.V.; Investigation, A.S.C.; R.M.; F.G.; I.A. and N.V.; Methodology, A.S.C.; R.M.; F.G.; I.A. and N.V.; Project administration, N.V.; Supervision, N.V.; Writing–original draft, A.S.C.; Writing–review & editing, F.G.; I.A. and N.V. All authors have read and agreed to the published version of the manuscript.

References

1. Zeng, L.; Li, W.; Chen, C.S. Breast cancer animal models and applications. *Zool. Res.* **2020**, *41*, 477–494. [CrossRef] [PubMed]
2. Beltrán Hernández, I.; Kromhout, J.Z.; Teske, E.; Hennink, W.E.; Van Nimwegen, S.A.; Oliveira, S. Molecular targets for anticancer therapies in companion animals and humans: What can we learn from each other? *Theranostics* **2021**, *11*, 3882–3897. [CrossRef] [PubMed]
3. Zappulli, V.; De Zan, G.; Cardazzo, B.; Bargelloni, L.; Castagnaro, M. Feline mammary tumours in comparative oncology. *J. Dairy Res.* **2005**, *72*, 98–106. [CrossRef]
4. Feline Mammary Tumors|Veterinary Medical Center. Available online: https://vet.osu.edu/vmc/companion/our-services/ oncology-and-hematology/common-tumor-types/feline-mammary-tumors (accessed on 27 May 2021).
5. Almeida, F.; Gameiro, A.; Correia, J.; Ferreira, F. Histone Deacetylase Inhibitors and Microtubule Inhibitors Induce Apoptosis in Feline Luminal Mammary Carcinoma Cells. *Animals* **2021**, *11*, 502. [CrossRef] [PubMed]
6. Figueira, A.C.; Gomes, C.; Mendes, N.; Amorim, I.; De Matos, A.J.F.; Dias-Pereira, P.; Gärtner, F. An in vitro and in vivo characterization of the cadherin-catenin adhesion complex in a feline mammary carcinoma cell line. *Clin. Diagn. Pathol.* **2016**, *1*. [CrossRef]
7. Correia, A.; Silva, D.; Correia, A.; Vilanova, M.; Gärtner, F.; Vale, N. Study of new therapeutic strategies to combat breast cancer using drug combinations. *Biomolecules* **2018**, *8*, 175. [CrossRef] [PubMed]
8. Ishida, J.; Konishi, M.; Ebner, N.; Springer, J. Repurposing of approved cardiovascular drugs. *J. Transl. Med.* **2016**, *14*, 269. [CrossRef]
9. Bertolini, F.; Sukhatme, V.P.; Bouche, G. Drug repurposing in oncology—Patient and health systems opportunities. *Nat. Rev. Clin. Oncol.* **2015**, *12*, 732–742. [CrossRef]
10. Han, K.; Jeng, E.E.; Hess, G.T.; Morgens, D.W.; Li, A.; Bassik, M.C. Synergistic drug combinations for cancer identified in a CRISPR screen for pairwise genetic interactions. *Nat. Biotechnol.* **2017**, *35*, 463–474. [CrossRef]
11. Foucquier, J.; Guedj, M. Analysis of drug combinations: Current methodological landscape. *Pharmacol. Res. Perspect.* **2015**, *3*, 149. [CrossRef]

12. Jia, J.; Zhu, F.; Ma, X.; Cao, Z.W.; Li, Y.X.; Chen, Y.Z. Mechanisms of drug combinations: Interaction and network perspectives. *Nat. Rev. Drug Discov.* **2009**, *8*, 111–128. [CrossRef]
13. Comprehensive Cancer Information-National Cancer Institute. Available online: https://www.cancer.gov/ (accessed on 27 May 2021).
14. DrugBank Online|Database for Drug and Drug Target Info. Available online: https://go.drugbank.com/ (accessed on 23 July 2021).
15. Li, P.; Zhong, D.; Gong, P. Synergistic effect of paclitaxel and verapamil to overcome multi-drug resistance in breast cancer cells. *Biochem. Biophys. Res. Commun.* **2019**, *516*, 183–188. [CrossRef]
16. Cheng, R.; Liu, Y.-J.; Cui, J.-W.; Yang, M.; Liu, X.-L.; Li, P.; Wang, Z.; Zhu, L.-Z.; Lu, S.-Y.; Zou, L.; et al. Aspirin regulation of c-myc and cyclinD1 proteins to overcome tamoxifen resistance in estrogen receptor-positive breast cancer cells. *Oncotarget* **2017**, *8*, 30252. [CrossRef] [PubMed]
17. Coulson, R.; Liew, S.H.; Connelly, A.A.; Yee, N.S.; Deb, S.; Kumar, B.; Vargas, A.C.; O'Toole, S.A.; Parslow, A.C.; Poh, A.; et al. The angiotensin receptor blocker, Losartan, inhibits mammary tumor development and progression to invasive carcinoma. *Oncotarget* **2017**, *8*, 18640–18656. [CrossRef] [PubMed]
18. Valdés-Abadía, B.; Morán-Zendejas, R.; Rangel-Flores, J.M.; Rodríguez-Menchaca, A.A. Chloroquine inhibits tumor-related Kv10.1 channel and decreases migration of MDA-MB-231 breast cancer cells in vitro. *Eur. J. Pharmacol.* **2019**, *855*, 262–266. [CrossRef] [PubMed]
19. Neoplasma. 2003, Volume 50, pp. 148–151. Available online: http://www.elis.sk/index.php?page=shop.product_details&flypage= flypage.tpl&product_id=889&category_id=31&option=com_virtuemart&vmcchk=1&Itemid=1 (accessed on 23 July 2021).
20. Wang, X.; Wei, S.; Zhao, Y.; Shi, C.; Liu, P.; Zhang, C.; Lei, Y.; Zhang, B.; Bai, B.; Huang, Y.; et al. Anti-proliferation of breast cancer cells with itraconazole: Hedgehog pathway inhibition induces apoptosis and autophagic cell death. *Cancer Lett.* **2017**, *385*, 128–136. [CrossRef]
21. Lv, Q.; Wang, D.; Yang, Z.; Yang, J.; Zhang, R.; Yang, X.; Wang, M.; Wang, Y. Repurposing antitubercular agent isoniazid for treatment of prostate cancer. *Biomater. Sci.* **2018**, *7*, 296–306. [CrossRef]
22. Sánchez, C.A.; Rodriguez, E.; Varela, E.; Zapata, E.; Páez, A.; Massó, F.A.; Montaño, L.F.; Maure-Lóopez, R. Statin-induced inhibition of MCF-7 breast cancer cell proliferation is related to cell cycle arrest and apoptotic and necrotic cell death mediated by an enhanced oxidative stress. *Cancer Investig.* **2008**, *26*, 698–707. [CrossRef]
23. Silva, S.; Alves, C.; Duarte, D.; Costa, A.; Sarmento, B.; Almeida, A.J.; Gomes, P.; Vale, N. Model Amphipathic Peptide Coupled with Tacrine to Improve Its Antiproliferative Activity. *Int. J. Mol. Sci.* **2020**, *22*, 242. [CrossRef]
24. Uyama, R.; Hong, S.H.; Nakagawa, T.; Yazawa, M.; Kadosawa, T.; Mochizuki, M.; Tsujimoto, H.; Nishimura, R.; Sasaki, N. Establishment and characterization of eight feline mammary adenocarcinoma cell lines. *J. Vet. Med. Sci.* **2005**, *67*, 1273–1276. [CrossRef]
25. Longley, D.B.; Harkin, D.P.; Johnston, P.G. 5-Fluorouracil: Mechanisms of action and clinical strategies. *Nat. Rev. Cancer* **2003**, *3*, 330–338. [CrossRef]
26. Hassan, B.B.; Elshafae, S.M.; Supsavhad, W.; Simmons, J.K.; Dirksen, W.P.; Sokkar, S.M.; Rosol, T.J. Feline Mammary Cancer: Novel Nude Mouse Model and Molecular Characterization of Invasion and Metastasis Genes. *Vet. Pathol.* **2017**, *54*, 32–43. [CrossRef] [PubMed]
27. Ribeiro, A.S.; Albergaria, A.; Sousa, B.; Correia, A.L.; Bracke, M.; Seruca, R.; Schmitt, F.C.; Paredes, J. Extracellular cleavage and shedding of P-cadherin: A mechanism underlying the invasive behaviour of breast cancer cells. *Oncogene* **2010**, *29*, 392–402. [CrossRef] [PubMed]
28. Ribeiro, A.S.; Sousa, B.; Carreto, L.; Mendes, N.; Nobre, A.R.; Ricardo, S.; Albergaria, A.; Cameselle-Teijeiro, J.F.; Gerhard, R.; Söderberg, O.; et al. P-cadherin functional role is dependent on E-cadherin cellular context: A proof of concept using the breast cancer model. *J. Pathol.* **2013**, *229*, 705–718. [CrossRef] [PubMed]
29. Zhang, Y.; Cao, Y.; Sun, X.; Feng, Y.; Du, Y.; Liu, F.; Yu, C.; Jin, F. Chloroquine (CQ) exerts anti-breast cancer through modulating microenvironment and inducing apoptosis. *Int. Immunopharmacol.* **2017**, *42*, 100–107. [CrossRef] [PubMed]
30. Diasio, R.B.; Harris, B.E. Clinical Pharmacology of 5-Fluorouracil. *Clin. Pharmacokinet.* **1989**, *16*, 215–237. [CrossRef]
31. Wohlhueter, R.M.; McIvor, R.S.; Plagemann, P.G.W. Facilitated transport of uracil and 5-fluorouracil, and permeation of orotic acid into cultured mammalian cells. *J. Cell. Physiol.* **1980**, *104*, 309–319. [CrossRef]
32. Vieira, A.F.; Paredes, J. P-cadherin and the journey to cancer metastasis. *Mol. Cancer* **2015**, *14*, 1–12. [CrossRef] [PubMed]
33. Mendonsa, A.M.; Na, T.Y.; Gumbiner, B.M. E-cadherin in contact inhibition and cancer. *Oncogene* **2018**, *37*, 4769–4780. [CrossRef]

9

The Role of lncRNA in the Development of Tumors, including Breast Cancer

Beata Smolarz [1,*], Anna Zadrożna-Nowak [2] and Hanna Romanowicz [1]

[1] Laboratory of Cancer Genetics, Department of Pathology, Polish Mother's Memorial Hospital Research Institute, Rzgowska 281/289, 93-338 Lodz, Poland; hanna-romanowicz@wp.pl

[2] Department of Chemotherapy, Copernicus Memorial Hospital, Medical University of Lodz, 93-513 Lodz, Poland; anna.m.zadrozna@gmail.com

* Correspondence: beata.smolarz@iczmp.edu.pl

Abstract: Long noncoding RNAs (lncRNAs) are the largest groups of ribonucleic acids, but, despite the increasing amount of literature data, the least understood. Given the involvement of lncRNA in basic cellular processes, especially in the regulation of transcription, the role of these noncoding molecules seems to be of great importance for the proper functioning of the organism. Studies have shown a relationship between disturbed lncRNA expression and the pathogenesis of many diseases, including cancer. The present article presents a detailed review of the latest reports and data regarding the importance of lncRNA in the development of cancers, including breast carcinoma.

Keywords: tumors; breast cancer; lncRNA; expression

---

1. lncRNA—History

The history of lncRNA, or long noncoding RNA, dates back to the early 21st century. In 2001, two groundbreaking works were published—the first in Nature and the second in Science—which presented 96% [1] and 100% of the human genome, respectively [2]. The final sequence of the human genome was released in 2003. In what came as a surprise to the world of science, only a small percentage (1.2%) of human genetic material was found to encode proteins. The remaining ~99% are noncoding DNA, of which 24% are intron DNA and 75% are intergenic DNA [3].

In 2012, the ENCODE (Encyclopedia of DNA Elements) consortium showed that, despite only a small number of genes encoding proteins, human genetic material is 93% transcribed, of which 39% of transcripts correspond to introns and UTR sequences of protein-coding genes, 1% to exons, and 54% to noncoding genes [3]. These findings contributed to the development of interest in noncoding sequences and their transcripts, initially thought to be merely "junk DNA".

The first long noncoding RNAs, treated at the time of discovery as mRNA, were the *H19* and *Xist* genes. The *H19* gene was discovered while studying the phenomenon of genomic imprinting. Genomic imprinting (parental genomic stigma) is associated with methylation and, consequently, the exclusion of a single maternal or paternal allele of a given gene in ova or sperm cells, respectively. This phenomenon, occurring during gametogenesis, preserves the variability of organisms [4]. The *H19* gene was identified in the 1980s on chromosome 7 of a mouse [5], where it formed a cluster together with the insulin-like growth factor gene *Igf2* [5,6]. The *H19* gene was inherited from the mother, and the *Igf2* gene was inherited from the father [3,5,6]. In contrast to the *Igf2* gene, which encodes the protein, the *H19* gene was transcribed but not translated [3].

The nucleotide sequence of the *H19* gene was conserved in mammalian genetic material. However, the described gene had mRNA features—being transcribed by RNA polymerase II, spliced, and located in the cytoplasm—and was initially recognized as such a molecule [3,7]. It garnered renewed interest from scientists after the discovery of another gene that does not encode a protein—the *Xist* gene. It is now known that the product of the *H19* gene is a suppressor of tumors.

The *Xist* gene belongs to a gene complex in a region of the X chromosome called the XIC (X-inactivation center). This complex is involved in the process of disabling one of the X chromosomes in women (or other female mammals), thus equalizing gene expression in women and men [8]. This process was first described by geneticist Mary Lyon and is often referred to, in her honor, as Lyonization or Lyon's law [9]. The exclusion of one of the X chromosomes in a woman's cells occurs at random during embryogenesis [8].

The *Xist* gene is crucial for the proper conduct of this phenomenon. In the first stage, it is expressed on the X chromosome, intended for inactivation. The product of the *Xist* gene—long noncoding RNA—then flattens the "selected" X chromosome, inducing the connection of subsequent factors (e.g., PCR2 complex), which leads to a change in chromatin conformation and, as a result of repression of most genes, formation of an inactive Barr body [3,8]. This function of disabling the entire chromosome is unique in the world of lncRNA.

2. lncRNA—Characteristics

Long noncoding RNA are molecules with a length of more than 200 base pairs. These molecules are transcribed by RNA polymerase II, occasionally by RNA polymerase III, and also, in the plant kingdom, by RNA polymerases IV and V [3]. Many lncRNAs have a 5′ cap, which makes their RNA structure more stable, with the exception of lncRNA derived from larger molecules (such as intronic lncRNA and circRNA) [3]. Stabilization of the lncRNA structure is also influenced by polyadenylation at the 3′ end, but this only occurs in certain parts of the molecule. Some lncRNAs may occur in both forms, i.e., either with or without a polyadenylated 3′ end (known as bimorphic lncRNA) [3].

Long noncoding RNAs contain many exon regions, which allow for the creation of diverse forms of this RNA family as a result of splicing. These diverse forms may perform different functions, including those of clinical importance [3]. In addition, the genes of these noncoding ribonucleic acids have a structure similar to protein-coding genes (PCGs), but the level of lncRNA gene expression is much lower. Lower expression may be due to the difference in the structure of lncRNA gene promoters and enhancers (especially in the context of epigenetic histone changes), which reduces the severity of the transcription process and results in lower stability of the lncRNA molecule compared with the mRNA molecule [3].

The stability of lncRNA molecules depends on their type. The lncRNA intron and promoter-related lncRNA are less stable than the intergenic, antisense, or end-related 3′ UTR [3,10].

Single-exon transcripts (a type of nuclear lncRNA) are considered unstable. In human cells, antisense lncRNA has been shown to be more stable than mRNA (half-lives of 3.9 vs. 3.2 h, respectively), and intronic lncRNAs have the form of both stable transcripts (with half-lives above 3 h) and unstable transcripts ($t1/2 < 1$ h), with an average half-life of 2.1 h [3,10]. The recently discovered circular RNA (circRNA) is a highly stable molecule with a half-life of approximately 19–24 h [3,11]. However, half-life times are estimates, due to the fact that lncRNA is very susceptible to cellular stress, so these times may vary depending on the conditions of the experiment. In vivo testing is necessary [3].

The expression of specific lncRNAs is characteristic of individual tissues and even cells [3,12]. Only a small number of lncRNAs are common throughout the body (e.g., MALAT1); however, these are usually found in high concentrations [13]. Long noncoding RNAs typical of tissues or cells show significantly lower expression [13]. Studies have shown that diseases associated with single-nucleotide polymorphisms within lncRNA genes and their promoters are associated with a changed expression of these lncRNAs, which would confirm their importance in disease pathogenesis. In addition, the specificity of lncRNA expression can testify to their key role in regulating the functioning of organisms, as well as in repairing pathological processes [14].

Long noncoding RNAs, unlike mRNA, are found in the cell nuclei, cytoplasm, and mitochondria; simultaneously in the nuclei and cytoplasm; only in the nuclei; or only in the cytoplasm [15]. Thanks to this distribution, lncRNAs are able to perform a variety of functions affecting mRNA stability, translation, and cell signaling pathways. Nuclear lncRNAs also perform functions affecting chromatin, transcription, RNA treatment, and the cytoplasm. Changes in the environment or infections can force lncRNAs from one cellular component to another [15]. In addition, lncRNA is a dynamic, adaptable molecule that can take a secondary structure. Thanks to its flexible design and the versatility of lncRNA functions, specific cellular decomposition—particularly in the nucleus—as well as interaction with proteins are made possible [3]. The conformation of lncRNAs allows them to avoid the evolutionary limitation of poor interspecies conservation. On the other hand, low conservation of the lncRNA sequence likely enables the variability of the structure, and with it, the function and specialization lncRNAs as a regulator [3,16].

Long noncoding RNAs are the largest group of ribonucleic acids and remain the least understood. Figure 1 presents the classification of lncRNA. It seems important to divide the classes by genome location; however, to understand the functions of lncRNAs, it is easier to distinguish them into cis- and trans-interacting classes (according to Kopp, F. and Mendell, J.) [17].

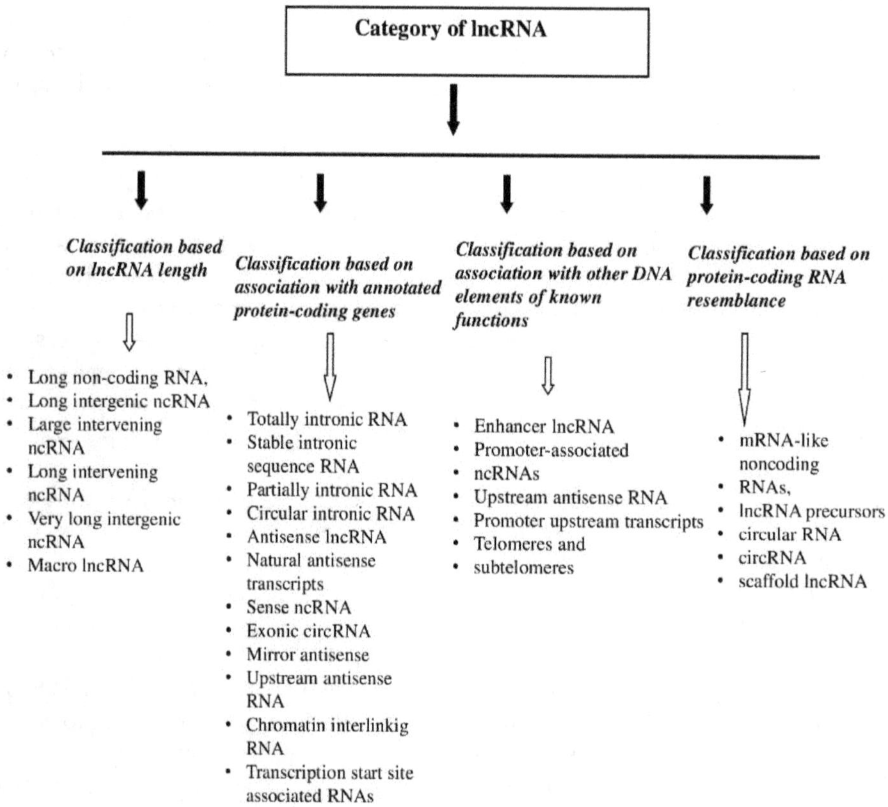

Figure 1. Classification of lncRNA.

3. lncRNA—Functions

The cis method indicates the effect of lncRNA on the expression of adjacent genes. The best example of cis action is the Xist transcript function described above [17]. The demonstration of gene expression, in this case the silencing of the entire chromosome, is evidently influenced by the transcript itself inducing the connection of protein complexes. However, cis regulation can occur independently of the lncRNA transcript.

In some cases, as in the case of Igfr2 paternal silencing, the overlap of the Airn sequence (antisense Igfr2 RNA noncoding) with the Igfr2 gene promoter has an impact on the adjacent gene, which impairs the connection of RNA Polymerase II and, as a result, the transcription process [17,18].

In a study by Latos et al., it was shown that a full Airn transcript is not needed to switch off the Igfr2 gene, but only an antisense sequence complementary to the Igfr2 gene promoter [18].

In contrast, Eingreitz et al. demonstrated that the cis regulation of the *Sfmbt2* gene was dependent not on the preserved sequence of Blustr lncRNA, but on the length of its transcription (the longer the transcription activity in the Blustr locus, the greater the expression of Sfmbt2), as well as the splicing of Blustr associated with the 5′ end [17,19]. The authors of the study assume that the altered transcription or splicing changes the chromatin conformation in the promoter region of the *Sfmbt2* gene and weakens the connection to the RNA polymerase promoter.

Sigova et al. described another mechanism of the influence of lncRNA on gene expression, this time through so-called trapping of transcription factors [20]. The authors noted that transcription factors can attach to both proximal promoter sequences and distal transcribed DNA elements, as well as the resulting RNA. In their study, the authors demonstrated that the transcription factor YY1 (YingYang1) attaches to DNA regulators and to RNA [20]. Reducing transcription resulted in YY1 being suppressed, and RNA connection increased YY1 activity in regulatory regions. Thus, it was suggested that RNA affects the function of transcription factors on a feedback basis and contributes moderately to the regulation of gene expression [17,20].

Another concept of cis regulation, as yet supported by little evidence [17,19], assumes that the DNA elements of the lncRNA gene are responsible for regulating the expression of adjacent genes. In the Eingreitz et al. study cited by Kopp and Mendell, decreased expression of adjacent genes for the lncRNA studied was demonstrated after several of its promoters had been removed. Reduced expression of adjacent genes was not achieved during lncRNA transcription at an earlier stage [17].

To summarize the above-described mechanisms of gene expression regulation in the cis manner, lncRNA affects the transcription process directly, acting as an enhancer, by "stopping" transcription factors, and by affecting chromatin looping and gene methylation (using epigenetic complexes such as PCR2) [21].

Trans regulation, in turn, is about controlling the expression of distant genes. Long noncoding RNAs can regulate these genes by affecting their promoters and enhancers, or via proteins associated with these regions, and, together with the attached proteins, by affecting chromatin conformation and polymerase activity [17].

Some lncRNAs are elements of complexes necessary for transcription or splicing. By facilitating the transport of these structures to the areas of the transcribed genes, they affect the structure of the cell nucleus [17]. In addition, lncRNAs bind proteins that combine with RNAs or RNA itself, e.g., microRNAs [17]. They regulate not only transcription, but also the post-transcription processes. Two of the first transfunctional lncRNAs discovered were the HOTAIR and MALAT1 transcripts, which, as further research has shown, play a significant role in the carcinogenesis process.

4. lncRNA and Malignant Tumors

The characteristics of long noncoded RNA described above—such as tissue or cellular specificity and the regulation of gene expression at the transcriptional and post-transcriptional levels—indicate that lncRNAs may be important in the formation of malignant tumors. Studies have shown that lncRNAs affect the pathways of division, growth, and cell differentiation, and are also involved in cellular death processes [21,22]. Modifications to these processes may lead to carcinogenesis [22]. Moreover, some lncRNAs are regulated by oncogene products or cancer transformation suppressors, which means that they are believed to indirectly perform tumorigenic functions (Table 1) [22].

Table 1. Long noncoding RNAs involved in cancer.

lncRNA	Genomic Location	Expression in Patients	Function in Tumorigenesis
PCGEM1	2q32.2	Increased in prostate cancer	oncogene
MALAT1	11q13.1	Increased in colon, lung, and liver cancers	oncogene
MEG3	14q32.2	Down-regulated in multiple cancers	tumor suppressor
HOTAIR	12q13.13	Increased in primary breast tumors and metastases, GIST, and pancreatic cancers	oncogene

Modern sequencing methods revealed different expressions of individual lncRNAs in cancerous tissues compared with healthy tissues [23]. The first observed transcripts of altered expression in the tissue of a malignant tumor—prostate cancer—were PCA3 and PCGEM1. PCA3 currently functions as a cancer marker [22]. The previously mentioned MALAT1 was also discovered in cancerous tissue as one of the first lncRNAs. Of prognostic significance, its altered expression was discovered in the tissues of lung cancer [24]. It is now known that altered expression of this transcript occurs in many cancers, which may indicate its importance in the process of cellular proliferation [25].

Altered lncRNA expression is not the only disorder of these molecules that occurs in cancerous tissues. Many lncRNA genes have been found in regions where somatic changes in the number of DNA copies (SNCA) occur in the form of deletion or amplification. These aberrations are extremely common in cancer cells [22]. Long noncoding RNAs also encounter single-nucleotide polymorphisms [22], and their transcription is regulated by factors that control the main cellular processes of homeostasis—including oncogenes and tumor suppressors—with the best examples being p53 and MYC factors.

DNA damage, a specific accumulation of which is observed in cancer cells, causes activation of the transcription factor p53. This factor, depending on the degree of DNA damage, induces apoptosis or halts the cell cycle for the duration of repair. One element of the proapoptotic pathway or the suspension of cell division is an increase in lncRNA transcription through the p53 factor.

The resulting transcripts are involved in the regulation of these pathways and thus modulate responses to cellular stress [22,26,27]. On the other hand, some lncRNAs affect p53 function by interacting with the gene enhancers of this protein [28]. Finally, the MEG3 transcript—a reduced expression of which has been found in many malignancies [22]—activates factor p53 itself [26,29].

The MYC transcription factor is an oncogene involved in the processes of cell proliferation, metabolism, and growth; angiogenesis; and metastasis. The transcriptionally active region of the MYC locus is one of the most commonly amplified in malignant neoplasms [22].

There are also many lncRNA genes in the region that, like the MYC oncogene, are translated more intensively [22]. Some of these lncRNAs regulate expression of the MYC gene in a cis manner [22]. On the other hand, expression of lncRNAs from the described region, involved in repression of the genes regulating the cell cycle according to MYC, is modified by the aforementioned proto-oncogene [22,30,31].

Studies have shown that the expression of oncogene and tumor transformation suppressors in malignant tumor tissues is increased and decreased, respectively [32].

This suggests that the interaction between lncRNAs and oncogenes or tumor suppressors is an important mechanism that contributes to the initiation of carcinogenesis. Another important mechanism seems to be the effect of lncRNAs on chromatin-modulating complexes through epigenetic changes, as an accumulation of epigenetic DNA modifications is very common in malignant tumors [33]. A well-understood epigenetic complex is PCR2 (polycomb repressive complex 2), which reduces gene expression by trimming histones (H3K27). Research indicates that many long noncoding RNAs affects PCR2 function [34].

An example of a lncRNA connecting to the PCR2 complex is the aforementioned trans-acting HOTAIR. Overexpression of this transcript occurs in many malignant tumors [35] including breast cancer [36], and is associated with poor prognosis. HOTAIR hyperactive complex with PCR2 causes increased gene suppression, contributing to the formation of metastases [37]. The mechanism described is an example of the agonist action of lncRNAs and chromatin modulating complexes. Some lncRNAs also exert antagonistic effects [22].

Long noncoding RNA can also affect cell homeostasis by post-transcriptional regulation; mRNA splicing, processing, and translation; or post-translational protein modification [22]. In addition, it has an impact on mRNA by binding microRNAs, reducing the amount of free short RNA and thereby reducing their impact on encoding transcripts [22].

The proper functioning of the cell is conditioned by the balance of metabolic processes. Studies show that lncRNAs are involved in the basic pathways of cellular metabolism, including in cancer cells, e.g., in the production of ATP under hypoxic conditions via HIF-1alpha factor or the Warburg effect [26].

A characteristic feature of malignant tumors is the ability to bypass immune control. Reports indicate that lncRNAs are involved in regulating the immune response by modifying the activity of immunocompetent cells [38]. For this reason, lncRNAs appear likely to be involved in the formation of immunomicelles of malignant tumors, even improving their defenses against the immune system [26,39].

It was mentioned above that overexpression of the HOTAIR transcript, which connects to the PCR2 complex, contributes to the formation of metastasis. Long noncoding RNAs also support the metastatic process by participating in epithelial–mesenchymal transition (EMT), as well as in signaling pathways associated with the activation of cancer stem cells [26]. Given the importance of lncRNAs in carcinogenesis, as well as the proven altered expression of these molecules in the tissue of malignant tumors, it seems natural to assess whether lncRNAs may represent new predictive factors. Over the past decade, much research has been conducted to analyze this problem, primarily in China.

In 2016, Serghiou et al. published a systematic review and meta-analysis of 111 studies assessing the effects of different lncRNAs on prognosis in malignancies: 83% of studies determined the effect of lncRNA on overall survival (OS) of patients, 32% on recurrence-free survival (RFS), 9% on disease-specific survival (DSS), 8% on metastasis-free survival (MFS), and 5% on progression-free survival (PFS) [40]. The study looked at 18 malignancies (almost half of which were gastrointestinal malignancies), primarily gastric cancer (16 studies), colorectal cancer (15 studies), and lung cancer (15 studies) [40].

In 96% of the studies analyzed, there was a statistically significant relationship between lncRNA expression and prognosis in malignancies. The vast majority of studies concerned HOTAIR and MALAT1 transcripts, the overexpression of which was associated with worse prognoses [40]. However, the authors of the publication point out that their work had many limitations.

5. lncRNA and Breast Cancer

Systematic reviews and meta-analyses were also conducted to assess the effect of altered lncRNA expression on prognosis in breast cancer alone.

Tian et al. analyzed 70 publications that examined the prognostic significance of the expression of 48 transcripts present in breast cancer tissues (in single blood tests) of 9307 patients [41].

The most commonly rated lncRNAs were MALAT1, HOTAIR, CCAT2, and MEG3.

In addition to the effect of lncRNAs on prognosis, the relationship between lncRNA expression and individual clinicopathological factors of breast cancer was assessed (Table 2).

This meta-analysis indicated that overexpression of CCAT2, MALAT1, and NEAT1 transcripts was associated with a shorter overall survival (OS) (hazard ratio, HR = 1.29, 95% CI: 1.03–1.63, $p = 0.03$; HR = 2.78, 95% CI: 1.95–3.97, $p < 0.01$; and HR = 1.65, 95% CI: 1.08–2.54, $p = 0.02$, respectively), and MEG3 transcript overexpression was associated with longer OS (HR = 0.47, 95% CI: 0.37–0.71, $p < 0.01$) [41].

Table 2. Summary of lncRNAs related to clinicopathological features and survival of breast carcinoma.

Clinicopathological Features	lncRNA
PR status	MALAT1
HER status	TUSC7
Histological grade	MEG3
TNM stage	NEAT1, TP73-AS1
survival	-
shorter overall survival	CCAT2, MALAT1, NEAT1
longer overall survival	MEG3
overall survival (better prognosis)	FGF14-AS2, AFAP1-AS1, EPB41L4A-AS2, BC040587, EGOT, GAS6-AS1, FENDRR
overall survival (worse prognosis)	BCAR4, HOTTIP, CCAT1, Z38, TUNAR, CRNDE, HULC, MVIH, TP73-AS1, linc-ITGB1, PVT1, UCA1, OR3A4, DANCR, LINP1, SNHG15, SUMO1P3
metastasis-free survival	CCAT2, HOTAIR, BCAR4
disease-free survival	MALAT1, HOTTIP, MVIH, LINC00978, linc-ITGB1, MEG3, GAS6-AS1, HOTAIR, LINP1
progression-free survival	MALAT1, MEG3, HOTAIR, RFS, CCAT1, MEG3, FENDRR

A correlation was also seen between CCAT2 and HOTAIR overexpression and shorter metastasis-free time (MFS) (respectively, HR = 1.18, 95% CI: 1.02–1.36, p = 0.03; and HR = 1.90, 95% CI: 1.41–2.55, $p < 0.01$) [41]. Of the remaining lncRNAs, altered expression of 24 transcripts had an impact on OS; overexpression of seven of them (FGF14-AS2, AFAP1-AS1, EPB41L4A-AS2, BC040587, EGOT, GAS6-AS1, and FENDRR) was associated with better OS, while overexpression of the remaining 17 (BCAR4, HOTTIP, CCAT1, Z38, TUNAR, CRNDE, HULC, MVIH, TP73-AS1, linc-ITGB1, PVT1, UCA1, OR3A4, DANCR, LINP1, SNHG15, and SUMO1P3) was associated with worse prognosis [42]. In addition, the expression of nine transcripts (MALAT1, HOTTIP, MVIH, LINC00978, linc-ITGB1, MEG3, GAS6-AS1, HOTAIR, and LINP1) had an impact on DFS, MALAT1, MEG3 and HOTAIR expression on RFS, CCAT1, MEG3 and FENDRR expression on PFS and BCAR4 expression on MFS [41].

Only ten transcripts (MALAT1, MEG3, CCAT2, BCAR, TUSC7, TP73-AS1, NEAT1, TUG1, HOTAIR, and CRNDE) were evaluated in the meta-analysis in the context of clinicopathological factors.

This analysis showed that MALAT1 overexpression was significantly correlated with the presence of a progesterone receptor, and TUSC7 overexpression with HER2 receptor [41]. MEG3 overexpression was associated with a lower histological grade (G) malignancy, overexpression of NEAT1 and TP73-AS1, and with a higher stage of breast cancer according to the TNM classification [41] (Table 2). Of the remaining 38 transcripts studied, only four transcripts did not in any way affect the presence of clinicopathological agents [41].

The latest literature data indicate that lncRNAs are transcribed from cancer risk loci and that these transcripts can play important roles in tumorigenesis [42,43]. Betts et al. used RNA sequences to identify two estrogen-regulated lncRNAs (CUPID1 and CUPID2) that might contribute to the risk of developing breast cancer by modulating pathway selection of double-strand break repair (DSB) [44]. Studies demonstrated that CUPID1 and CUPID2 are important to homologous recombinational repair (HRR). Repair by recombination enables removal of a number of serious DNA damages including, first of all, double-strand breaks. These breaks may cause a loss of some chromosomes and induce translocation of genetic material between them. Moreover, they are strong inducers of programmed cell death. As demonstrated in the work of Betts and colleagues, the loss of CUPID1 and CUPID2 expression results in reduced DNA end resection and defects in pRPA and RAD51 recruitment, leading to reduced HR DNA repair, favoring 53BP1 recruitment and selecting

NHEJ as a DNA repair pathway. The role of BRCA1 and 53BP1 and related partners in selection of a DNA repair pathway remains to be elucidated [45].

The credible causal variants (CCVs) at 11q13 fall within estrogen-regulated enhancers of two lncRNAs: CUPID1 and CUPID2. Fachal et al. defined CCVs within each signal (7394CCVs/196). CCVs are located in noncoding genomic regions [46] and reduce CUPID1/2 expression by inhibiting chromatin looping. CUPID1/2 play a role in modulating the choice of the pathway for repairing of double-stranded DNA breaks by promoting repair based on homologous recombination, providing a reliable mechanism by which CCVs alter the risk of breast cancer.

Marjaneh et al. demonstrated that CCV is enriched with exons but not in introns or mencRNA promoters, suggesting that genetic variants may alter the structure and/or function of mencRNAs [47].

Breast cancer is a heterogeneous disease with at least five molecular subtypes, including luminal A, luminal B, basal-like, HER2-enriched, and normal-like. These five molecular subtypes are usually stratified according to their mRNA profile patterns; however, lncRNA is increasingly used for this purpose.

NORAD and HCG11 are highly similar lncRNAs that contain binding sites for PUMILIO proteins. PUMILIO acts on hundreds of target mRNAs, helping to modulate gene expression. Mathias et al. analyzed NORAD and HCG11 expression levels in luminal A and basal-like breast cancer subtypes and the regulatory networks associated with these lncRNAs [48]. NORAD was upregulated in luminal A, while HCG11 was upregulated in the basal-like subtype. An increased NORAD expression is associated with reduced disease-free survival in basal-like patients, suggesting that its prognostic value may vary from subtype to subtype. The biological pathways observed for the HCG11 network are associated with epithelial–mesenchymal transition. NORAD-related pathways appear to be associated with the transformation of luminal epithelial cells.

Mathias and colleagues revealed that LINC01871 is associated with activation of the immune response and favorable overall survival in basal-like samples. EBLN3P is associated with immune response suppression and progression in the luminal B subtype, and MEG3, XXYLT1-AS2, and LINC02613 are associated with activation of immune response in luminal A, HER2-enriched, and normal-like subtypes, respectively. Further research is needed to better understand the role of lncRNAs as regulators of the immune response to provide new perspectives on diagnosis, prognosis, and therapeutic targets for the molecular subtypes of BRCA [49].

The latest scientific reports indicate that psoriasis-susceptibility-related RNA gene induced by stress (PRINS) is a novel lncRNA which is underexpressed in breast cancer in the Cancer Genome Atlas (TCGA). Chehade et al. showed that PRINS is underexpressed in primary breast cancer relative to normal breast tissues. Further research to investigate its molecular and intracellular effects is warranted to establish PRINS as a biomarker of functional importance in breast cancer [50].

Long noncoding RNAs are becoming understood as key players in the pathogenesis of cancer. Many lncRNAs have been shown to play a direct role in cancer cell proliferation, cancer progression, and/or metastasis. The specific tissue expression of lncRNA makes them exciting candidates for the development of diagnostic markers or presumed therapeutic targets for systemic treatment. The ability to target lncRNAs at different functional levels provides a wide range of therapeutic options. Targeted approaches may include nucleic acid-based drugs, small molecule inhibitors, and gene-editing methods. Targeted methods based on RNA are evolving rapidly to potentially cure various pathologies. Recent clinical success and FDA approval of antisense drugs for spinal muscular atrophy and Duchenne muscular dystrophy have led to various preclinical studies targeting lncRNAs using nucleic acid-based therapies. Further functional studies using appropriate preclinical models will confirm the importance of several lncRNA species in cancer pathogenesis, leading to a broad examination of this class of molecules as viable therapeutic targets in many types of cancer [51].

6. lncRNA—T-UCRs

Of those lncRNAs whose expression is altered in the tissues of malignant tumors, including breast cancer, some transcripts arise from so-called ultraconservative regions (UCRs). UCRs are genomic sequences that have survived evolution and are 100% compatible between the orthologous regions of humans, mice, and rats [3,52]. Of the 481 UCRs discovered, 111 coincide with sequences of genes encoding a human protein (exonic UCRs), 256 bear no resemblance to either the coding sequence or the resulting mRNA (nonexonic UCRs), and, for the remaining 114, insufficient evidence has been obtained to determine whether they are transcribed (possibly exonic UCRs) [52]. Of all known UCRs, 39% are intergenically located, 43% are found in intron sequences (including one hundred nonexonic UCRs), and 15% are in exon sequences [3]. Nonexonic UCRs, both intronic and intergenic, often form clusters near the genes of transcription factors and developmental proteins, but are also often found in so-called "gene deserts", i.e., long, noncoding sections of DNA [53].

The importance of UCRs is not fully understood, but Bejerano et al. indicated possible functions of transcriptional regulators, including alternative splicing, RNA and DNA binding, and regulation of distal gene enhancers associated with development [52]. Jarroux et al. give an example of a transcript T-UCR (Evf2) that behaves like a decoy for the DLX1 transcription factor, as well as for a chromatin-modulating complex similar to the SWI-/SNF BRG1 gene, eventually withholding transcription [3].

7. T-UCRs and Malignant Tumors

The importance of T-UCRs in the process of carcinogenesis also remains unknown, although they are associated with oncogenes and suppressors of tumor transformation; participate in the apoptosis, proliferation, and migration of cancer cells; and also seem to regulate microRNA functions [43,54].

Moreover, studies have shown that transcription of certain T-UCRs is induced by hypoxia [55]. Despite the lack of relevant literature, there is evidence of a changed expression of T-UCRs in malignant tumor tissues.

One of the first studies confirming the presence of a changed number, compared with healthy tissues, of numerous T-UCRs in cancerous tissues—including cancer cells of chronic lymphocytic leukemia and tissues of colorectal and hepatocellular carcinoma—was that of Calin et al., published in 2007 [53,55]. In 2010, a changed expression of T-UCRs was also discovered in neuroblastoma tissues [56].

In 2012, a reduced amount of UC.73 and UC.388 was shown in the tissues of colorectal cancer, indicating the likely prognostic significance of these transcripts [57]. Subsequent years brought further evidence of deregulation of transcription of ultraconservative regions in prostate cancer [58], pancreatic cancer [59], cervical cancer [60], bladder cancer [61,62], gastric cancer [63,64], and lung cancer [65]. In the case of breast cancer, only two studies have been developed to analyze the expression and prognostic significance of T-UCRs—specifically, uc.63 and uc.38. The authors of the other three publications focus on determining the importance of single-nucleotide polymorphisms in ultraconservative regions and lncRNA genes.

8. T-UCRs and Breast Cancer

Marini et al. (2017) published a paper in which they determined uc.63 lncRNA expression in cultured breast cancer cell lines, compared with that of healthy breast tissue. Uc.63 is an ultraconserved region located in the third intron of the exportin 1 (*XPO1*) gene—a protein that exports certain molecules from the nucleus to the cytoplasm [66].

Transcription of uc.63 is induced by hypoxia [55]. The authors of the study observed a significant variety of uc.63 expression profiles in breast cancer cell lines. After rejecting the lines with low and very high expression of the study transcript, a cell line with high transcript concentration, from advanced breast cancer, was selected. In order to determine the probable biological function of the uc.63 transcript, silencing of the studied region was performed in the selected cell line.

The exclusion of uc.63 led to an increase in cancer cell death, which was diagnosed after observation of an increased number of cells in the G0/G1 phase, a reduction of cells in the G2/M phase, and detection of an increased concentration of the markers of apoptosis, PARP-1 and caspase-3 [66]. The above observations may indicate the importance of uc.63 in regulating the cycle of breast cancer cells [66]. The authors also point out that deregulation of *XPO1* gene transcription did not affect either uc.63 expression or cancer cell function [66].

To determine the prognostic significance of the altered expression of uc.63 in this malignant tumor, the authors performed bioinformatic analysis of the data of more than 2000 breast cancer samples from the Cancer Genome Atlas portal.

This analysis concluded that overexpression of uc.63 is associated with a reduction in disease-free time (DFS) in the luminal subtype A of breast cancer, but only in its more aggressive form [66].

Again, this correlation was independent of xpo1 gene expression [66].

In conclusion, the authors of the study suggest that uc.63 may act as an oncogene, and its overexpression may contribute to the survival and growth of breast cancer cells [66]. In addition, the authors point to the potential function of uc.63 as a predictor in luminal A breast cancer [66].

In a study by Zhang et al., uc.38 expression was evaluated in 100 breast cancer tissue samples and breast cancer cell lines, compared with normal tissues and cells of normal breast epithelium, respectively. This study showed that uc.38 expression was significantly reduced in cancer tissues [67]. As a result of the analysis of the relationship between the expression level of uc.38 and clinical and pathological factors, a correlation was observed between the reduced concentration of the uc.38 transcript and the higher stage of the cancer in question, according to TNM classification and the larger diameter of the primary tumor [67].

The above study also revealed a reduced expression of uc.38 in breast cancer cell lines compared with normal breast epithelial cells, which, the authors believe, may indicate an important role of uc.38 in the formation of the primary tumor and its progression [67].

An in vitro analysis was then carried out, which looked at the effect of increased or decreased expression of uc.38 on the breast cancer cell cycle.

This analysis noted that overexpression of uc.38 was associated with a significant reduction in cell proliferation, a decrease in the ability of cells to form colonies, and an increase in the number of cells subjected to apoptosis [67]. In contrast, reduced expression uc.38 had the opposite effect—increased proliferation, greater colony formation, and fewer apoptotic cells [67].

The evaluation of uc.38 expression and its consequences, as described above, are part one of a two-part study by Zhang et al.

In part two, the authors focused on the alleged regulation of the *PBX1* (pre-B-cell leukemia homeobox 1) gene by the lncRNA uc.38. PBX1 is a transcription factor whose overexpression is associated with poor prognosis in luminal breast cancers and promotion of metastasis [68]. This study showed that overexpression of uc.38 was accompanied by a lower concentration of PBX1 protein, and a reduced expression of uc.38 with an increased concentration of PBX1 protein [67].

The above data suggest that uc.38 controls PBX1 expression at the post-transcriptional translation level [67]. Further analyses indicated that the uc.38 transcript was present mainly in the cell nucleus, which, according to the authors, may demonstrate the role of uc.38 in regulating gene expression at the nuclear level [67].

As a result of RNA immunoprecipitation with PBX1 antibodies, an interaction between this transcription factor and lncRNA was demonstrated. Subsequent experiments demonstrated the dynamics of change in PBX1 protein concentration depending on the level of uc.38 expression: The silencing of lncRNA transcription resulted in an increase in PBX1 concentration [67]. Based on the above observations, the authors concluded that the transcript uc.38 not only had an effect on the PBX1 transcription factor, but also accelerated its degradation when uc.38 was present at an elevated concentration [67]. This relationship is an important part of the cell cycle; further studies demonstrated that PBX1 overexpression fosters the proliferation of breast cancer cells and halts the apoptotic process. The silencing effect of lncRNA uc.38 overexpression on the PBX1 transcription factor in turn contributed to cellular death induction [67]. The authors of this publication also analyzed the effects of uc.38 overexpression on breast cancer in vivo. After 4 weeks of follow-up, primary tumors were found in mice with uc.38 overexpression to have significantly lower volume and weight compared with primary tumors in control mice. In addition, the mice in the study group had significantly longer overall survival (OS) [67].

9. Conclusive Summary

Recent studies confirm assumptions about the great importance of both ultraconservative regions and other types of lncRNAs in pathogenesis and the course of malignant tumors, including breast cancer. The diagnostic, predictive, and even therapeutic potential of these unique molecules seems undeniable. While previously considered to be noncoding, they are in fact a matrix for the synthesis of short peptides [69]. These peptides are encoded in the sequence of short open reading frames (sORF) of lncRNA genes [70]. Recent reports indicate that these peptides play a significant role in the carcinogenesis process, providing new hope for breakthroughs in the search for effective anticancer treatment [71].

Author Contributions: Conceptualization, B.S., A.Z.-N. and H.R.; writing—original draft preparation, B.S.; writing—review and editing, B.S.; revision and proofreading, B.S. All authors have read and agreed to the published version of the manuscript.

References

1. Lander, E.S.; Linton, L.M.; Birren, B.; Nusbaum, C.; Zody, M.C.; Baldwin, J.; Devon, K.; Dewar, K.; Doyle, M.; FitzHugh, W.; et al. Inter-national human genome sequencing consortium. Initial sequencing and analysis of the human ge-nome. *Nature* **2001**, *409*, 860–921.
2. Venter, J.C.; Adams, M.D.; Myers, E.W.; Li, P.W.; Mural, R.J.; Sutton, G.G.; Smith, H.O.; Yandell, M.; Evans, C.A.; Holt, R.A.; et al. The sequence of the human genome. *Science* **2001**, *291*, 1304–1351. [CrossRef] [PubMed]
3. Jarroux, J.; Morillon, A.; Pinskaya, M. Discovery, and Classification of lncRNAs. *Adv. Exp. Med. Biol.* **2017**, *1008*, 1–46.
4. Marciniak, M. Imprinting genomowy u ssaków: Najnowsze doniesienia. *Postępy Biol. Komórki* **2008**, *35*, 243–257.
5. Bartolomei, M.S.; Zemel, S.; Tilghman, S.M. Parental imprinting of the mouse H19 gene. *Nature* **1991**, *351*, 153–155. [CrossRef] [PubMed]
6. Barlow, D.P.; Stöger, R.; Herrmann, B.G.; Saito, K.; Schweifer, N. The mouse insulin-like growth factor type-2 receptor is imprinted and closely linked to the Tme locus. *Nature* **1991**, *349*, 84–87. [CrossRef]
7. Brannan, C.I.; Dees, E.C.; Ingram, R.S.; Tilghman, S.M. The product of the H19 gene may function as an RNA. *Mol. Cell. Biol.* **1990**, *10*, 28–36. [CrossRef]
8. XIST Gene—GeneCards|XIST RNA Gene. Weizmann Institute of Science. Available online: https://www.genecards.org/cgi- bin/carddisp.pl?gene=XIST&keywords=xist (accessed on 4 August 2021).
9. Lyon, M.F. Gene action in the X-chromosome of the mouse (*Mus musculus* L.). *Nature* **1961**, *190*, 372–373. [CrossRef]
10. Ayupe, A.C.; Tahira, A.C.; Camargo, L.; Beckedorff, F.C.; Verjovski-Almeida, S.; Reis, E.M. Global analysis of biogenesis, stability and sub-cellular localization of lncRNAs mapping to intragenic re-gions of the human genome. *RNA Biol.* **2015**, *12*, 877–892. [CrossRef]
11. Enuka, Y.; Lauriola, M.; Feldman, M.E.; Sas-Chen, A.; Ulitsky, I.; Yarden, Y. Circular RNAs are long-lived and display only minimal early alterations in response to a growth factor. *Nucleic Acids Res.* **2016**, *44*, 1370–1383. [CrossRef]
12. Ward, M.; McEwan, C.; Mills, J.D.; Janitz, M. Conservation and tissue-specific transcription patterns of long noncoding RNAs. *J. Hum. Transcr.* **2015**, *1*, 2–9. [CrossRef]
13. Jiang, C.; Li, Y.; Zhao, Z.; Lu, J.; Chen, H.; Ding, N.; Wang, G.; Xu, J.; Li, X. Identifying and functionally characterizing tissue-specific and ubiquitously expressed human lncRNAs. *Oncotarget* **2016**, *7*, 7120–7133. [CrossRef]

14. Kumar, V.; Westra, H.J.; Karjalainen, J.; Zhernakova, D.V.; Esko, T.; Hrdlickova, B.; Almeida, R.; Zhernakova, A.; Reinmaa, E.; Võsa, U.; et al. Human disease-associated genetic variation impacts large intergen-ic non-coding RNA expression. *PLoS Genet.* **2013**, *9*, 1. [CrossRef] [PubMed]
15. Giannakakis, A.; Zhang, J.; Jenjaroenpun, P.; Nama, S.; Zainolabidin, N.; Aau, M.Y.; Yarmishyn, A.A.; Vaz, C.; Ivshina, A.V.; Grinchuk, O.V.; et al. Contrasting expression patterns of coding and noncoding parts of the human genome upon oxidative stress. *Sci. Rep.* **2015**, *5*, 9737. [CrossRef] [PubMed]
16. Johnsson, P.; Lipovich, L.; Grandér, D.; Morris, K.V. Evolutionary conservation of long non-coding RNAs; sequence, structure, function. *Biochim. Biophys. Acta* **2014**, *1840*, 1063–1071. [CrossRef] [PubMed]
17. Kopp, F.; Mendell, J.T. Functional classification and experimental dissection of long noncoding RNAs. *Cell* **2018**, *172*, 393–407. [CrossRef] [PubMed]
18. Latos, P.A.; Pauler, F.M.; Koerner, M.V.; Şenergin, H.B.; Hudson, Q.J.; Stocsits, R.R.; Allhoff, W.; Stricker, S.H.; Klement, R.M.; Warczok, K.E.; et al. Airn tran-scriptional overlap, but not its lncRNA products, induces imprinted Igf2r silencing. *Science* **2012**, *338*, 1469–1472. [CrossRef]
19. Engreitz, J.M.; Haines, J.E.; Perez, E.M.; Munson, G.; Chen, J.; Kane, M.; McDonel, P.E.; Guttman, M.; Lander, E.S. Local regulation of gene expression by lncRNA promoters, transcription and splicing. *Nature* **2016**, *539*, 452–455. [CrossRef]
20. Sigova, A.A.; Abraham, B.J.; Ji, X.; Molinie, B.; Hannett, N.M.; Guo, Y.E.; Jangi, M.; Giallourakis, C.C.; Sharp, P.A.; Young, R.A.; et al. Transcription factor trapping by RNA in gene regulatory elements. *Science* **2015**, *350*, 978–981. [CrossRef]
21. Schmitt, A.M.; Chang, H.Y. Long noncoding RNAs in cancer pathways. *Cancer Cell* **2016**, *29*, 452–463. [CrossRef]
22. Huarte, M. The emerging role of lncRNAs in cancer. *Nat. Med.* **2015**, *21*, 1253–1261. [CrossRef]
23. Iyer, M.K.; Niknafs, Y.S.; Malik, R.; Singhal, U.; Sahu, A.; Hosono, Y.; Barrette, T.R.; Prensner, J.R.; Evans, J.R.; Zhao, S.; et al. The landscape of long noncoding RNAs in the human transcriptome. *Nat. Genet.* **2015**, *47*, 199–208. [CrossRef]
24. Ji, P.; Diederichs, S.; Wang, W.; Böing, S.; Metzger, R.; Schneider, P.M.; Tidow, N.; Brandt, B.; Buerger, H.; Bulk, E.; et al. MALAT-1, a novel noncoding RNA, and thymosin beta4 predict metastasis and survival in early-stage non-small cell lung cancer. *Oncogene* **2003**, *22*, 8031–8041. [CrossRef] [PubMed]
25. Gutschner, T.; Hämmerle, M.; Diederichs, S. MALAT1—A paradigm for long noncoding RNA function in cancer. *J. Mol. Med.* **2013**, *91*, 791–801. [CrossRef] [PubMed]
26. Jiang, M.C.; Ni, J.J.; Cui, W.Y.; Wang, B.Y.; Zhuo, W. Emerging roles of lncRNA in cancer and therapeutic opportunities. *Am. J. Cancer Res.* **2019**, *9*, 1354–1366.
27. Hung, T.; Wang, Y.; Lin, M.F.; Koegel, A.K.; Kotake, Y.; Grant, G.D.; Horlings, H.M.; Shah, N.; Umbricht, C.; Wang, P.; et al. Extensive and coordinated transcription of noncoding RNAs within cell-cycle promoters. *Nat. Genet.* **2011**, *43*, 621–629. [CrossRef]
28. Léveillé, N.; Melo, C.A.; Rooijers, K.; Díaz-Lagares, A.; Melo, S.A.; Korkmaz, G.; Lopes, R.; Moqadam, F.A.; Maia, A.R.; Wijchers, P.J.; et al. Genome-wide profiling of p53-regulated enhancer RNAs uncovers a subset of enhancers controlled by a lncRNA. *Nat. Commun.* **2015**, *6*, 6520. [CrossRef]
29. Zhou, Y.; Zhong, Y.; Wang, Y.; Zhang, X.; Batista, D.L.; Gejman, R.; Ansell, P.J.; Zhao, J.; Weng, C.; Klibanski, A. Activation of p53 by MEG3 non-coding RNA. *J. Biol. Chem.* **2007**, *282*, 24731–24742. [CrossRef]
30. Kim, T.; Jeon, Y.J.; Cui, R.; Lee, J.H.; Peng, Y.; Kim, S.H.; Tili, E.; Alder, H.; Croce, C.M. Role of MYC-regulated long noncoding RNAs in cell cycle regulation and tumorigenesis. *J. Natl. Cancer Inst.* **2015**, *107*, 4. [CrossRef] [PubMed]
31. Hart, J.R.; Roberts, T.C.; Weinberg, M.S.; Morris, K.V.; Vogt, P.K. MYC regulates the non-coding transcriptome. *Oncotarget* **2014**, *5*, 12543–12554. [CrossRef] [PubMed]
32. Sánchez, Y.; Segura, V.; Marín-Béjar, O.; Athie, A.; Marchese, F.P.; González, J.; Bujanda, L.; Guo, S.; Matheu, A.; Huarte, M. Genome-wide analysis of the human p53 transcriptional network unveils a lncRNA tumour suppressor signature. *Nat. Commun.* **2014**, *5*, 5812. [CrossRef] [PubMed]
33. Dawson, M.A.; Kouzarides, T. Cancer epigenetics: From mechanism to therapy. *Cell* **2012**, *150*, 12–27. [CrossRef]
34. Marchese, F.P.; Huarte, M. Long non-coding RNAs and chromatin modifiers: Their place in the epigenetic code. *Epigenetics* **2014**, *9*, 21–26. [CrossRef] [PubMed]
35. Zhang, J.; Zhang, P.; Wang, L.; Piao, H.L.; Ma, L. Long non-coding RNA HOTAIR in carcinogenesis and metastasis. *Acta Biochim. Biophys. Sin.* **2014**, *46*, 1–5. [CrossRef] [PubMed]

36. Gupta, R.A.; Shah, N.; Wang, K.C.; Kim, J.; Horlings, H.M.; Wong, D.J.; Tsai, M.C.; Hung, T.; Argani, P.; Rinn, J.L.; et al. Long non-coding RNA HOTAIR reprograms chromatin state to promote cancer me-tastasis. *Nature* **2010**, *464*, 1071–1076. [CrossRef]
37. Tsai, M.C.; Manor, O.; Wan, Y.; Mosammaparast, N.; Wang, J.K.; Lan, F.; Shi, Y.; Segal, E.; Chang, H.Y. Long noncoding RNA as modular scaffold of histone modification complexes. *Science* **2010**, *329*, 689–693. [CrossRef]
38. Heward, J.A.; Lindsay, M.A. Long non-coding RNAs in the regulation of the immune response. *Trends Immunol.* **2014**, *35*, 408–419. [CrossRef]
39. Jiang, R.; Tang, J.; Chen, Y.; Deng, L.; Ji, J.; Xie, Y.; Wang, K.; Jia, W.; Chu, W.M.; Sun, B. The long noncoding RNA lnc-EGFR stimulates T-regulatory cells differentiation thus promoting hepatocellu-lar carcinoma immune evasion. *Nat. Commun.* **2017**, *8*, 15129. [CrossRef]
40. Serghiou, S.; Kyriakopoulou, A.; Ioannidis, J.P. Long noncoding RNAs as novel predictors of survival in human cancer: A systematic review and meta-analysis. *Mol. Cancer* **2016**, *15*, 50. [CrossRef] [PubMed]
41. Tian, T.; Wang, M.; Lin, S.; Guo, Y.; Dai, Z.; Liu, K.; Yang, P.; Dai, C.; Zhu, Y.; Zheng, Y.; et al. The Impact of lncRNA Dysregulation on Clinicopathology and Survival of Breast Cancer: A Systematic Review and Meta-analysis. Molecular therapy. *Nucleic Acids* **2018**, *12*, 359–369. [CrossRef] [PubMed]
42. Jendrzejewski, J.; He, H.; Radomska, H.S.; Li, W.; Tomsic, J.; Liyanarachchi, S.; Davuluri, R.V.; Nagy, R.; de la Chapelle, A. The polymorphism rs944289 predisposes to papillary thyroid carcinoma through a large intergenic noncoding RNA gene of tumor suppressor type. *Proc. Natl. Acad. Sci. USA* **2012**, *109*, 8646–8651. [CrossRef] [PubMed]
43. Pasmant, E.; Sabbagh, A.; Vidaud, M.; Bièche, I. ANRIL, a long, noncoding RNA, is an unex-pected major hotspot in GWAS. *FASEB J.* **2011**, *25*, 444–448. [CrossRef]
44. Betts, J.A.; Marjaneh, M.M.; Al-Ejeh, F.; Lim, Y.C.; Shi, W.; Sivakumaran, H.; Tropée, R.; Patch, A.M.; Clark, M.B.; Bartonicek, N.; et al. Long Noncoding RNAs CUPID1 and CUPID2 Mediate Breast Cancer Risk at 11q13 by Modulating the Response to DNA Damage. *Am. J. Hum. Genet.* **2017**, *101*, 255–266. [CrossRef]
45. Daley, J.M.; Sung, P. 53BP1, BRCA1, and the choice between recombination and end joining at DNA double-strand breaks. *Mol. Cell. Biol.* **2014**, *34*, 1380–1388. [CrossRef]
46. Fachal, L.; Aschard, A.; Beesley, J.; Barnes, D.R.; Allen, J.; Kar, S.; Pooley, K.A.; Dennis, J.; Michailidou, K.; Turman, C.; et al. Fine mapping of 150 breast cancer risk regions identifies 191 likely target genes. *Nat. Genet.* **2020**, *52*, 56–73. [CrossRef]
47. Marjaneh, M.M.; Beesley, J.; O'Mara, T.A.; Mukhopadhyay, P.; Koufariotis, L.T.; Kazakoff, S.; Hussein, N.; Fachal, L.; Bartonicek, N.; Hillman, K.M. French Non-coding RNAs underlie genetic predis-position to breast cancer. *Genome Biol.* **2020**, *21*, 7. [CrossRef]
48. Mathias, C.; Pedroso, G.A.; Pabst, F.R.; de Lima, R.S.; Kuroda, F.; Cavalli, I.J.; de Oliveira, J.C.; de Souza Fonseca Ribeiro, E.M.; Gradia, D.F. So alike yet so different. Differential expres-sion of the long non-coding RNAs NORAD and HCG11 in breast cancer subtypes. *Genet. Mol. Biol.* **2021**, *44*, e20200153. [CrossRef] [PubMed]
49. Mathias, C.; Muzzi, J.C.D.; Antunes, B.B.; Gradia, D.F.; Castro, M.A.A.; de Oliveira, J.C. Un-raveling immune-related lncRNAs in breast cancer molecular subtypes. *Front. Oncol.* **2021**, *11*, 692170. [CrossRef]
50. Chehade, M.; Bullock, M.; Moore, K.; Hutvagner, G.; Sidhu, S.B. The long non-coding RNA psoriasis susceptibility-associated RNA induced by stress (PRINS) as a tumour suppressor and potential biomarker in invasive breast cancer. *Abstr. J. Breast Surg.* **2020**, *90*, 21.
51. Arun, G.; Diermeier, S.D.; Spector, D.L. Therapeutic targeting of long non-coding RNAs in cancer. *Trends Mol. Med.* **2018**, *24*, 257–277. [CrossRef] [PubMed]
52. Bejerano, G.; Pheasant, M.; Makunin, I.; Stephen, S.; Kent, W.J.; Mattick, J.S.; Haussler, D. Ultracon-served elements in the human genome. *Science* **2004**, *304*, 1321–1325. [CrossRef]
53. Calin, G.A.; Liu, C.G.; Ferracin, M.; Hyslop, T.; Spizzo, R.; Sevignani, C.; Fabbri, M.; Cimmino, A.; Lee, E.J.; Wojcik, S.E.; et al. Ultraconserved regions encoding ncRNAs are altered in human leukemias and carcinomas. *Cancer Cell* **2007**, *12*, 215–229. [CrossRef] [PubMed]
54. Terracciano, D.; Terreri, S.; de Nigris, F.; Costa, V.; Calin, G.A.; Cimmino, A. The role of a new class of long noncoding RNAs transcribed from ultraconserved regions in cancer. Biochimica et biophysica acta. *Rev. Cancer* **2017**, *1868*, 449–455.
55. Ferdin, J.; Nishida, N.; Wu, X.; Nicoloso, M.S.; Shah, M.Y.; Devlin, C.; Ling, H.; Shimizu, M.; Kumar, K.; Cortez, M.A.; et al. HINCUTs in cancer: Hypoxia-induced noncoding ultraconserved tran-scripts. *Cell Death Differ.* **2013**, *20*, 1675–1687. [CrossRef] [PubMed]
56. Mestdagh, P.; Fredlund, E.; Pattyn, F.; Rihani, A.; Van Maerken, T.; Vermeulen, J.; Kumps, C.; Menten, B.; De Preter, K.; Schramm, A.; et al. An integrative genomics screen uncovers ncRNA T-UCR functions in neuroblastoma tumours. *Oncogene* **2010**, *29*, 3583–3592. [CrossRef]

57. Sana, J.; Hankeova, S.; Svoboda, M.; Kiss, I.; Vyzula, R.; Slaby, O. Expression levels of transcribed ultraconserved regions uc.73 and uc.388 are altered in colorectal cancer. *Oncology* **2012**, *82*, 114–118. [CrossRef]
58. Hudson, R.S.; Yi, M.; Volfovsky, N.; Prueitt, R.L.; Esposito, D.; Volinia, S.; Liu, C.G.; Schetter, A.J.; Van Roosbroeck, K.; Stephens, R.M.; et al. Transcription signatures en-coded by ultraconserved genomic regions in human prostate cancer. *Mol. Cancer* **2013**, *12*, 13. [CrossRef]
59. Jiang, J.; Azevedo-Pouly, A.C.; Redis, R.S.; Lee, E.J.; Gusev, Y.; Allard, D.; Sutaria, D.S.; Badawi, M.; Elgamal, O.A.; Lerner, M.R.; et al. Globally increased ultraconserved noncoding RNA expression in pancreatic adenocarcinoma. *Oncotarget* **2016**, *7*, 53165–53177. [CrossRef]
60. Li, Q.; Li, X.; Wang, C. Uc.206 regulates cell proliferation and apoptosis by targeting P53 in cervical cancer cells. *Neoplasma* **2016**, *63*, 411–418. [CrossRef]
61. Olivieri, M.; Ferro, M.; Terreri, S.; Durso, M.; Romanelli, A.; Avitabile, C.; De Cobelli, O.; Messere, A.; Bruzzese, D.; Vannini, I.; et al. Long non-coding RNA containing ultraconserved genomic region 8 promotes bladder cancer tumorigenesis. *Oncotarget* **2016**, *7*, 20636–20654. [CrossRef]
62. Sekino, Y.; Sakamoto, N.; Goto, K.; Honma, R.; Shigematsu, Y.; Sentani, K.; Oue, N.; Teishima, J.; Matsubara, A.; Yasui, W. Transcribed ultraconserved region Uc.63+ promotes resistance to docet-axel through regulation of androgen receptor signaling in prostate cancer. *Oncotarget* **2017**, *8*, 94259–94270. [CrossRef] [PubMed]
63. Honma, R.; Goto, K.; Sakamoto, N.; Sekino, Y.; Sentani, K.; Oue, N.; Yasui, W. Expression and function of Uc.160+, a transcribed ultraconserved region, in gastric cancer. *Gastric Cancer* **2017**, *20*, 960–969. [CrossRef] [PubMed]
64. Pang, L.; Li, Q.; Zhang, Y.; Deng, B.; Wu, F.; Wang, J.; Wu, K.; Ding, Y.; Yu, D. Transcribed ultraconserved noncoding RNA uc.160 acts as a negative regulator in gastric cancer. *Am. J. Transl. Res.* **2018**, *10*, 2822–2833.
65. Zhou, J.; Wang, C.; Huang, C.; Ding, Z.; Shi, M. TUCR.454 inhabits metastasis in lung cancer cells. *Int. J. Clin. Exp. Pathol.* **2018**, *11*, 1289–1296.
66. Marini, A.; Lena, A.M.; Panatta, E.; Ivan, C.; Han, L.; Liang, H.; Annicchiarico-Petruzzelli, M.; Di Daniele, N.; Calin, G.A.; Candi, E.; et al. Ultraconserved long non-coding RNA uc.63 in breast cancer. *Oncotarget* **2017**, *8*, 35669–35680. [CrossRef] [PubMed]
67. Zhang, L.X.; Xu, L.; Zhang, C.H.; Lu, Y.H.; Ji, T.H.; Ling, L.J. uc.38 induces breast cancer cell apoptosis via PBX1. *Am. J. Cancer Res.* **2017**, *7*, 2438–2451.
68. Magnani, L.; Ballantyne, E.B.; Zhang, X.; Lupien, M. PBX1 genomic pioneer function drives ERα signaling underlying progression in breast cancer. *PLoS Genet.* **2011**, *7*, e1002368. [CrossRef]
69. Anderson, D.M.; Anderson, K.M.; Chang, C.L.; Makarewich, C.A.; Nelson, B.R.; McAnally, J.R.; Kasaragod, P.; Shelton, J.M.; Liou, J.; Bassel-Duby, R.; et al. A micropeptide encoded by a putative long noncoding RNA regulates muscle performance. *Cell* **2015**, *160*, 595–606. [CrossRef] [PubMed]
70. Andrews, S.J.; Rothnagel, J.A. Emerging evidence for functional peptides encoded by short open reading frames. *Nat. Rev. Genet.* **2014**, *15*, 193–204. [CrossRef]
71. Wu, P.; Mo, Y.; Peng, M.; Tang, T.; Zhong, Y.; Deng, X.; Xiong, F.; Guo, C.; Wu, X.; Li, Y.; et al. Emerging role of tumor-related functional peptides encoded by lncRNA and circRNA. *Mol. Cancer* **2020**, *19*, 22. [CrossRef]

10

Development of Dl1.72, a Novel Anti-DLL1 Antibody with Anti-Tumor Efficacy against Estrogen Receptor-Positive Breast Cancer

Gabriela Silva [1,*,†], Joana Sales-Dias [1,2,†], Diogo Casal [3,4], Sara Alves [3,5], Giacomo Domenici [1,2], Clara Barreto [1,6,‡], Carolina Matos [1], Ana R. Lemos [1,2], Ana T. Matias [4], Khrystyna Kucheryava [1], Andreia Ferreira [4], Maria Raquel Moita [1,2], Sofia Braga [4,6], Catarina Brito [1,2], M. Guadalupe Cabral [4], Cristina Casalou [4,§], Duarte C. Barral [4], Pedro M. F. Sousa [1,2], Paula A. Videira [7], Tiago M. Bandeiras [1,2] and Ana Barbas [1,||]

1 iBET, Instituto de Biologia Experimental e Tecnológica, Apartado 12, 2781-901 Oeiras, Portugal; jsdias@ibet.pt (J.S.-D.); giacomo.domenici@ibet.pt (G.D.); clara.barreto@medicina.ulisboa.pt (C.B.); carolina.matos@ibet.pt (C.M.); ar.lemos@ibet.pt (A.R.L.); kkucheryava@ibet.pt (K.K.); mraquelmoita@ibet.pt (M.R.M.); anabrito@ibet.pt (C.B.); pedrosousa@ibet.pt (P.M.F.S.); tiagob@ibet.pt (T.M.B.); ana.barbas@bayer.com (A.B.)

2 Instituto de Tecnologia Química e Biológica António Xavier, Universidade Nova de Lisboa, Av. da República, 2780-157 Oeiras, Portugal

3 Departamento de Anatomia, NOVA Medical School (NMS), Universidade NOVA de Lisboa, 1150-082 Lisbon, Portugal; diogo.casal@nms.unl.pt (D.C.); sara.p.alves@chlc.min-saude.pt (S.A.)

4 iNOVA4Health, CEDOC, NOVA Medical School (NMS), Universidade NOVA de Lisboa, 1150-082 Lisbon, Portugal; ana.matias@nms.unl.pt (A.T.M.); andreia.ferreira@nms.unl.pt (A.F.); sofia.braga@jmellosaude.pt (S.B.); guadalupe.cabral@nms.unl.pt (M.G.C.); cristina.casalou@ucd.ie (C.C.); duarte.barral@nms.unl.pt (D.C.B.)

5 Serviço de Anatomia Patológica, Centro Hospitalar de Lisboa Central-Hospital de São José, 1150-199 Lisbon, Portugal

6 Unidade de Mama, Instituto CUF de Oncologia, 1998-018 Lisbon, Portugal

7 UCIBIO, Departamento Ciências da Vida, Faculdade de Ciências e Tecnologia, Universidade NOVA de Lisboa, 2829-516 Caparica, Portugal; p.videira@fct.unl.pt

* Correspondence: gabrielasilva@ibet.pt;

† These authors share first authorship.

‡ Current address: Instituto de Medicina Molecular, Faculdade de Medicina, Universidade de Lisboa, 1649-028 Lisbon, Portugal.

§ Current address: Charles Institute of Dermatology, UCD School of Medicine, University College Dublin, Belfield, Dublin4, Ireland.

|| Current address: Bayer Portugal, 2790-143 Carnaxide, Portugal.

Simple Summary: Over 70% of breast cancers (BCs) are estrogen receptor-positive (ER^+). The development of endocrine therapy has considerably improved patient outcomes. However, there is a clinical need for novel effective therapies against ER^+ BCs, since many of these do not respond to standard therapy, and more than one-third of responders acquire resistance, experience relapse and metastasize. The Notch ligand Delta-like 1 (DLL1) is a key player in ER^+ BC development and aggressiveness. Contrary to complete Notch pharmacological inhibitors, antibody-targeting of individual Notch components is expected to have superior therapeutic efficacy and be better tolerated. In this study, we developed and characterized a novel specific anti-DLL1 antibody with efficacy in inhibiting BC cell proliferation, mammosphere formation and angiogenesis, as well as anti-tumor and anti-metastatic efficacy in an ER^+ BC mouse model without side effects. Thus, our data suggest that this anti-DLL1 antibody is a promising candidate for ER^+ BC treatment.

Abstract: The Notch-signaling ligand DLL1 has emerged as an important player and promising therapeutic target in breast cancer (BC). DLL1-induced Notch activation promotes tumor cell proliferation, survival, migration, angiogenesis and BC stem cell maintenance. In BC, DLL1 overexpression is associated with poor prognosis, particularly in estrogen receptor-positive (ER^+) subtypes. Directed therapy in early and advanced BC has dramatically changed the natural course of ER^+ BC; however, relapse is a major clinical issue, and new therapeutic strategies are needed. Here, we report the development and characterization of a novel monoclonal antibody specific to DLL1. Using phage display technology, we selected an anti-DLL1 antibody fragment, which was converted into a full human IgG1 (Dl1.72). The Dl1.72 antibody exhibited DLL1 specificity and affinity in the low nanomolar range and significantly impaired DLL1-Notch signaling and expression of Notch target genes in ER+ BC cells. Functionally, in vitro treatment with Dl1.72 reduced MCF-7 cell proliferation, migration, mammosphere formation and endothelial tube formation. In vivo, Dl1.72 significantly inhibited tumor growth, reducing both tumor cell proliferation and liver metastases in a xenograft mouse model, without apparent toxicity. These findings suggest that anti-DLL1 Dl1.72 could be an attractive agent against ER+ BC, warranting further preclinical investigation.

Keywords: ER+ breast cancer; Notch signaling; DLL1; monoclonal antibody; cell proliferation; angiogenesis; tumor growth

---

1. Introduction

Breast cancer (BC) is the most frequent cancer in women and the second leading cause of cancer deaths in women worldwide [1]. BC is a highly heterogeneous and multifactorial disease that can be classified into four subtypes (Luminal A/B, human epidermal growth factor receptor 2 (HER2)-positive and triple-negative), based on the expression of the estrogen receptor (ER), progesterone receptor (PR) and HER2 [1,2]. Clinical outcomes differ greatly between subtypes, and most BC deaths arise from distant metastasis in the liver, bone and lung [3]. ER+ BC accounts for more than 70% of all BC cases. The development of endocrine therapies such as tamoxifen and fulvestrant has considerably improved the outcomes of ER+ BC patients [4]. Nonetheless, approximately one-third of patients do not respond to initial therapy, and a large proportion of tumors acquire resistance, recur, and undergo metastasis [2,5,6]. Therefore, there is an urgent need to develop new therapeutic strategies to improve the prognosis of patients with ER+ BC.

In this regard, the Notch signaling pathway appears as an attractive alternative therapeutic target in BC. This pathway is a cell–cell communication system that is crucial for embryonic development and post-natal tissue homeostasis and regeneration [7]. Mammalian Notch signaling relies on four receptors (Notch1–4) and five activating ligands: Delta-like (DLL) 1, 3 and 4 and Jagged (JAG) 1 and 2 [8,9]. Notch ligands are transmembrane proteins with an extracellular domain (ECD) that contains an N-terminal domain, a highly conserved Delta/Serrate/LAG-2 region and several epidermal growth factor (EGF)-like repeats [8,9]. Binding of the ECD of one of the ligands to one of the receptors present in an adjacent cell triggers sequential proteolytic cleavages that release the Notch intracellular domain (NICD) in the cytoplasm. The NICD then translocates to the nucleus, where it interacts with DNA-binding proteins, leading to the transcription of Notch target genes (e.g., *HEY* family), which regulate many cellular processes [10]. The activation of Notch signaling varies remarkably depending on pathway component expression, signal dose and cell context [11]. The dysregulation of Notch signaling, by virtue of abnormal expression of its receptors and/or ligands, has been reported in more than 50% of BCs [12], and aberrant Notch signaling is implicated in essentially all hallmarks of cancer [13] and drug resistance [6,14,15].

The human Notch ligand DLL1 is overexpressed in BC tumors and is associated with poor prognosis in patients with ER+ BCs [16,17]. We and others have shown that DLL1 contributes to BC tumor biology through the promotion of cancer cell colony formation, cell proliferation, survival, migration, and invasion, BC stem cell (BCSC) function, metastases formation and angiogenesis [17–19]. Moreover, recently, DLL1+ cells have been shown to bear similarities to CSCs by showing a high tumor-initiating capacity as well as the ability to drive metastasis and chemoresistance in aggressive luminal breast tumors [20]. These multiple roles of DLL1 in BC support the development of specific anti-DLL1 therapies for ER+ BC treatment. DLL1-targeting therapies are expected to provide clinical benefits when used alone and in combination with conventional chemotherapy, or as an alternative therapeutic strategy in the case of endocrine resistance.

In this study, we characterized the in vitro and in vivo BC anti-tumorigenic effect of a novel anti-DLL1 antibody, the Dl1.72, developed using phage display technology. Biophysical characterization of Dl1.72 showed that it binds to human DLL1 with nanomolar affinity, displaying no binding for other human Notch ligands. Cellular assays using MCF-7 ER^+ BC cells revealed that Dl1.72 impaired DLL1-Notch signaling and reduced cancer cell proliferation and migration as well as the BCSC population. In addition, endothelial cell tube formation ability was impaired by Dl1.72, suggesting a potential anti-angiogenic effect of this mAb. Finally, using a human ER^+ BC xenograft model, we verified that Dl1.72 remarkably inhibited tumor growth, reducing both tumor cell proliferation and liver metastasis, without associated toxicity. Together, these observations suggest that anti-DLL1 Dl1.72 could be an attractive tool against ER^+ BC and warrant further preclinical investigation of this mAb against ER^+ BC.

2. Materials and Methods

2.1. Cell Culture and Reagents

HEK293E6 [21] and MCF-7 (ATCC, Manassas, VA, USA, HTB-22) cells were cultured as previously described [18]. CHO-K1 cells (ATCC, CCL-61) were cultured in DMEM F12 media (#12634010) containing 10% heat-inactivated fetal bovine serum (FBS, #10270-106) plus 100 μg/mL penicillin and streptomycin (#15140163) (all from Gibco Thermo Fisher Scientific, Waltham, MA, USA). HUVEC cells (C-003-5C) were cultured in Medium 200 (M-200-500) plus large vessel endothelial supplement (A14608-01) (all from Life Technologies, Waltham, MA, USA) and used until passage four. All cells were cultured at 37 °C, 5% CO_2, according to the supplier's instructions, and tested for the absence of mycoplasma. Culture media was replaced every 2–3 days. The Notch pathway signaling inhibitor DAPT (Sigma-Aldrich, St. Louis, MO, USA, D5942) was used at 5 μM. DMSO (Sigma-Aldrich, #472301) was used as a control for DAPT in vitro exposure in a final dilution more than 1/1000.

2.2. Phage Display Screening, Antibody Generation and Characterization

Selection of anti-DLL1 single-chain variable fragments (scFvs) by phage display and generation of anti-DLL1 Dl1.72 were performed as described previously [22].

For Dl1.72 production, HEK293E6 suspension cells were transfected with 0.5 mg/L of the respective LC and HC plasmids. An isotype-matched negative control mAb (Ctr Ab) was also produced in a similar mode [22]. The secreted mAbs were purified in endotoxin-free conditions and analyzed by sodium dodecyl sulfate–polyacrylamide gel electrophoresis (SDS–PAGE), analytical size exclusion chromatography and Western blotting, as described in [22]. Protein concentration was determined by the Bradford method and spectrophotometry at 280 nm. Purity was estimated from SDS–PAGE by densitometry analysis using ImageJ/Fiji software [23], and endotoxin content was measured using the Endosafe-PTS system (Charles River, Boston, MA, USA, PTS2001F). Dl1.72 reactivity and specificity were evaluated by ELISA (see Table S1 for proteins used) and flow cytometry, as described in [22]. Binding kinetic characterization of D11.72 interaction with untagged rhDLL1, containing the full ECD [22], was performed by Surface Plasmon Resonance (SPR) Horseradish Peroxidase conjugation of anti-DLL1 Dl1.72, and Ctr Ab was performed using the EZ-Link™ Plus Activated Peroxidase kit (Thermo Scientific, Waltham, MA, USA, #31488); the resulting conjugates were analyzed by SDS–PAGE, Western blotting and ELISA. For details, see Supplementary Materials.

2.3. Notch Reporter Assay

MCF-7 cells (1.25×10^5 cells/mL) were co-transfected with 750 ng of Notch firefly luciferase reporter (4xCSL, Addgene, Watertown, MA, USA, #41726) along with 10 ng of pRL-SV40 vector encoding renilla luciferase (Promega, Madison, WI, USA, #E2231) using GeneJuice transfection reagent (Merck-Millipore, Darmstadt, Germany, #70967), according to the manufacturer's instructions. Cells were then plated in 96-well plates either not coated (control) or pre-coated with rhDLL1- Fc or Fc control protein in the absence or presence of either Dl1.72, Ctr Ab (1, 2.5, 5, 10 and 20 μg/mL each), DAPT or an equivalent amount of vehicle (DMSO. Luciferase activities were measured in whole cell lysates 28 h after culture using the Dual Luciferase assay kit (Promega, #E1910), following the kit's instructions, in a plate reader MultiskanTM FC (Thermo Scientific). Firefly luciferase activities were normalized to renilla luciferase units in the same samples. Three to four replicates were analyzed for each condition. Results were calculated relative to cells plated in the control uncoated wells, which were set as 1.

2.4. *Real-Time RT-qPCR*

Cells were plated on culture plates either not coated (control) or pre-coated with rhDLL1-Fc, for the induction of DLL1-Notch target genes, or Fc protein in the absence or presence of Dl1.72, Ctr Ab, DAPT, or DMSO, as indicated elsewhere. Total RNA was extracted using the RNeasy Mini kit (Qiagen, La Jolla, CA, USA, #50974104), and cDNA was generated from equal amounts of RNA by reverse transcription using the Advantage RT-for-PCR kit (Clontech Laboratories, Mountain View, CA, USA, # 639506), as per the manufacturer's instructions. The expression of *HEY-1*, *HEY-L*, *HPRT1*, *RPL22*, *SOX2* and *SOX9* genes was quantified on Roche LightCycler 480 equipment using SYBR Green I Master Kit (Roche, Bazel, Switzerland). mRNA transcripts were normalized to housekeeping genes *HPRT1* and *RPL22* levels in the same sample, and the results were calculated as fold change relative to control cells, as previously described [24]. The primers used in these assays are listed in Table S2.

2.5. *MCF-7 Cell Growth, Scratch Wound Healing, and Mammosphere Formation Assays*

Cells were seeded at 3–4 $\times$ 10^4 cells/cm^2 in 24-well plates (500 μL/well) or 96-well plates (100 μL/well) either not coated or pre-coated with rhDLL1-Fc or Fc proteins, as indicated above. Cells were left untreated or were treated with either Dl1.72, Ctr Ab (both at 10 μg/mL), DAPT, or DMSO and incubated for 70–76 h. After incubation, cell growth was determined using the MTT (3-(4,5-dimethylthiazolyl-2)-2,5-diphenyltetrazolium bromide) colorimetric method (96-well plates) or by microscopy using the trypan blue exclusion method (24-well plates), as previously described [18,25]. Each condition was tested in triplicate (trypan blue exclusion) or quadruplicate (MTT) for all assays. Growth media was replaced with fresh media containing the specific treatment every 48 h.

For the wound healing assay, MCF-7 cells (2.5–4 $\times$ 10^4 cells/cm^2) seeded in 24-well plates were treated 16 h later with Abs or left untreated as above and cultured for 48–52 h until 90% confluence. Thereafter, cell monolayers were scratched, washed and incubated in complete media with the respective treatments. Images of 3 different areas of the wound of each scratch were taken at 0 and 72 h after the scratches were made with a Leica DMI6000 microscope (5$\times$ objective). The wound widths were determined using ImageJ/Fiji software, as described in [18].

The mammosphere (MS) formation assay was performed as indicated in [22].

2.6. *HUVEC Tube Formation, Cell Growth, and Viability Assays*

Tube formation assay was performed using the Angiogenesis starter kit from Life Technologies (#A1460901) following the manufacturer's instructions, with Geltrex from the kit or Matrigel (BD Biosciences, San Jose, CA, USA, #356230). Briefly, HUVEC at 80% confluence were collected using trypsin/EDTA and trypsin neutralizing solution (Lonza, Basel, Switzerland, CC-5012 and CC-5002, respectively) and seeded at 4 $\times$ 10^3 cells/cm^2 in T-25 tissue culture flasks in medium 200 with large vessel endothelial supplement. After 6 h, cells were left untreated (control) or were treated with either Dl1.72, Ctr Ab (10 μg/mL each), DAPT or DMSO and incubated for 3 days until 80% confluence. Afterwards, cells were collected and seeded on a layer of solidified Geltrex or Matrigel at a density of 2.5 $\times$ 10^4 cells/cm^2 in complete media (250 μL/well of 24-well tissue culture plates) and incubated at 37 °C for 16–18 h. Pictures of cells stained with Calcein AM (Corning, NY, USA, #354216, 2 μg/mL in PBS plus Ca^{++} and Mg^{++}, 250 μL/well, 30 min at 37 °C) were taken using a phase-contrast inverted microscope (5× objective). At least four independent images were acquired per condition. Morphology of the tube network formation, including the number of nodes and meshes, and total branching length were quantified using the ImageJ Angiogenesis Analyzer plugin [26]. The growth and viability of cells at the end of the treatments were evaluated by microscopy using the trypan blue exclusion method, as described above.

2.7. Human Breast Tumor Samples

Formalin-fixed, paraffin-embedded (FFPE) ER^+ BC 2.5 μm tissue sections ($N = 9$) were obtained from surgical BC specimens, selected by pathologists from the Hospital Professor Doutor Fernando Fonseca (HFF, Amadora-Sintra, Portugal). The study was approved by the ethics committees from NOVA Medical School, Faculdade de Ciências Médicas, Universidade NOVA de Lisboa, and HFF (ref. 98/2019/CEFCM). All participants gave informed consent, and this study was performed in accordance with the ethical standards outlined in the 1964 Declaration of Helsinki. The clinicopathological characteristics of BC samples used in the study are described in Table S3.

2.8. MCF-7 Breast Cancer Xenograft Model

All animal experiments were conducted with approval from the national regulatory authority, Direção Geral de Alimentação e Veterinária (DGAV) (ref. 0421/000/000/2017) and the Institutional Ethics Committee (CEFCM 07/2016) and performed according to their guidelines and under the rules of the Federation for Animal Science Associations (FELASA). Five-week-old female NOD scid gamma (NSG) female mice (Charles River Laboratories) were used for this study and maintained under pathogen-free conditions. Four days prior to tumor cell implantation, estrogen pellets (0.36 mg/pellet 90 day release, Innovative Research of America, 0.36 mg/pellet 90-day release, Innovative Research of America, Sarasota, FL, USA, #NE-121) were implanted subcutaneously (s.c.) in the mice dorsal neck region using a sterilized trocar. Xenografts were initiated by s.c. implanting 2×10^6 MCF-7 cells in 100 μL of PBS:matrigel (1:1 ratio, BD Biosciences, #356230) into the mammary fat pad of each tested mouse (2 mammary fat pad injections/mouse) using an established protocol [27]. After fifteen days, mice were weighed and injected intraperitoneally (i.p.) with Dl1.72, Ctr Ab (each at 10 mg/kg of mice body weight (BW), $n = 5$ mice per each group) or an equal volume of vehicle PBS ($n = 6$ mice). Treatment was repeated twice a week for 12 weeks. Animals were monitored daily for clinical symptoms and adverse effects. Tumor growth and mouse weight were determined weekly. Tumor volume was estimated by measuring tumor length (L) and width (W) with a digital caliper and by applying the following formula: ($\pi \times L \times W2$)/6. Twelve weeks after the beginning of treatment, mice were sacrificed and their blood, tumor, liver and kidney were collected for analysis.

2.9. Serology

Mice blood withdrawal was performed by cardiac puncture to tubes. To stop coagulation, 10 units of heparin per mL of blood were added to collection tubes. Blood was centrifuged at 2000× *g* for 10 min at 4 °C, and serum was immediately collected. Urea, creatinine and alanine aminotransferase (ALT) serum levels were determined by DNAtech (Lisbon, http://www.dnatech.pt/web/, accessed on 18 October 2019).

2.10. Histological and Immunohistochemical Analysis

Immunohistochemical (IHC) staining of FFPE human ER^+ BC tissue section specimens was performed as previously specified [28]. Stained samples were scored for both signal intensity and abundance of positive cells using ImageJ/Fiji software using a macro developed by the authors (https://github.com/ClaraBarreto/Dl1.72.git, accessed on 22

July 2021). Staining intensity was measured using the scale 0–3, with 0 being negative and 3 being very high expression. The H-score was calculated by multiplying intensity with abundance using the following formula: $(1 \times (\% \text{ cells } 1+) + 2 \times (\% \text{ cells } 2+) + 3 \times (\% \text{ cells } 3+))$. Scoring was done independently by three researchers.

Mice tumor, liver, and kidney tissues were fixed in formalin (10%), embedded in paraffin and cut into 4 μm sections on a microtome (Leica, Wetzlar, Germany). The sections were stained with hematoxylin-eosin (H&E) [29] or immunostained with the pan-cytokeratin AE1/AE3/PCK26 antibody cocktail (#760-2135) for the identification of human epithelial cells or anti-human Ki67 (#05298512001) for detection of proliferating cells. IHC was performed by BenchMark ULTRA—Automated IHC and in situ hybridization slide staining systems (Ventana, Roche), as described in [30]. Stained images were scanned using NanoZoomer—SQ Digital Slide Scanner (Hamamatsu, Japan). The tumor area was determined from the largest tumor sections stained with H&E and AE1/AE3/PCK26 Ab and metastasis of BC cell in liver sections stained with AE1/AE3/PCK26 Ab using the imageJ/Fiji software. The percentage of proliferating cells from tumor sections stained with Ki67 Ab was determined by ImageJ/Fiji software with the ImmunoRatio plugin [31]. Proliferation and metastasis analysis were done by examining multiple random fields of view (FOVs) for each sample. Histological analyses was independently evaluated by two pathologists, and immunostaining analysis by at least two researchers. For details on IHC staining, see Supplementary Materials.

2.11. *Analysis of Tumor Cell Apoptosis by TUNEL*

Mice tumor sections prepared as above were deparaffinized with Xylene (3 min, 3 times) and rehydrated in 100% ethanol (3 min, 2 times), 95% ethanol (3 min), 70% ethanol (3 min) and ddH_2O (10 min). For antigen retrieval, samples were soaked in Citrate Buffer, pH 6, heated in a microwave until liquid boiled, and cooled down for 20 min. Then, samples were washed with Tris-buffered saline containing 0.05% Tween-20 (5 min, 3 times) and incubated with proteinase K (Merck Millipore, # 21627, 20 μg/mL, 15 min, RT). Then, the ApopTag red in situ apoptosis detection kit (Merck Millipore, # S7165) procedure for fluorescent staining of paraffin-embedded tissue samples was followed according to the manufacturer's instructions. Samples were mounted in ProLong Gold antifade reagent with DAPI for nuclei staining (Invitrogen, Waltham, MA, USA, #P36931). Images were acquired on a Leica DMI 6000-inverted microscope equipped with a Leica DFC360 FX camera, using a 20x HCX PL FLUOTAR objective, controlled with the Leica Application Suite × software. Images were analyzed with the ImageJ/Fiji software. The percentage of apoptotic cells was determined by counting 10 independent FOVs, performed by independent researchers.

2.12. *Statistical Analysis*

Results are presented as mean ± standard deviation (SD) or mean ± standard error of the mean (SEM) for the mice studies (see Figure 1e). Statistical analyses were performed using Graphpad Prism 8 software. The significance of differences was analyzed using the Student *t*-test and the non-parametric Mann–Whitney test for normally and non-normally distributed datasets, respectively. One-way analysis of variance (ANOVA) with Tukey's test was used to determine differences between tumor growth datasets. p values < 0.05 were considered statistically significant.

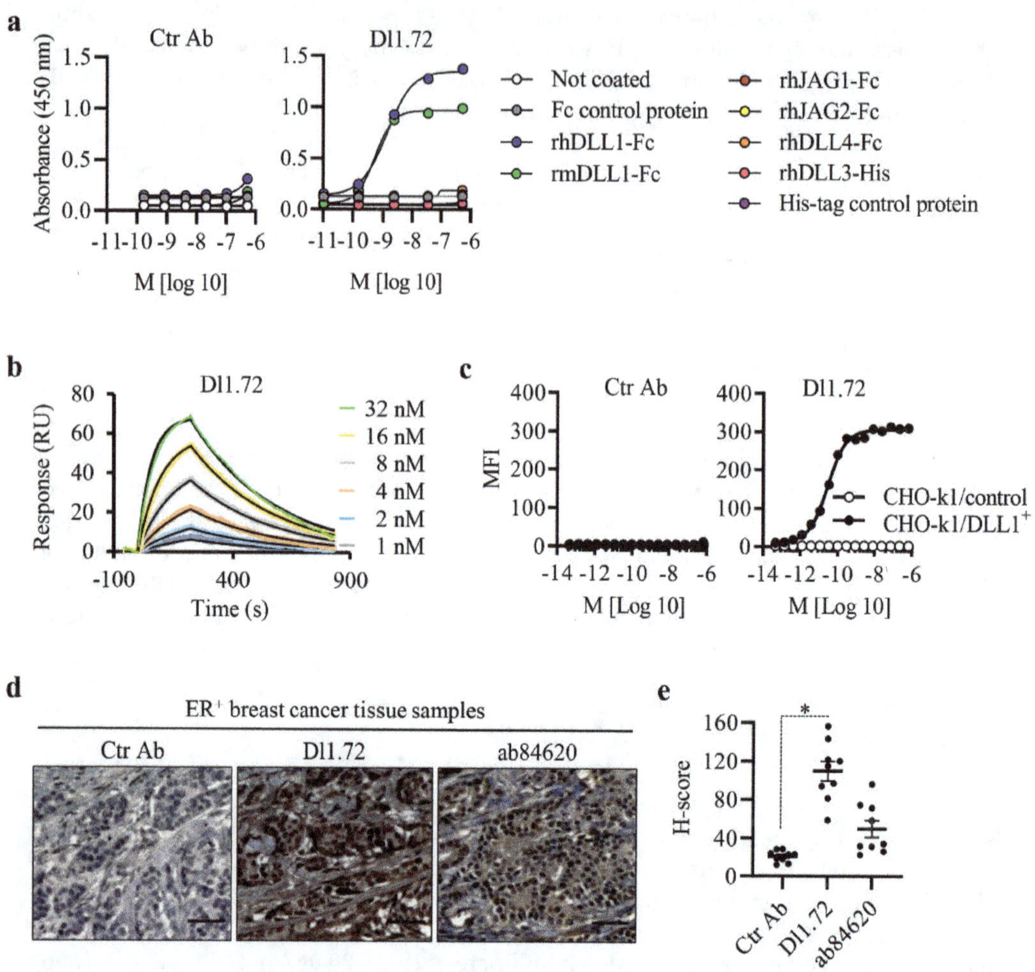

Figure 1. Anti-DLL1 Dl1.72 binding affinity and specificity to DLL1. (**a**) ELISA measuring Dl1.72 and isotope-matched negative control (Ctr Ab) binding to recombinant human (rh) Notch ligands rhDLL1-Fc, rhDLL3-His, rhDLL4-Fc, rhJAG1-Fc and rhJAG2-Fc, and murine DLL1 (rmDLL1). Uncoated wells and wells coated with Fc protein or an unrelated His-tag protein were used as negative controls. (**b**) Surface plasmon resonance was used to determine the Dl1.72 binding affinity to rhDLL1 (without Fc portion). Representative curves from one assay run with three technical replicates are shown. RU, response units. (**c**) Binding of Dl1.72 to cell surface DLL1. CHO-k1 cells overexpressing rhDLL1 on the cellular surface (CHO-k1/DLL1$^+$, filled circles) and CHO-k1 control cells not expressing hDLL1 (open circles) were incubated with Dl1.72 or Ctr Ab, and Ab-antigen binding was determined by flow cytometry. MFI, mean fluorescence intensity. Graphs in (**a**,**c**) are representative of three independent assays. (**d**) Binding of Dl1.72 to human ER$^+$ BC tumor samples by IHC. Matched-tissue sections from ER$^+$ BC samples ($n = 9$) were stained individually with Dl1.72 or Ctr Ab, pre-conjugated with HRP, or with the commercial anti-DLL1 polyclonal ab84620 followed by anti-rabbit HRP-conjugated secondary antibody as a control for DLL1 detection and tissue distribution. Representative IHC images from matched samples at disease stage T1 are shown. Brown color indicates DLL1 staining and blue nuclei counterstaining with hematoxylin. (**e**) Quantification of the mean value (± SEM) of each immunoreactive score. Scale bars, 50 µm. *, $p < 0.05$ (Mann–Whitney test).

3. Results

3.1. Characterization of the Generated Anti-DLL1 Dl1.72 Antibody That Specifically Interacts with DLL1

Using Phage display technology to generate synthetic mAbs with blocking activity against DLL1 [22], we identified our scFv lead candidate, which was converted into the anti-DLL1 Dl1.72 full IgG1 antibody. Dl1.72 was produced in mammalian cells in parallel with a control isotype IgG1 mAb (Ctr Ab). The purified mAbs have the expected sizes of approximately 50 kDa for IgG HC and 25 kDa for IgG LC, with a purity > 90% and less than

0.16 EU/mg. To evaluate Dl1.72 binding ability for its cognate antigen, we performed a dose-dependent ELISA of Dl1.72 or Ctr Ab with a fixed concentration of rhDLL1-Fc. Cross-reactivity to murine DLL1 (rmDLL1 presents more than 85% sequence identity to hDLL1) was also evaluated. As a negative control, Dl1.72 was incubated with Fc protein. Dl1.72 bound to both purified human and murine DLL1 proteins but not to the Fc control protein, with no binding of Ctr Ab (Figure 1a). Specificity testing by ELISA in the same conditions showed Dl1.72 does not bind to any other human Notch ligand (rhDLL3, rhDLL4, rhJAG1 and rhJAG2) (Figure 1a). The calculated half-maximal effective concentration (EC_{50}) of Dl1.72 to purified rhDLL1 was found to be 1.15 $\pm$ 0.16 nM (Table 1). The binding kinetics of Dl1.72 interaction with rhDLL1 were measured by surface plasmon resonance (Figure 1b). The kinetic affinity (K_D) of the interaction between D11.72 and rhDLL1 was calculated to be 4.78 $\pm$ 1.05 nM (Table 1).

Table 1. Estimated EC_{50} values and affinity constants of anti-DLL1 Dl1-72 mAb towards DLL1. Data are mean value $\pm$ SD of three independent ELISA and flow cytometry assays and three replicates from the SPR assays.

ELISA	Flow Cytometry		SPR	
EC_{50} (nM)	EC_{50} (nM)	K_D (nM)	k_a (s^{-1})	k_d (M^{-1} s^{-1})
1.15 $\pm$ 0.16	2.07×10^{-2} $\pm 1.20 \times 10^{-2}$	4.78 $\pm$ 1.05	5.44×10^{5} $\pm 8.21 \times 10^{4}$	2.60×10^{-3} $\pm 2.50 \times 10^{-4}$

To verify the binding ability of Dl1.72 to cell surface hDLL1, CHO-K1 cells over-expressing hDLL1 and control cells without hDLL1 [22] were incubated with various concentrations of Dl1.72 or Ctr Ab, and binding was analyzed by flow cytometry. Dl1.72 bound strongly to DLL1-overexpressing cells but not to cells not expressing DLL1. Ctr Ab showed no effective binding to both cell lines (Figure 1c). The EC_{50} of the interaction between Dl1.72 and cells overexpressing hDLL1 was calculated to be 20.7 pM, on average (Table 1). This EC_{50} value is more than 50-fold lower than the one obtained with the immobilized pure protein by ELISA, suggesting that the native protein conformation in the cells as well as the amino acid residues recognized by Dl1.72 are more accessible in the cell surface DLL1.

We next examined the ability of Dl1.72 to recognize and bind to endogenous human DLL1 by immunohistochemistry using cross-sections of breast tissues from patients with ER^+ BC. Matched BC tissue samples were incubated with Dl1.72, Ctr Ab or a commercially available rabbit anti-DLL1 antibody (ab84620), used as a control for DLL1 detection and to confirm tissue distribution, as previously reported [17]. Mammary tissues, especially BC tissues, contain significant amounts of human IgGs [32]. Thus, Dl1.72 and Ctr Ab were previously conjugated with HRP for these assays. Our results showed high binding levels of Dl1.72 to ER^+ BC tissues, contrary to Ctr Ab. Moreover, Dl1.72 and ab84620 presented similar IHC staining patterns to the same tissue samples, suggesting that both Abs are binding to the same antigen, i.e., DLL1 (Figures 1d and S1). Quantification of the intensity and abundance of each Ab staining showed that Dl1.72 presented a higher immunoreactivity score in comparison with ab84620 (Figure 1e). Altogether, these results suggest that anti-DLL1 Dl1.72 binds specifically to endogenous DLL1 in BC tissue samples.

3.2. *Anti-DLL1 Dl1.72 Inhibits DLL1-Notch Signaling in ER^+ Breast Cancer Cells*

DLL1-Notch signaling has been implicated in the oncogenic capacities of MCF-7 ER^+ BC cells [18]. Accordingly, this BC cell line was chosen to examine Dl1.72 capacity to impair DLL1-Notch signaling by luciferase Notch reporter assay and evaluating the expression levels of the Notch target genes *HEY-1* and *HEY-L*, which are significantly induced by DLL1 [18]. Dl1.72-treated cells showed significant dose-dependent inhibition of DLL1-Notch signaling when compared to control cells not treated or treated with Ctr Ab (Figure 2a). Similar to DAPT, Dl1.72 at 10–20 µg/mL almost completely inhibited Notch signaling activation by rhDLL1. As expected, Fc control protein had no effect in the Notch reporter activity (Figure 2a).

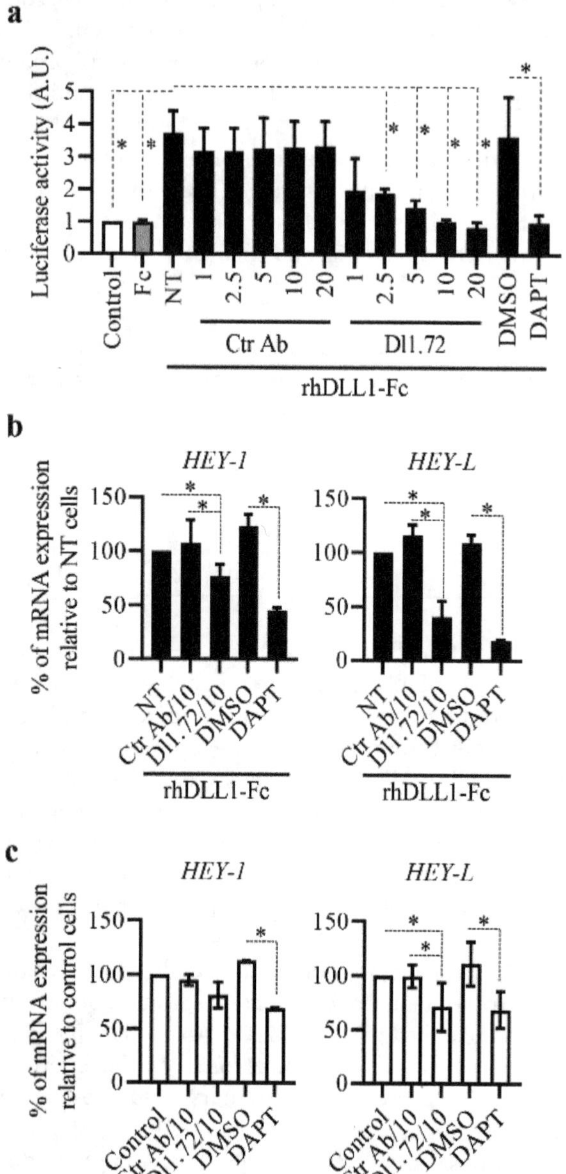

Figure 2. Anti-DLL1 Dl1.72 impairs DLL1-Notch signaling in MCF-7 cells. (**a**) Notch luciferase reporter assay. Cells transfected with the Notch firefly luciferase reporter were cultured for 28 h in uncoated (control) wells or wells pre-coated with Fc control protein or rhDLL1-Fc in the absence (NT) or presence of the indicated concentration (µg/mL) of Dl1.72, Ctr Ab, the pan-Notch inhibitor DAPT (5 µM) or DMSO (DAPT vehicle). The graph shows luciferase activity (mean ± SD, $n = 3$) compared to control unchallenged cells. (**b**) Effect of Dl1.72 on the levels of *HEY-1* and *HEY-L* induced by DLL1. Cells were cultured in wells pre-coated with rhDLL1-Fc proteins and not treated (NT) or treated with Dl1.72, Ctr Ab (10 µg/mL each), DAPT or DMSO. After 17–20 h, the transcript levels of Notch-dependent genes *HEY-1* and *HEY-L* were determined by RT-qPCR. Graphs show the mean percentage (±SD, $n = 3$) of *HEY-1* and *HEY-L* mRNAs relative to untreated cells. (**c**) Effect of Dl1.72 on the basal levels of *HEY-1* and *HEY-L*. MCF-7 cells were cultured in the absence (control) or presence of Dl1.72, Ctr Ab (10 µg/mL each), DMSO or DAPT, and the transcript levels were determined as above. Graphs show the mean percentage (±SD, $n > 3$) of *HEY-1* and *HEY-L* mRNAs relative to unstimulated control cells. *, $p < 0.05$ (two-tailed paired Student t-test).

Consistent with the impairment of Notch reporter activity, Dl1.72 decreased the induction levels of *HEY-1* and *HEY-L* by DLL1 in a dose-dependent manner (Figure S2). At 10 μg/mL, this mAb reduced the levels of DLL1-induced *HEY-1* and *HEY-L* by 20% and 60%, respectively (Figure 2b) when compared to control cells not treated or treated with Ctr Ab. Furthermore, DAPT reduced *HEY-1* and *HEY-L* levels by 55% and 80%, respectively, in response to the ligand (Figure 2b). Assessment of the effect of Dl1.72 in the mRNA levels of these genes in unstimulated MCF-7 cells showed Dl1.72 at 10 μg/mL decreased the expression of basal *HEY-L* at levels comparable with DAPT (30% reduction on average when compared to control cells) but had no significant effect on those of *HEY-1* (Figure 2c). Altogether, these results show that anti-DLL1 Dl1.72 is able to impair DLL1-Notch signaling.

3.3. Anti-DLL1 Dl1.72 Decreases MCF-7 ER$^+$ Breast Cancer Cell Proliferation, Migration and Mammosphere Formation

We have shown that siRNA-mediated DLL1 downregulation decreases MCF-7 cell proliferation and migration, whereas incubation with DLL1 increases them [18]. Following the findings described above, showing that Dl1.72 impairs DLL1-Notch signaling in MCF-7 cells, we next evaluated the Dl1.72 ability to impair DLL1-induced MCF-7 cell proliferation, using the MTT assay and trypan blue exclusion methods. In agreement with our previous results [18], MCF-7 cells exposed to DLL1 alone or in the presence of Ctr Ab or DMSO showed a significant increase in cell growth (45% and 100% increase by MTT and trypan blue exclusion, respectively) compared to control cells or cells treated with Fc control protein. In contrast, treatment with Dl1.72 mAb reduced MCF-7 cell growth induced by DLL1 by approximately 50% (Figure 3a,b). DLL1-induced cell growth was partially inhibited by DAPT (Figure 3a,b). Dl1.72 also delayed the proliferation of unstimulated cells by 25% on average compared to control cells, as determined by trypan blue exclusion by microscopy (Figure 3c). The reduction was comparable with that obtained with DAPT. Trypan blue exclusion showed similar low levels of non-viable cells in all tested conditions, suggesting that Dl1.72 indeed impaired cell proliferation.

The ability of Dl1.72 to impair MCF-7 migratory capability was assessed in scratch wound-healing assays. Dl1.72 resulted in a significant delay in wound closure in MCF-7 cells (20% reduction on average) compared to control cells not treated or treated with Ctr Ab (Figure 3d,e), suggesting that this mAb impairs MCF-7 cell migration.

Breast cancer stem cells (BCSCs), which have tumor initiation potential, have emerged as drivers of tumor chemoresistance, recurrence and metastasis in BC [33–35]. Given that DLL1-Notch signaling in ER$^+$ BCs promotes BCSC function [17], we next examined the potential of Dl1.72 to influence the BCSC subpopulation of MCF-7 cells. To assess this, we employed the mammosphere (MS) formation assay, a functional 3D-BCSC cell culture-based assay commonly used to evaluate in vitro the amount of BCSC within a heterogeneous cell population [36]. The amount of MS formed correlates with the content of BCSCs. The results obtained in these assays showed that Dl1.72 impaired the number of the MS formed by approximately 30% and 38% compared to control cells not treated or treated with Ctr Ab, respectively (Figure 3f,g). The effect was comparable to that obtained with DAPT. To confirm that MS resulted from the expansion of the BCSC subpopulation, we evaluated the expression levels of the stemness-related genes *SOX2* and *SOX9*, involved in the maintenance and expansion of BCSCs [34,35], in the formed MS and in the original MCF-7 cells growing in parallel as 2D monolayers. As compared to the parental cells cultured in 2D, MS presented three- and nine-fold increased levels of *SOX2* and *SOX9*, respectively (Figure S3a), similar to what was reported previously [34,35].

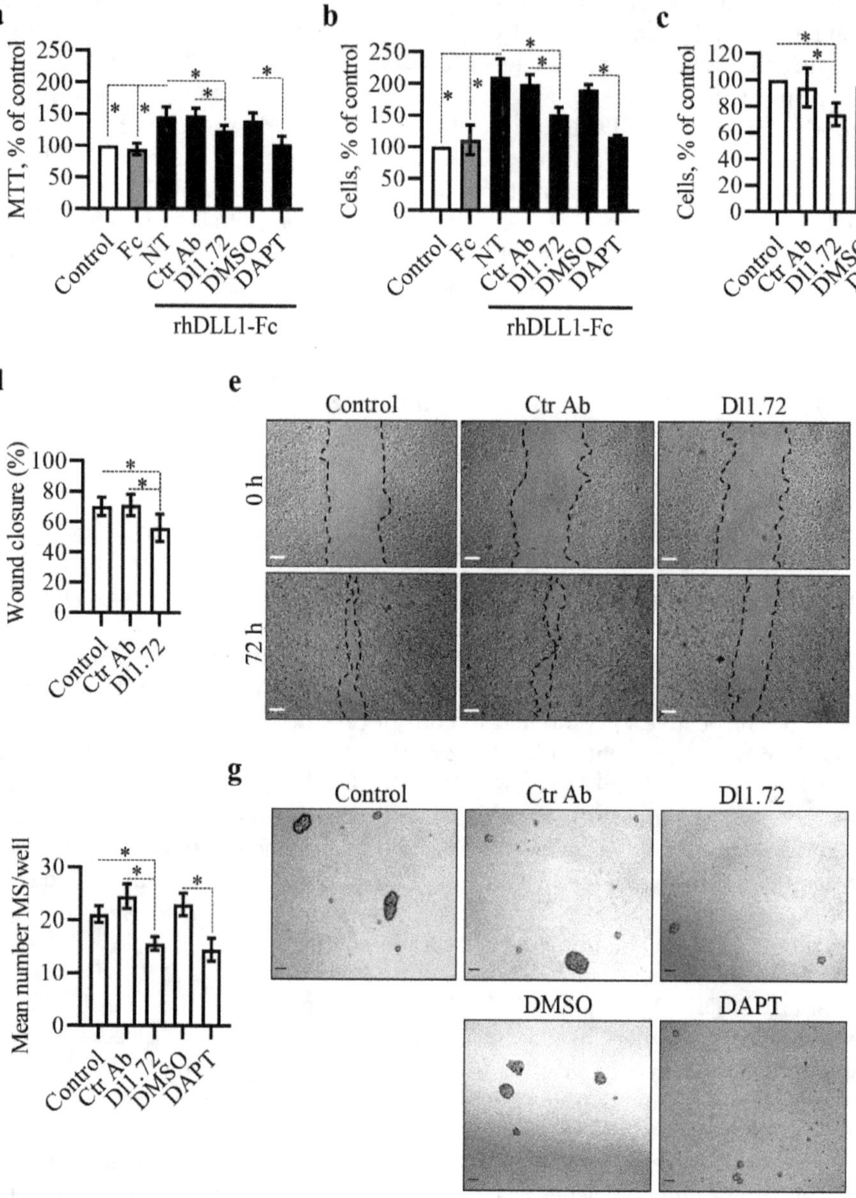

Figure 3. Anti-DLL1 Dl1.72 impairs MCF-7 cell proliferation, migration and mammosphere formation. (**a**,**b**) Effect of Dl1.72 in MCF-7 cell proliferation induced by DLL1. Cells were cultured in uncoated wells (control) or wells coated with Fc or rhDLL1-Fc proteins in the absence (NT) or presence of Dl1.72, Ctr Ab (10 µg/mL), DAPT or DMSO, and cell growth was analyzed after 72 h by the (**a**) MTT method and (**b**) trypan blue exclusion microscopy. Values were calculated as percentages relative to those obtained in control cells. The graphs represent mean percentage (±SD, $n = 4$). (**c**) Effect of Dl1.72 on cell proliferation in the absence of DLL1-induced proliferation. At 16 h following seeding, cells were left untreated or treated, as indicated above, and cell growth was analyzed after 72 h by trypan blue exclusion microscopy. The graph shows the mean percentage (±SD, $n = 6$) of cells relative to control untreated cells. (**d**,**e**) MCF-7 cells seeded and treated as in (**c**) were scratched at 90% confluence, and wound closure was evaluated by microscopy. (**d**) Mean percentage values (±SD, $n = 3$) of wound closure at 72 h after wounding. (**e**) Representative images taken at the indicated times post-wounding from the three independent experiments. Scale bars, 200 µm. (**f**,**g**) Effect of Dl1.72 on MCF-7 BCSC population. Single cell suspensions were plated in mammosphere (MS) formation medium in ultra-low attachment plates and not treated (control) or treated as in (**c**). (**f**) Graph shows mean number (±SD, $n = 5$) of MS after 5 days of culture. (**g**) Representative images from experiments. Scale bars, 50 µm. *, $p < 0.05$ (two-tailed paired Student *t*-test).

Next, we investigated whether DLL1 has a role in *SOX2* or *SOX9* expression. MCF-7 cells plated in rhDLL1-Fc coated plates showed a clear increase in *SOX9* (five-fold induction on average) but not *SOX2*, when compared to control cells not treated or treated with Fc control protein (Figure S3b). We further confirmed these results by challenging DLL1-exposed MCF-7 cells to Dl1.72 and DAPT. In line with an impairment of DLL1-Notch signaling (Figure 2), Dl1.72 reduced the expression levels of *SOX9* induction by DLL1 by approximately 55% when compared to untreated control cells or cells exposed to the same concentration of Ctr Ab (Figure S3c). Inhibition of Notch signaling with DAPT nearly eliminated DLL1-induced *SOX9* expression (Figure S3c). To our knowledge, this is the first report showing that the DLL1 Notch mediates *SOX9* expression in BC cells.

Overall, these results indicate that anti-DLL1 Dl1.72 can impair oncogenic features of ER^+ BC MCF-7 cells, such as cell proliferation, migration and the maintenance of the BCSC subpopulation, possibly through *SOX9* modulation.

3.4. Anti-DLL1 Dl1.72 Impairs the Angiogenic Potential of Human Vascular Endothelial Cells

Previous studies have shown that DLL1 plays a critical role in tumor angiogenesis [17,37]. We therefore investigated whether Dl1.72 exerts anti-angiogenic effects. For this, we used the HUVEC tube formation assay, a rapid and quantitative in vitro method that measures the ability of vascular endothelial cells to form capillary-like structures on an extracellular matrix substrate widely used as a screening assay for angiogenic or anti-angiogenic agents [38]. Our results showed that Dl1.72 treatment impaired the pro-angiogenic potential of HUVEC cells, in comparison to control cells not treated or treated with Ctr Ab, as evidenced by a significant reduction in the number of capillary-like structures (total branching length and meshes/cavities) as well as the number of nodes (Figure 4a–d). DAPT severely affected the tube network performance of HUVEC cells (Figure 4a–d). To further confirm these findings, we aimed to exclude the possibility that the in vitro anti-angiogenic effects were caused by a Dl1.72-induced reduction in HUVEC cell proliferation and viability. Assessment of cell proliferation and viability in these assays showed that Dl1.72 treatment had no effect on these biological functions of HUVEC cells (Figure 4e,f). Moreover, analysis of the mRNA levels of *HEY-1* and *HEY-L* in HUVEC cells showed that Dl1.72 significantly reduced the levels of *HEY-L* (50% reduction, on average), compared to the untreated control cells or cells treated with Ctr Ab, but not the levels of *HEY-1*. DAPT reduced *HEY-L* and *HEY-1* levels by approximately 60% and 30%, respectively (Figure 4g). Of note, *HEY-L* has been shown to promote tumor angiogenesis [39].

Altogether, these results show that anti-DLL1 Dl1.72 impairs Notch signaling in HUVEC cells and suggest it has antiangiogenic activity, without affecting HUVEC viability.

3.5. Anti-DLL1 Dl1.72 Inhibits Tumor Growth in a MCF-7 ER^+ Breast Cancer Xenograft Mice Model

We next investigated in vivo the ability of Dl1.72 to inhibit tumor growth of human ER^+ BC in a MCF-7 xenograft mice model, to address the tumorigenic role of DLL1 in human BCs [17] (Figure 5a). Treatment with Dl1.72 significantly impaired tumor growth (Figure 5b–d). Analysis of the largest tumor cross-sections stained with the pan-cytokeratin AE1/AE3 antibody, an epithelial cell marker that stains MCF-7 tumor cells, confirmed a significant decrease in tumor sizes in mice treated with Dl1.72 (Figure 5e,f). Histological analysis showed that tumors from control mice treated with PBS or Ctr Ab presented more necrotic areas within the tumor when compared to mice treated with Dl1.72 and were more prone to invade adjacent tissues, such as muscle and fat, than tumors treated with Dl1.72 (Figure 5g, upper panels). Conversely, there was more fibro-fatty infiltration of the tumor regions in mice treated with Dl1.72 (Figure 5g, lower panels). No body weight loss (Figure S4a) or signs of animal distress were observed. Organ function analysis using measurement of the levels of ALT, urea and creatinine in the sera of these mice showed similar levels of these parameters among all groups (Figure S4b). Consistent with these results, histological analysis of liver and kidney sections from mice treated with Dl1.72,

PBS or Ctr Ab showed no signs of tissue damage (Figure S4c). The inhibition of tumor growth of MCF-7 xenografts by Dl1.72 and its safety profile were validated in a second in vivo assay (Figure S5). Collectively, these results show that anti-DLL1 Dl1.72 inhibits tumor growth and is well tolerated.

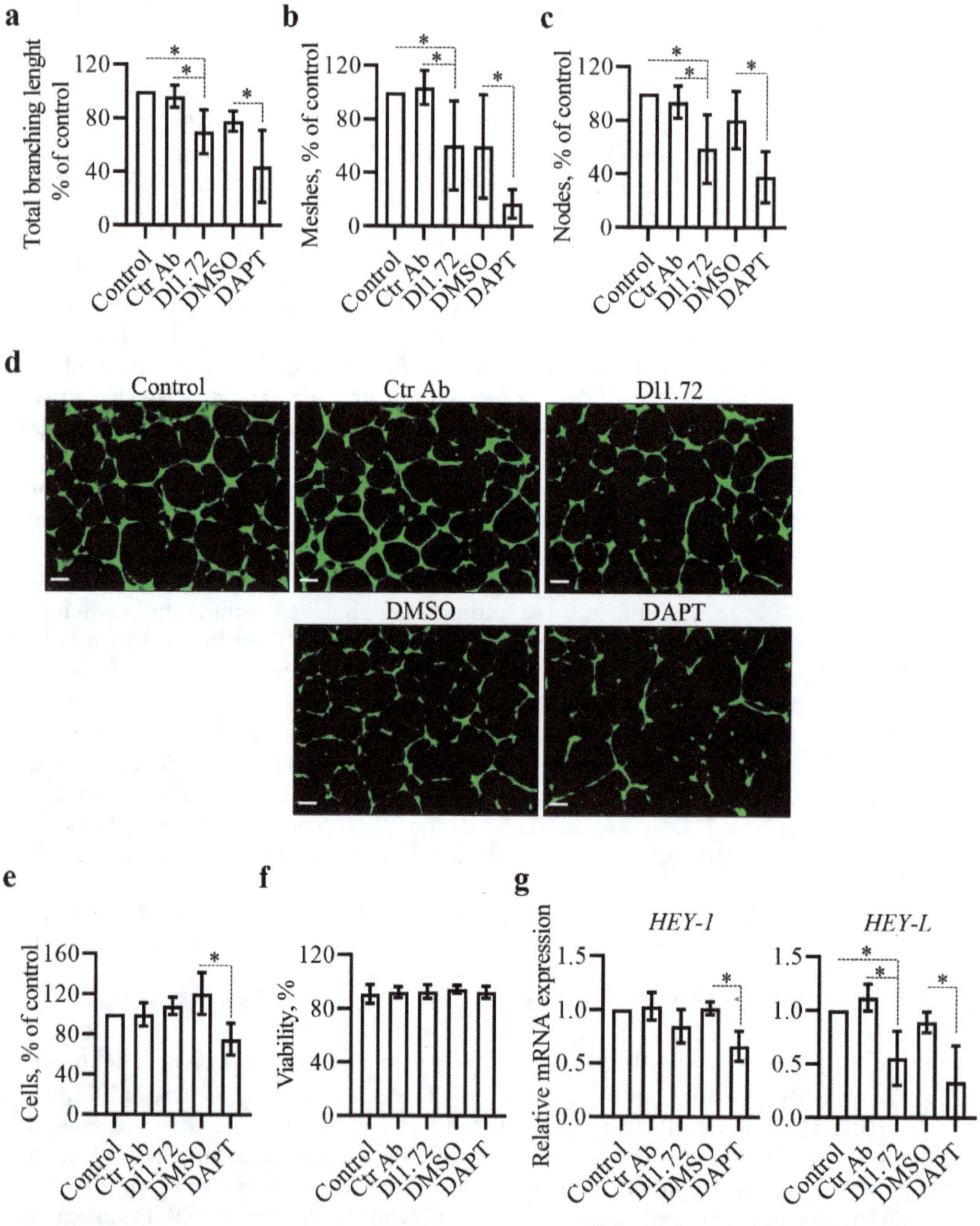

Figure 4. Anti-DLL1 Dl1.72 impairs the angiogenic potential of HUVEC cells. HUVEC cells were cultured in the absence (control) or presence of Dl1.72, Ctr Ab (10 µg/mL each), DAPT or DMSO for 70–76 h until 80% confluence, collected and plated on matrigel or geltrex to evaluate (**a–d**) HUVEC tube-network forming ability performance. The graphs in (**a–c**) show mean percentage values (±SD, $n = 6$) of total branching length, meshes/cavities, and nodes. (**d**) Representative images of calcein-stained cells. Scale bars, 200 µm. Mean percentage of (**e**) cells and (**f**) viability relative to control untreated cells (±SD) from five independent assays performed as described above. (**g**) Gene expression profile of Notch-target genes *HEY-1* and *HEY-L* in HUVEC cells treated as above was determined by RT-qPCR. Graphs show mean mRNA fold change relative to control cells (±SD, $n = 4$). *, $p < 0.05$ (two-tailed paired Student *t*-test).

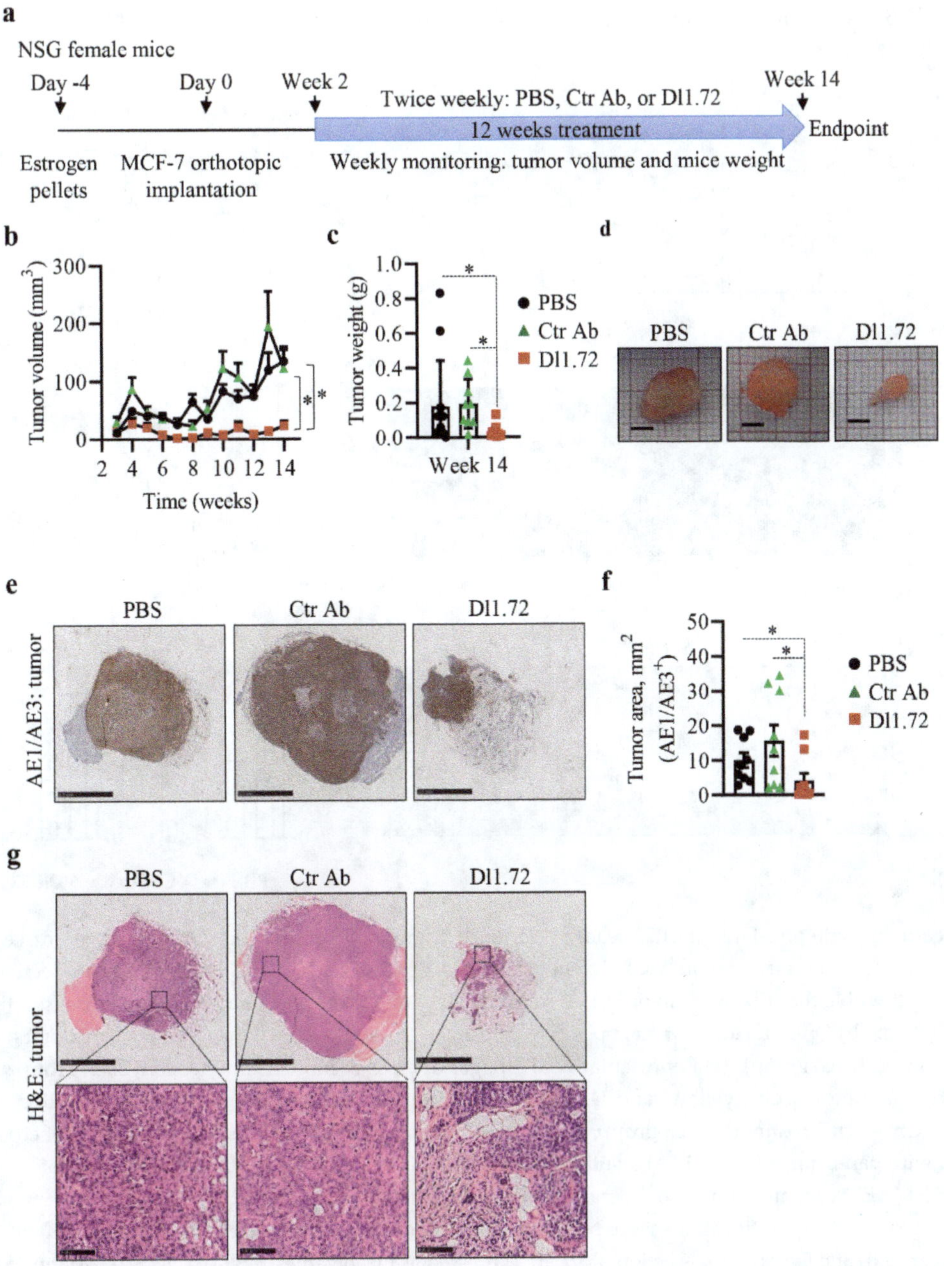

Figure 5. Anti-DLL1 Dl1.72 decreases tumor growth in a MCF-7 xenograft mice model. (**a**) Schematic representation of mice tumor induction and treatment with either PBS (control vehicle) or with 10 mg per kg of isotype-matched Ctr Ab or Dl1.72 for 12 weeks. (**b**) Tumor growth was evaluated by caliper (PBS, $n = 12$; Ctr Ab, $n = 9$; Dl1.72, $n = 10$). (**c**) Weight of tumors from each group immediately after resection. (**d**) Representative whole tumor images from each group. (**e**) Representative IHC images of the largest cross-sections of tumors from each group stained with the pan-cytokeratin AE1/AE3 Ab, specific to human epithelial cells. Scale bars, 2.5 mm. (**f**) Quantification of tumor area determined by AE1/AE3 staining ($n = 9$ tumors/group). (**g**) Representative hematoxylin and eosin (H&E) stained images of tumor cross-sections of each group. Scale bars, 2.5 mm (top image) and 100 µm (bottom image). Data are expressed as mean values ± SEM. *, $p < 0.05$ by one-way ANOVA with Tukey's multiple comparisons test in (**a**) and the Mann–Whitney test in (**c**,**f**).

Since DLL1 promotes tumor cell proliferation [17], and Dl1.72 decreases MCF-7 cell proliferation in vitro (Figure 3a–c), we assessed tumor cell proliferation in tumor sections stained with Ki67 antibody. Our results showed that tumors from mice treated with Dl1.72 presented a significant decrease of proliferating tumor cells (approximately 60% reduction of Ki67$^+$ cells) in comparison to tumors from control mice treated with PBS or Ctr Ab (Figure 6a,b).

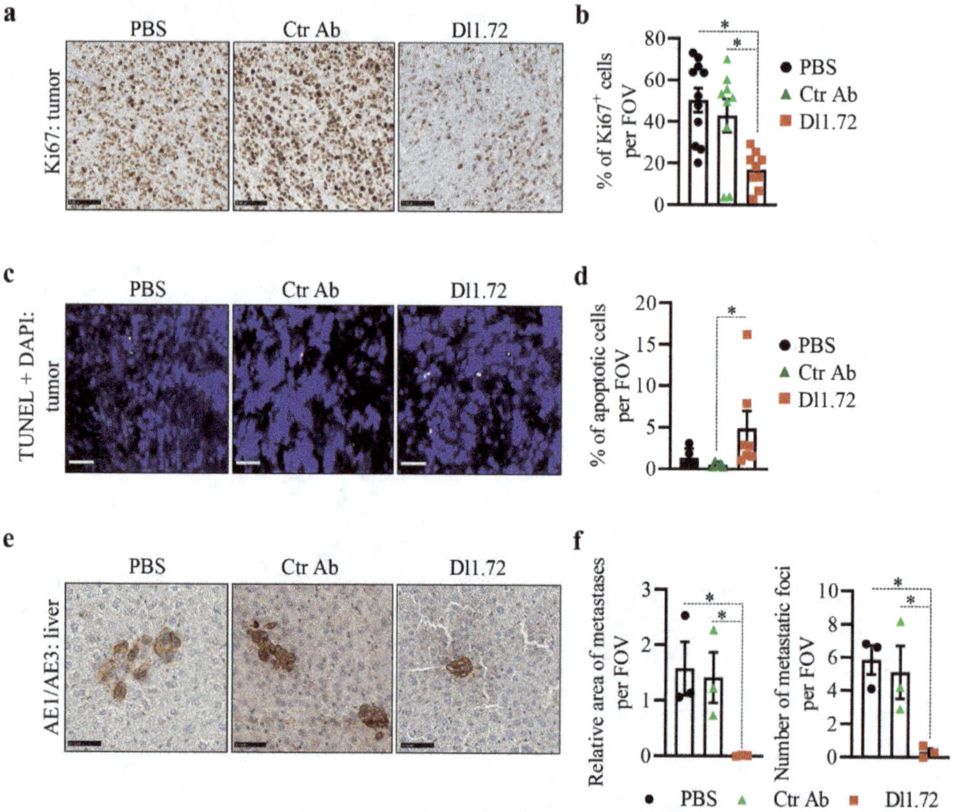

Figure 6. Treatment with anti-DLL1 Dl1.72 leads to reduced tumor cell proliferation, increased tumor cell apoptosis and impaired liver micrometastases in MCF-7 xenografts. (**a**) Representative IHC images of cross-sectioned tumors from mice treated with either PBS, Ctr Ab or Dl1.72 twice weekly for 12 weeks stained with Ki67 (proliferation marker). Scale bars, 100 μm. (**b**) Quantification of Ki67 positive cells from the stained sections (PBS, n = 11 tumors; Ctr Ab and Dl1.72, n = 9 tumors/each group). (**c**) Representative IF images of cross-sectioned tumors from each group stained with TUNEL method (apoptotic cells, yellow) and DAPI (nuclei, blue). Scale bars, 50 μm. (**d**) Quantification of apoptotic cells (PBS and Ctr Ab, n = 5 tumors/each group; Dl1.72, n = 7 tumors). (**e**) IHC representative images of cross-sectioned livers stained with pan-cytokeratin AE1/AE3 antibody. Scale bars, 100 μm. (**f**) Quantification of liver relative areas (mm^2) occupied by AE1/AE3$^+$ cells and number of liver micrometastatic foci (i.e., number of AE1/AE3$^+$ areas) of indicated groups (n = 3 tumors/group). All quantifications were performed in ten random fields of view (FOVs) at 10x magnified images from each tumor (**b**,**d**) and liver (**f**) cross-section. Data are expressed as mean values ± SEM. *, $p < 0.05$ (Mann–Whitney test).

The observation that DLL1 downregulation induces apoptosis of MCF-7 cells [18] prompted us to next evaluate apoptosis in tumor sections, using the TUNEL method. We verified that 12 weeks after the initiation of the treatments, tumors from mice treated with Dl1.72 showed a significant increase in the percentage of apoptotic cells compared to tumors from control mice that received PBS or Ctr Ab (Figure 6c,d), even though these events were not very frequent (mean 5% apoptotic cells/field in Dl1.72 tumors from treated mice).

Histological analysis of H&E-stained livers suggested the presence of tumor cell micrometastasis in control mice treated with PBS and Ctr Ab but not in mice treated with Dl1.72 mAb. To determine if this was the case, the presence of liver metastases was then evaluated by IHC in mouse liver sections stained with AE1/AE3 antibody. These results showed that Dl1.72 treatment significantly reduced liver metastasis, as determined by the number of metastatic foci and area of metastasis, when compared to livers from mice treated with PBS or Ctr Ab (Figure 6e,f and Figure S6), suggesting Dl1.72 has the capacity to reduce metastasis of ER$^+$ BCs.

Collectively, our results show that anti-DLL1 Dl1.72 mAb is effective in inhibiting ER^+ tumor growth and metastases.

4. Discussion

Notch signaling is a well-established oncogenic player in BC [13], and its ligand DLL1 has been shown to be overexpressed in BC tumors. Moreover, recent studies have demonstrated that it is involved in tumor progression, metastasis, chemoresistance, and poor patient survival in ER^+ BCs [16–18,20,40]. Given the relevance of Notch signaling components in multiple aspects of BC biology, various strategies have been pursued to develop therapeutic agents to block the Notch signaling pathway in BC [41]. Gamma-secretase inhibitors (GSIs), small compounds that prevent the release of the NICD [10], were the first and most extensively explored inhibitors of the Notch pathway. While extensive clinical testing showed GSIs have anti-tumor efficacy, these induce severe gastrointestinal tract toxicity in patients, likely due to complete Notch signaling inhibition, limiting their therapeutic benefits [41]. These results demonstrated the need for a specific targeted approach, for example by using anti-Notch signaling component Abs. Over the last decade, Abs have become an important component in the arsenal of cancer therapeutics [42]. Antibodies targeting individual Notch receptors and ligands (i.e., JAG1, DLL4) have been developed, showing anti-tumor efficacy against different types of cancers in preclinical studies, with manageable toxicity profiles [41,43–48]. The ER^+ BC is the most common BC subtype and is treated with anti-estrogenic drugs such as tamoxifen and fulvestrant, presenting a good prognosis. However, a large proportion of ER^+ BCs develop endocrine resistance, leading to treatment failure, tumor recurrence and eventually metastasis, which dramatically decreases life expectancy [5]. Motivated by these observations and the accumulating evidence suggesting DLL1 drives ER^+ BC pathogenesis and aggressiveness, we developed specific DLL1 targeting mAbs, which could show activity against this type of BC.

Here we report the development and characterization of Dl1.72, a novel anti-DLL1 mAb selected by phage display. This mAb binds to DLL1 protein with a calculated kinetic affinity of 4.78 nM, but not to the other human ligands of the Notch pathway, and recognizes cellular DLL1 in DLL1-overexpressing cells and ER^+ BC tumor tissues. Dl1.72 is able to inhibit Notch signaling in MCF-7 ER^+ BC and HUVEC cells. Moreover, in vitro studies using MCF-7 cells showed that Dl1.72 reduced their cell proliferation and wound closure capacities. These results are in line with our previous data showing that DLL1 promotes MCF-7 proliferation and migration [18]. It is likely that the wound healing impairment by Dl1.72 is due mostly to reduced cell proliferation, given the low migration capacity of these cells [18,49]. Importantly, treatment with Dl1.72 reduced MCF-7 MS forming ability, suggesting that it may be able to reduce the BCSC subpopulation of MCF-7 cells. This finding is in accordance with the enrichment of DLL1 in BCSCs [20] and the reduction of BCSC number and function in ER^+ BC cells upon the loss of DLL1 [17] and Notch signaling blockade [46]. This is particularly relevant since BCSCs, which have tumor initiation potential, have emerged as drivers of tumor chemoresistance, recurrence and metastasis in BC [33,40]. Interestingly, we also found that Dl1.72 reduced the expression of *SOX9*, driven by DLL1. *SOX9* expression was induced in the MCF-7 MS in our assays, compared to cells growing in 2D, and it was reported to be involved in BC stemness induction as well as playing various pro-oncogenic roles in BC, including in the ER^+ subtype [34,50]. Based on these observations, it is tempting to speculate that Dl1.72 anti-BCSC activity in MCF-7 cells involves the regulation of *SOX9*. However, this needs to be properly assessed in future studies. Data showing that $DLL1^+$ BC tumor cells display CSC characteristics [20], together with our findings showing that DLL1 controls the expression of *SOX9*, supports the importance of these studies, which may provide additional insights into the mechanisms underlying DLL1's key oncogenic role in BC. *SOX9* is a direct target of Notch signaling [50] and is regulated by DLL1 in other cell types such as pancreatic cells [51], but to our knowledge no previous information is available on the specific role of DLL1 in *SOX9* expression in the context of BC.

DLL1 was previously shown to be involved in BC angiogenesis [17]. As such, we explored the possibility that Dl1.72 mAb could inhibit angiogenesis. Using HUVEC cells as a model, we found that inhibition of the Notch-dependent gene *HEY-L* by Dl1.72 mAb was associated with the reduction of their angiogenic potential. Strikingly, the reduction in angiogenesis potential in vitro by Dl1.72 mAb was not accompanied by an increased cell cytotoxicity, which clearly points to a potential anti-angiogenic effect and is not related to the reduction in cell viability/increased HUVEC cell cytotoxicity. These results are consistent with a role of DLL1-Notch signaling in the promotion of angiogenesis [17,37]. Considering the reported angiogenic role of *HEY-L* in BC [39], our results may suggest a potential link between *HEY-L* downregulation by Dl1.72 and its anti-angiogenic potential, which should be assessed by future studies.

In vivo studies demonstrated that Dl1.72 mAb severely impaired tumor growth of MCF-7 xenografts without detectable associated side effects. Tumor growth inhibition by Dl1.72 was significantly associated with reduction of tumor cell proliferation and apoptosis. These results are consistent with studies showing that DLL1 downregulation impairs tumor growth and tumor cell proliferation in xenografts [17] and MCF-7 proliferation and apoptosis [18], suggesting that decreased proliferation and induction of apoptosis accounted, at least partially, for the Dl1.72 anti-tumor effects. Moreover, our in vitro data showing that Dl1.72 has anti-BCSC activity and anti-angiogenic potential support the hypothesis that these effects of Dl1.72 can also contribute to its anti-tumor activity. It is important to point out that Dl1.72 recognizes murine DLL1, and that DLL1 is important for endothelial cell branching and sprouting [37]. Accordingly, it is conceivable that targeting murine DLL1, namely in the tumor microenvironment, could also account for the anti-tumorigenic effects herein observed in the MCF-7 xenograft mouse model. Importantly, in addition to tumor growth inhibition, we found that Dl1.72 mAb decreased the formation of liver metastases. Over 90% of deaths of BC patients are due to metastases, and liver metastases can potentially occur in aggressive ER^+ BCs, which are associated with decreased BC patient survival [5]. Considering the role of DLL1 cells in the regulation of BCSCs in ER^+ tumors [17] and recent findings showing $DLL1^+$ tumor cells confer chemoresistance to conventional therapy [20], our findings strengthen the interest in evaluating the anti-cancer potential of Dl1.72 mAb in aggressive metastatic models of ER^+ BC tumors to further evaluate its therapeutic potential, both as monotherapy or in combination with standard endocrine therapy.

5. Conclusions

In conclusion, the present study describes the development and characterization of a novel anti-DLL1 mAb with potent anti-tumor activity in an ER^+ BC mouse model, without detectable side effects. Given the growing body of evidence showing the crucial role of DLL1 in the aggressive phenotypes of this BC type and its association with high mortality in BC patients, Dl1.72 may prove to be a promising tool for clinical development of a treatment for patients with aggressive ER^+ BCs, as well as for drug-resistant ER^+ BCs.

Supplementary Materials: Figure S1: Binding of Dl1.72 to human ER^+ BC tumor samples by IHC, Figure S2: Dose-response effect of anti-DLL1 Dl1.72 in the expression levels of Notch-dependent genes induced by the ligand in MCF-7 cells, Figure S3: DLL1 induces the expression of the stemness-associated gene *SOX9* in MCF-7 cells and anti-DLL1 Dl1.72 impairs DLL1-mediated *SOX9* expression, Figure S4: Anti-DLL1 Dl1.72 toxicity and safety assessment in vivo, Figure S5: Second experiment to validate tumor growth inhibition by anti-DLL1 Dl1.72 in a MCF7 xenograft mice model, Figure S6: Anti-DLL1 Dl1.72 impairs the occurrence of BC liver micrometastases in a MCF-7 xenograft mice model, Table S1: Recombinant Notch ligands and control proteins used for plate coating in ELISA, Table S2: Primers used for transcript amplification, Table S3: Clinicopathological characteristics of breast cancer tissue samples obtained from the pathology department of Hospital Professor Doutor Fernando Fonseca (HFF).

Author Contributions: Conceptualization, G.S., J.S.-D., G.D., M.G.C., C.C., P.M.F.S., P.A.V., T.M.B. and A.B.; methodology, G.S., J.S.-D., S.A., G.D., C.B. (Clara Barreto), C.B. (Catarina Brito), M.G.C., D.C.B., P.M.F.S., P.A.V., T.M.B. and A.B.; software, C.B. (Clara Barreto); validation, G.S., M.G.C. and P.M.F.S.; formal analysis, G.S., J.S.-D., D.C., G.D., C.B. (Clara Barreto), C.M., A.R.L., A.T.M., K.K., A.F., M.R.M. and P.M.F.S.; investigation, G.S., J.S.-D., D.C., S.A., G.D., C.B. (Clara Barreto), C.M., A.R.L., A.T.M., K.K., A.F., M.R.M., C.C., P.M.F.S. and P.A.V.; resources, S.B.; writing—original draft preparation, G.S. and J.S.-D.; writing—review and editing, G.S., J.S.-D., G.D., C.C., D.C.B., P.M.F.S., P.A.V. and A.B.; visualization, G.S., J.S.-D., D.C., S.A., G.D., C.B. (Clara Barreto), C.M., A.T.M. and M.R.M.; supervision, G.S., T.M.B. and A.B.; project administration, G.S. and A.B.; funding acquisition, G.S., G.D. and A.B. All authors have read and agreed to the published version of the manuscript.

References

1. Siegel, R.L.; Mph, K.D.M.; Jemal, A. Cancer statistics, 2019. *CA Cancer J. Clin.* **2018**, *69*, 7–34. [CrossRef]
1. Bettaieb, A.; Paul, C.; Plenchette, S.; Shan, J.; Chouchane, L.; Ghiringhelli, F. Precision medicine in breast cancer: Reality or utopia? *J. Transl. Med.* **2017**, *15*, 1–13. [CrossRef] [PubMed]
2. Wu, Q.; Li, J.; Zhu, S.; Wu, J.; Chen, C.; Liu, Q.; Wei, W.; Zhang, Y.; Sun, S. Breast cancer subtypes predict the preferential site of distant metastases: A SEER based study. *Oncotarget* **2017**, *8*, 27990–27996. [CrossRef] [PubMed]
3. Patel, H.K.; Bihani, T. Selective estrogen receptor modulators (SERMs) and selective estrogen receptor degraders (SERDs) in cancer treatment. *Pharmacol. Ther.* **2017**, *186*, 1–24. [CrossRef] [PubMed]
4. Rueda, O.M.; Sammut, S.-J.; Seoane, J.A.; Chin, S.-F.; Caswell-Jin, J.; Callari, M.; Batra, R.; Pereira, B.; Bruna, A.; Ali, H.R.; et al. Dynamics of breast-cancer relapse reveal late-recurring ER-positive genomic subgroups. *Nat. Cell Biol.* **2019**, *567*, 399–404. [CrossRef]
5. Bai, J.-W.; Wei, M.; Li, J.-W.; Zhang, G.-J. Notch Signaling Pathway and Endocrine Resistance in Breast Cancer. *Front. Pharmacol.* **2020**, *11*, 924. [CrossRef] [PubMed]
6. Bray, S. Notch signalling in context. *Nat. Rev. Mol. Cell Biol.* **2016**, *17*, 722–735. [CrossRef]
7. Cordle, J.; Johnson, S.; Tay, J.Z.Y.; Roversi, P.; Wilkin, M.B.; De Madrid, B.H.; Shimizu, H.; Jensen, S.; Whiteman, P.; Jin, B.; et al. A conserved face of the Jagged/Serrate DSL domain is involved in Notch trans-activation and cis-inhibition. *Nat. Struct. Mol. Biol.* **2008**, *15*, 849–857. [CrossRef]
8. Kershaw, N.J.; Church, N.L.; Griffin, M.; Luo, C.S.; Adams, T.; Burgess, A.W. Notch ligand delta-like1: X-ray crystal structure and binding affinity. *Biochem. J.* **2015**, *468*, 159–166. [CrossRef]
9. Kopan, R.; Ilagan, M.X.G. The Canonical Notch Signaling Pathway: Unfolding the Activation Mechanism. *Cell* **2009**, *137*, 216–233. [CrossRef]
10. Nandagopal, N.; Santat, L.A.; LeBon, L.; Sprinzak, D.; Bronner, M.E.; Elowitz, M.B. Dynamic Ligand Discrimination in the Notch Signaling Pathway. *Cell* **2018**, *172*, 869–880.e19. [CrossRef] [PubMed]
11. Pece, S.; Serresi, M.; Santolini, E.; Capra, M.; Hulleman, E.; Galimberti, V.; Zurrida, S.; Maisonneuve, P.; Viale, G.; Di Fiore, P.P. Loss of negative regulation by Numb over Notch is relevant to human breast carcinogenesis. *J. Cell Biol.* **2004**, *167*, 215–221. [CrossRef] [PubMed]
12. Aster, J.C.; Pear, W.S.; Blacklow, S.C. The Varied Roles of Notch in Cancer. *Annu. Rev. Pathol. Mech. Dis.* **2017**, *12*, 245–275. [CrossRef] [PubMed]
13. Simões, B.M.; O'Brien, C.S.; Eyre, R.; Silva, A.; Yu, L.; Sarmiento-Castro, A.; Alférez, D.G.; Spence, K.; Santiago-Gómez, A.; Chemi, F.; et al. Anti-estrogen Resistance in Human Breast Tumors Is Driven by JAG1-NOTCH4-Dependent Cancer Stem Cell Activity. *Cell Rep.* **2015**, *12*, 1968–1977. [CrossRef] [PubMed]
14. Nandi, A.; Chakrabarti, R. The many facets of Notch signaling in breast cancer: Toward overcoming therapeutic resistance. *Genes Dev.* **2020**, *34*, 1422–1438. [CrossRef]
15. Mittal, S.; Subramanyam, D.; Dey, D.; Kumar, R.V.; Rangarajan, A. Cooperation of Notch and Ras/MAPK signaling pathways in human breast carcinogenesis. *Mol. Cancer* **2009**, *8*, 1–12. [CrossRef] [PubMed]
16. Kumar, S.; Srivastav, R.K.; Wilkes, D.W.; Ross, T.; Kim, S.; Kowalski, J.; Chatla, S.; Zhang, Q.; Nayak, A.; Guha, M.; et al. Estrogen-dependent DLL1-mediated Notch signaling promotes luminal breast cancer. *Oncogene* **2018**, *38*, 2092–2107. [CrossRef]
17. Dias, J.S.; Silva, G.; Lamy, M.; Ferreira, A.; Barbas, A. The Notch ligand DLL1 exerts carcinogenic features in human breast cancer cells. *PLoS ONE* **2019**, *14*, e0217002. [CrossRef]
18. Shui, Y.; Yu, X.; Duan, R.; Bao, Q.; Wu, J.; Yuan, H.; Ma, C. miR-130b-3p inhibits cell invasion and migration by targeting the Notch ligand Delta-like 1 in breast carcinoma. *Gene* **2017**, *609*, 80–87. [CrossRef] [PubMed]

19. Kumar, S.; Nandi, A.; Singh, S.; Regulapati, R.; Li, N.; Tobias, J.W.; Siebel, C.W.; Blanco, M.A.; Klein-Szanto, A.J.; Lengner, C.; et al. Dll1+ quiescent tumor stem cells drive chemoresistance in breast cancer through NF-κB survival pathway. *Nat. Commun.* **2021**, *12*, 1–13. [CrossRef]
20. Durocher, Y.; Perret, S.; Kamen, A. High-level and high-throughput recombinant protein production by transient transfection of suspension-growing human 293-EBNA1 cells. *Nucleic Acids Res.* **2002**, *30*, E9. [CrossRef] [PubMed]
21. Sales-Dias, J.; Ferreira, A.; Lamy, M.; Domenici, G.; Monteiro, S.M.; Pires, A.; Lemos, A.R.; Kucheryava, K.; Nobre, L.S.; Sousa, P.M.; et al. Development of antibodies against the notch ligand Delta-Like-1 by phage display with activity against breast cancer cells. *New Biotechnol.* **2021**, *64*, 17–26. [CrossRef]
22. Schindelin, J.; Arganda-Carreras, I.; Frise, E.; Kaynig, V.; Longair, M.; Pietzsch, T.; Preibisch, S.; Rueden, C.; Saalfeld, S.; Schmid, B.; et al. Fiji: An open-source platform for biological-image analysis. *Nat. Methods* **2012**, *9*, 676–682. [CrossRef] [PubMed]
23. Silva, G.; Aboussekhra, A. p16INK4A inhibits the pro-metastatic potentials of osteosarcoma cells through targeting the ERK pathway and TGF-β1. *Mol. Carcinog.* **2015**, *55*, 525–536. [CrossRef] [PubMed]
24. Silva, G.; Cardoso, B.A.; Belo, H.; Almeida, A.M. Vorinostat induces apoptosis and differentiation in myeloid malignancies: Genetic and molecular mechanisms. *PLoS ONE* **2013**, *8*, e53766. [CrossRef] [PubMed]
25. Carpentier, G. Angiogenesis Analyzer for ImageJ—A comparative morphometric analysis of "Endothelial Tube Formation Assay" and "Fibrin Bead Assay". *Sci. Rep.* **2012**, *10*, 11568. [CrossRef] [PubMed]
26. Chakrabarti, R.; Kang, Y. Transplantable Mouse Tumor Models of Breast Cancer Metastasis. *Methods Mol. Biol.* **2015**, *1267*, 367–380. [CrossRef]
27. Loureiro, L.R.; Sousa, D.P.; Ferreira, D.; Chai, W.; Lima, L.; Pereira, C.; Lopes, C.B.; Correia, V.G.; Silva, L.M.; Li, C.; et al. Novel monoclonal antibody L2A5 specifically targeting sialyl-Tn and short glycans terminated by alpha-2–6 sialic acids. *Sci. Rep.* **2018**, *8*, 1–16. [CrossRef] [PubMed]
28. Fischer, A.H.; Jacobson, K.A.; Rose, J.; Zeller, R. Hematoxylin and Eosin Staining of Tissue and Cell Sections. *Cold Spring Harb. Protoc.* **2008**, *2008*, pdb-prot4986. [CrossRef]
29. Casal, D.; Iria, I.; Ramalho, J.S.; Alves, S.; Mota-Silva, E.; Mascarenhas-Lemos, L.; Pontinha, C.; Guadalupe-Cabral, M.; Silva, J.; Ferraz-Oliveira, M.; et al. BD-2 and BD-3 increase skin flap survival in a model of ischemia and Pseudomonas aeruginosa infection. *Sci. Rep.* **2019**, *9*, 7854. [CrossRef]
30. Tuominen, V.J.; Ruotoistenmäki, S.; Viitanen, A.; Jumppanen, M.; Isola, J. ImmunoRatio: A publicly available web application for quantitative image analysis of estrogen receptor (ER), progesterone receptor (PR), and Ki-67. *Breast Cancer Res.* **2010**, *12*, 1–12. [CrossRef]
31. Yang, B.; Ma, C.; Chen, Z.; Yi, W.; McNutt, M.A.; Wang, Y.; Korteweg, C.; Gu, J. Correlation of Immunoglobulin G Expression and Histological Subtype and Stage in Breast Cancer. *PLoS ONE* **2013**, *8*, e58706. [CrossRef]
32. de Angelis, M.; Francescangeli, F.; Zeuner, A. Breast Cancer Stem Cells as Drivers of Tumor Chemoresistance, Dormancy and Relapse: New Challenges and Therapeutic Opportunities. *Cancers* **2019**, *11*, 1569. [CrossRef] [PubMed]
33. Domenici, G.; Aurrekoetxea-Rodríguez, I.; Simões, B.M.; Rábano, M.; Lee, S.Y.; Millán, J.S.; Comaills, V.; Oliemuller, E.; López- Ruiz, J.A.; Zabalza, I.; et al. A Sox2–Sox9 signalling axis maintains human breast luminal progenitor and breast cancer stem cells. *Oncogene* **2019**, *38*, 3151–3169. [CrossRef] [PubMed]
34. Piva, M.; Domenici, G.; Iriondo, O.; Rábano, M.; Simões, B.M.; Comaills, V.; Barredo, I.; López-Ruiz, J.A.; Zabalza, I.; Kypta, R.; et al. Sox2 promotes tamoxifen resistance in breast cancer cells. *EMBO Mol. Med.* **2013**, *6*, 66–79. [CrossRef]
35. Dontu, G.; Abdallah, W.M.; Foley, J.M.; Jackson, K.W.; Clarke, M.F.; Kawamura, M.J.; Wicha, M.S. In vitro propagation and transcriptional profiling of human mammary stem/progenitor cells. *Genes Dev.* **2003**, *17*, 1253–1270. [CrossRef]
36. Napp, L.C.; Augustynik, M.; Paesler, F.; Krishnasamy, K.; Woiterski, J.; Limbourg, A.; Bauersachs, J.; Drexler, H.; Noble, F.L.; Limbourg, F. Extrinsic Notch Ligand Delta-Like 1 Regulates Tip Cell Selection and Vascular Branching Morphogenesis. *Circ. Res.* **2012**, *110*, 530–535. [CrossRef]
37. DeCicco-Skinner, K.L.; Henry, G.; Cataisson, C.; Tabib, T.; Gwilliam, J.C.; Watson, N.J.; Bullwinkle, E.M.; Falkenburg, L.; O'Neill, R.C.; Morin, A.; et al. Endothelial Cell Tube Formation Assay for the In Vitro Study of Angiogenesis. *J. Vis. Exp.* **2014**, e51312. [CrossRef]
38. Han, L.; Korangath, P.; Nguyen, N.K.; Diehl, A.; Cho, S.; Teo, W.W.; Cope, L.; Gessler, M.; Romer, L.; Sukumar, S. HEYL Regulates Neoangiogenesis Through Overexpression in Both Breast Tumor Epithelium and Endothelium. *Front. Oncol.* **2021**, *10*. [CrossRef]
39. Mavingire, N.; Campbell, P.; Wooten, J.; Aja, J.; Davis, M.B.; Loaiza-Perez, A.; Brantley, E. Cancer stem cells: Culprits in endocrine resistance and racial disparities in breast cancer outcomes. *Cancer Lett.* **2020**, *500*, 64–74. [CrossRef]

40. Lamy, M.; Ferreira, A.; Dias, J.S.; Braga, S.; Silva, G.; Barbas, A. Notch-out for breast cancer therapies. *New Biotechnol.* **2017**, *39*, 215–221. [CrossRef]
41. Lu, R.-M.; Hwang, Y.-C.; Liu, I.-J.; Lee, C.-C.; Tsai, H.-Z.; Li, H.-J.; Wu, H.-C. Development of therapeutic antibodies for the treatment of diseases. *J. Biomed. Sci.* **2020**, *27*, 1–30. [CrossRef]
42. Hoey, T.; Yen, W.-C.; Axelrod, F.; Basi, J.; Donigian, L.; Dylla, S.; Fitch-Bruhns, M.; Lazetic, S.; Park, I.-K.; Sato, A.; et al. DLL4 Blockade Inhibits Tumor Growth and Reduces Tumor-Initiating Cell Frequency. *Cell Stem Cell* **2009**, *5*, 168–177. [CrossRef]
43. Zheng, H.; Bae, Y.; Kasimir-Bauer, S.; Tang, R.; Chen, J.; Ren, G.; Yuan, M.; Esposito, M.; Li, W.; Wei, Y.; et al. Therapeutic Antibody Targeting Tumor- and Osteoblastic Niche-Derived Jagged1 Sensitizes Bone Metastasis to Chemotherapy. *Cancer Cell* **2017**, *32*, 731–747.e6. [CrossRef]
44. Masiero, M.; Li, D.; Whiteman, P.; Bentley, C.; Greig, J.; Hassanali, T.; Watts, S.; Stribbling, S.; Yates, J.; Bealing, E.; et al. Development of Therapeutic Anti-JAGGED1 Antibodies for Cancer Therapy. *Mol. Cancer Ther.* **2019**, *18*, 2030–2042. [CrossRef]
45. Sharma, A.; Paranjape, A.N.; Rangarajan, A.; Dighe, R.R. A Monoclonal Antibody against Human Notch1 Ligand–Binding Domain Depletes Subpopulation of Putative Breast Cancer Stem–like Cells. *Mol. Cancer Ther.* **2011**, *11*, 77–86. [CrossRef]
46. Qiu, M.; Peng, Q.; Jiang, I.; Carroll, C.; Han, G.; Rymer, I.; Lippincott, J.; Zachwieja, J.; Gajiwala, K.; Kraynov, E.; et al. Specific inhibition of Notch1 signaling enhances the antitumor efficacy of chemotherapy in triple negative breast cancer through reduction of cancer stem cells. *Cancer Lett.* **2013**, *328*, 261–270. [CrossRef] [PubMed]
47. Coleman, R.L.; Handley, K.F.; Burger, R.; Molin, G.Z.D.; Stagg, R.; Sood, A.K.; Moore, K.N. Demcizumab combined with paclitaxel for platinum-resistant ovarian, primary peritoneal, and fallopian tube cancer: The SIERRA open-label phase Ib trial. *Gynecol. Oncol.* **2020**, *157*, 386–391. [CrossRef] [PubMed]
48. Phannasil, P.; Thuwajit, C.; Warnnissorn, M.; Wallace, J.C.; Macdonald, M.J.; Jitrapakdee, S. Pyruvate Carboxylase Is Up-Regulated in Breast Cancer and Essential to Support Growth and Invasion of MDA-MB-231 Cells. *PLoS ONE* **2015**, *10*, e0129848. [CrossRef] [PubMed]
49. Jana, S.; Krishna, B.M.; Singhal, J.; Horne, D.; Awasthi, S.; Salgia, R.; Singhal, S.S. SOX9: The master regulator of cell fate in breast cancer. *Biochem. Pharmacol.* **2020**, *174*, 113789. [CrossRef]
50. Nakano, Y.; Negishi, N.; Gocho, S.; Mine, T.; Sakurai, Y.; Yazawa, M.; Abe, K.; Yagita, H.; Habu, S.; Kageyama, R.; et al. Disappearance of centroacinar cells in the Notch ligand-deficient pancreas. *Genes Cells* **2015**, *20*, 500–511. [CrossRef] [PubMed]

11

Predictors of Sentinel Lymph Node Metastasis in Postoperatively Upgraded Invasive Breast Carcinoma Patients

Chi-Chang Yu [1], Yun-Chung Cheung [2], Chuen Hsueh [3] and Shin-Cheh Chen [1,*]

1 Department of General Surgery, Chang Gung Memorial Hospital at Linkou, Chang Gung University, Taoyuan 333, Taiwan; kenneth0609@cgmh.org.tw
2 Department of Diagnostic Radiology, Chang Gung Memorial Hospital at Linkou, Chang Gung University, Taoyuan 333, Taiwan; alex2143@cgmh.org.tw
3 Department of Pathology, Chang Gung Memorial Hospital at Linkou, Chang Gung University, Taoyuan 333, Taiwan; ch9211@cgmh.org.tw
* Correspondence: chensc@adm.cgmh.org.tw;

Simple Summary: Routine sentinel lymph node (SLN) biopsy (SLNB) is not necessary for breast-conserving surgery (BCS)-treated ductal carcinoma in situ (DCIS) but is indicated for underestimated invasive carcinoma (IC) postoperatively. In this retrospective study, we aimed to investigate the factors contributing to SLN metastasis in underestimated IC patients with an initial diagnosis of DCIS by core needle biopsy. We found that only the features related to IC, including an IC tumor size (>0.5 cm) and the presence of LVI, could be used as risk predictors of SLN metastasis. In the absence of any predictors, the incidence of positive SLNs was very low (2.6%) in the total population and extremely low (1.3%) in the BCS subgroup. Therefore, we suggest that SLNB may be omitted in patients who initially underwent BCS without risk predictors on final pathological assessment. However, further prospective studies are warranted before its clinical application.

Abstract: Sentinel lymph node (SLN) biopsy (SLNB) usually need not be simultaneously performed with breast-conserving surgery (BCS) for patients diagnosed with ductal carcinoma in situ (DCIS) by preoperative core needle biopsy (CNB), but must be performed once there is invasive carcinoma (IC) found postoperatively. This study aimed to investigate the factors contributing to SLN metastasis in underestimated IC patients with an initial diagnosis of DCIS by CNB. We retrospectively reviewed 1240 consecutive cases of DCIS by image-guided CNB from January 2010 to December 2017 and identified 316 underestimated IC cases with SLNB. Data on clinical characteristics, radiologic features, and final pathological findings were examined. Twenty-three patients (7.3%) had SLN metastasis. Multivariate analysis indicated that an IC tumor size > 0.5 cm (odds ratio: 3.11, $p = 0.033$) and the presence of lymphovascular invasion (odds ratio: 32.85, $p < 0.0001$) were independent risk predictors of SLN metastasis. In the absence of any predictors, the incidence of positive SLNs was very low (2.6%) in the total population and extremely low (1.3%) in the BCS subgroup. Therefore, omitting SLNB may be an acceptable option for patients who initially underwent BCS without risk predictors on final pathological assessment. Further prospective studies are necessary before clinical application.

Keywords: breast cancer; ductal carcinoma in situ; underestimation; sentinel lymph node biopsy

---

1. Introduction

For patients with a suspicious lesion on breast imaging, the suggested initial diagnostic procedure is imaged-guided percutaneous biopsy rather than surgical biopsy, unless image-guided biopsy is not feasible [1]. Among the various biopsy results, ductal carcinoma in situ (DCIS) accounts for approximately 20% of the newly diagnosed breast cancers [2]. DCIS is a non-invasive breast cancer that occurs within the basement membrane and is defined as no contact with lymphatic vessels. Therefore, pure DCIS is thought to have no theoretical potential for regional lymph node metastasis. Nonetheless, the upgrading rate of DCIS to invasive breast carcinoma (IBC) at final postoperative pathology, initially diagnosed by preoperative percutaneous biopsy, is approximately 23–30% [3]. Associated risk factors for the underestimation of IBC include the biopsy device and guidance method, lesion size on image, tumor grading, mammographic features, and palpable mass [3].

For the diagnosis of lymph node stage in patients with early breast cancer and clinically negative axillary lymph nodes (ALNs), traditional ALN dissection [4–6] has been replaced by sentinel lymph node biopsy (SLNB) owing to its comparable accuracy, relative safety, and fewer complications. The reported incidence of sentinel lymph node (SLN) metastasis in patients with preoperative DCIS ranges from 0.9–15.6% [7–14]. Although several studies have analyzed the risk factors for subsequent SLN metastasis in patients with preoperative DCIS [7,9,12,14], no other clinicopathological findings or radiological features except for the IBC finding on final pathology, which was consistently confirmed as a factor related to SLN metastasis, were consistently identified by those studies.

According to the American Society of Clinical Oncology guidelines, for patients diagnosed with DCIS preoperatively, SLNB may be performed simultaneously with mastectomy, but it may not be performed for those who will undergo breast-conserving surgery (BCS) [4]. Most studies have discussed the incidence of SLN metastasis in patients diagnosed with DCIS preoperatively, later upgrading to IBC after surgery. These studies included a large number of cases of pure DCIS in the analysis of risk factors for SLN metastasis. Furthermore, the pathological characteristics are usually analyzed using specimens obtained by core needle biopsy (CNB) rather than complete specimens during surgery. However, insufficient tissue obtained by CNB is an important factor for lesions being underestimated as DCIS. In fact, a common clinical scenario is that the lesion is diagnosed as DCIS preoperatively and then diagnosed as IBC after BCS; therefore, SLNB should be subsequently performed following the current guidelines. Since the de-escalation of invasive axillary surgery in clinically node-negative patients with limited SLN metastases is a current trend [15,16]—and three prospective randomized trials, including SOUND, INSEMA, and BOOG13-084 are investigating whether SLNB can be avoided in early breast cancer patients treated with BCS [17–19]—it is necessary to consider whether SLNB is unavoidable for all patients with underestimated IBC diagnosed by CNB.

On the basis of these findings, what interested us was whether patients with underestimated IBC diagnosed by imaged-guided CNB must undergo subsequent SLNB examinations regardless of their objective conditions, especially for those who have undergone BCS. The primary objectives of this study were to determine the incidence of SLN metastasis in underestimated IBC patients with DCIS diagnosed by preoperative image-guided CNB and to identify specific clinical characteristics, radiologic features, and final pathological findings that could be predictors of SLN metastasis. A secondary objective was to identify patients who may be treatable without SLNB if the SLN metastasis rate is low.

2. Materials and Methods

2.1. Patients

We conducted a retrospective review of the electronic medical records in the database of the Department of Pathology at Chang Gung Memorial Hospital, collected between January 2010 and December 2017, and identified 1240 consecutive cases with a preoperative diagnosis of DCIS by image-guided CNB followed by subsequent surgery. The study was approved by the Institutional Review Board of Chang Gung Memorial Hospital, and the need for written informed consent was waived. A single breast cancer pathologist with 28 years of experience reviewed the 1240 CNB results. A total of 329 patients with IBC on the final pathology after subsequent surgery were identified. Nine patients with proven preoperative lymph node metastasis and four with no axillary staging were excluded. The details regarding the data selection are shown in Figure 1. A total of 316 underestimated IBC patients with preoperative DCIS diagnosed by image-guided CNB were finally included in the analysis. Data on clinical findings, patient demographics, radiologic findings, operation type, and pathological findings on final pathology of these cases were collected from the electronic database for analyses.

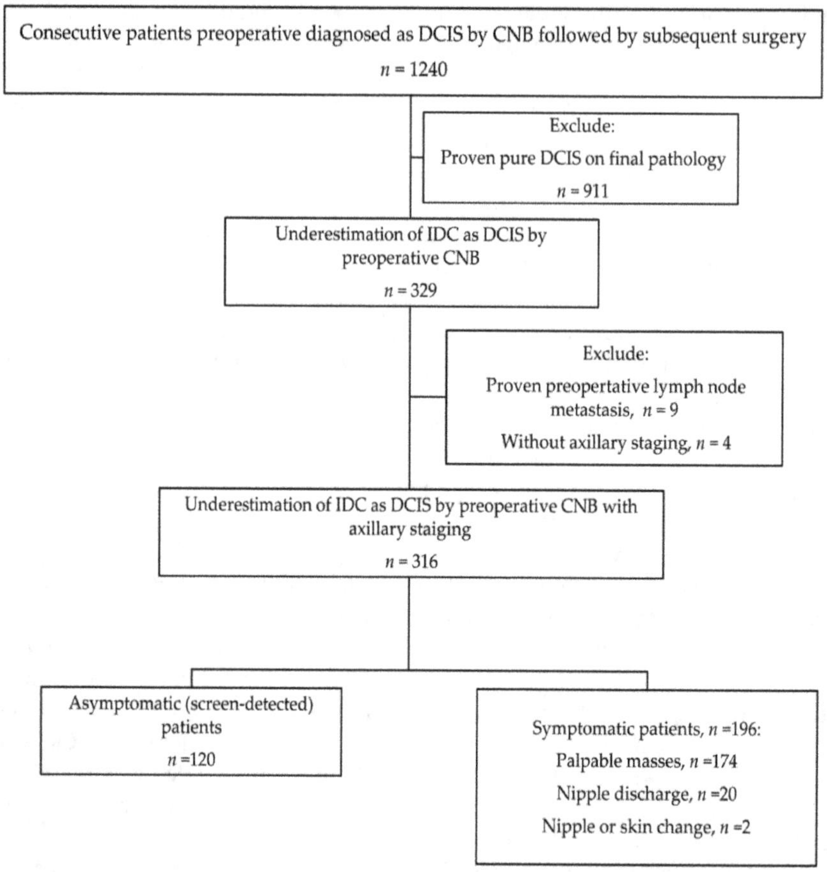

Figure 1. The flow diagram of the study. DCIS, ductal carcinoma in situ; CNB, core needle biopsy; IDC, invasive ductal carcinoma.

2.2. *Image-Guided Core Needle Biopsy Procedure*

Ultrasound-guided CNB was routinely performed for suspicious lesions to obtain a tissue diagnosis at our institution. Mammography-guided CNB was preserved for lesions that could only be detected on mammography. Therefore, ultrasound-guided CNB was performed in 275 patients (87.0%), and mammography-guided CNB was performed in 41 patients (13.0%). Ultrasound-guided CNB procedures were performed using a Bard Magnum (Covington, CA, USA) spring-loaded biopsy gun, with a 16-gauge biopsy needle in 267 (97.1%) cases and an 18-gauge biopsy needle in eight (2.9%) cases. Mammography-guided CNB procedures were conducted using mammography with an add-on unit (Lorad, Danbury, CT, USA), with the patient in either a sitting or lateral position, depending on the feasibility of localizing the lesions. Of the 41 mammography-guided CNB procedures, 38 (92.7%) were performed using vacuum-assisted biopsy devices (Vacora or Encor; Bard, Irvine, CA, USA), with a 7-gauge or 10-gauge biopsy needle, and three (7.3%) were performed using a Bard Magnum spring-loaded biopsy gun (Covington, CA, USA) with a 14-gauge biopsy needle. The median number of specimens obtained per lesion was 4 (range, 3–8) under ultrasound guidance and 12 (range, 3–20) under mammography guidance.

2.3. *Radiologic Features of Tumor*

Mammographic images of breast cancer were retrospectively reviewed on a high-resolution digital mammographic screen by a radiologist with 23 years of experience. Ultrasound images of breast cancer were retrospectively reviewed by a sonographer with

15 years of experience diagnosing breast cancer. Both mammography and ultrasound findings were classified according to the 5th edition of the Breast Imaging Reporting and Data System (BI-RADS) [20]. The interpretation of whether the lesion itself can be detected by mammography and/or breast ultrasound was determined by the radiologist and sonographer after discussion. In addition, breast cancer lesions were categorized into three morphologic groups based on mammography and ultrasound manifestations: mass with calcifications, mass without calcifications, and non-mass.

2.4. Surgical Procedure

Surgical management of breast cancer involves BCS or mastectomy. The choice of operation type is mainly based on the location, size of the tumor, and the patient's preference. Lymphatic mapping with sentinel lymph node identification was routinely performed using the radiocolloid technique, with subareolar or peritumor injection with technetium 99 m labeled sulfur colloid.

2.5. Pathological Assessment

SLNs and breast specimens were formalin-fixed, paraffin-embedded, and stained with hematoxylin and eosin (H&E). If no metastasis was detected with H&E staining for SLN analysis, immunohistochemical examination was performed using an anti-cytokeratin antibody. SLNs were classified as negative if they contained no tumor cells and positive if isolated tumor cells ($\leq$0.2 mm), micrometastases (>0.2 mm and $\leq$2 mm), or macrometastasis (>2 mm) were present.

The final pathological evaluation of resected breast specimens was reviewed to determine the histologic pattern, DCIS architecture pattern, DCIS and invasive ductal carcinoma (IDC) grade, number of foci of invasion, tumor size of DCIS and IDC, presence of tumor necrosis, presence of lymphovascular invasion (LVI), and immunohistochemistry (IHC) examinations of IBC (estrogen receptor [ER], progesterone receptor [PR], human epidermal growth factor receptor 2 [HER2], and Ki67 index). To identify LVI on H&E sections, we followed the criteria by Rosen PP [21]. First, we tended to focus more on peritumoral areas than intratumoral areas to look for LVI, since shrinkage artifacts resembling lymphatic channels often occurred in the latter. Secondly, true LVI usually did not conform to the shape of the space in which it was found. Thirdly, the space should be lined by endothelial cells to be qualified for a lymphatic channel. IHC stain is of great help in identifying a true lymphatic space and it has been suggested to be a supplementary study in the foregoing guidelines. The DCIS grade was classified as low, intermediate, or high according to the Van Nuys classification [22]. DCIS architecture patterns were classified according to their predominant microscopic growth pattern as comedo DCIS and non-comedo DCIS (including cribriform, solid, papillary, and micropapillary) [23]. Comedo necrosis is conventionally defined as a solid growth of pleomorphic tumor cells with high grade nuclei, central necrosis and sometimes active mitosis. However, there is no consensus regarding the size of the necrosis, which may occupy from 10% to 70% of the ductal diameter [24]. The best cutoff has been proposed to be 53% of the ductal diameter occupied by necrosis [25]. Although the interobserver variability of comedo necrosis is high, we still use the conventional definition to evaluate our cases because no general agreement on size has been established. All IBCs were graded according to the method of Elston and Ellis [26]. Positive ER and PR statuses were defined as tumors with 1% or more positively nuclear-stained cells [27]. HER2 status was considered negative when the IHC score was 0 or 1+. Fluorescence in situ hybridization (FISH) was mandatory in the case of a 2+ IHC score. HER2 positivity was defined as an IHC score of 3 (>10% of cells with strong intensity circumferential membrane staining) or FISH positivity. The cut-off point for Ki67 was 20%.

2.6. Statistical Analysis

To assess the association between the variables and the existence of positive SLN in the underestimation of IBC patients diagnosed with DCIS by an ultrasound- or mammography-guided CNB preoperatively, categorical variables were compared using Pearson's Chi-squared test, and continuous variables were assessed using the t-test. A logistic regression model was used for the multivariate analysis. Differences were considered statistically significant at $p \leq 0.05$. All statistical analyses were performed using the SPSS software (version 20.0; SPSS Inc., Chicago, IL, USA).

3. Results

3.1. Clinical Data

The clinicopathologic and radiologic findings are summarized in Table 1. All patients were female, and the median age of the patients was 53 years (range, 27–78 years). Thirty-one patients (9.8%) had a first-degree family history of breast cancer. Of the 316 tumors, 174 (55.1%) were clinically palpable, while the remaining 142 (44.9%) were not.

Table 1. Clinicopathologic findings and radiologic features of the entire cohort.

Variable	No. of Cases	%
Age (years), median (IQR)	53 (16)	
Lesion location		
Left breast	180	57.0
Right breast	136	43.0
First-degree family history of breast cancer		
Yes	31	9.8
No	285	90.2
Palpability		
Palpable	174	55.1
Non-palpable	142	44.9
Lesion-detecting imaging modality		
Ultrasonography only	44	13.9
Mammography only	36	11.4
Detected by both ultrasonography and mammography	236	74.7
Radiologic morphology		
Mass with calcifications	164	51.9
Mass without calcifications	85	26.9
Non-mass	67	21.2
Parenchymal density		
Entirely fatty	11	3.5
Scattered fibroglandular	52	16.5
Heterogeneously dense	179	56.6
Extremely dense	74	23.4
MMG-BI-RADS category		
0	49	15.5
1	6	1.9
2	26	8.2
4a	50	15.8
4b	71	22.5
4c	78	24.7
5	36	11.4
Ultrasound-BI-RADS category		
1	15	4.7
2	10	3.2
3	10	3.2
4a	82	25.9
4b	71	22.5
4c	78	24.7
5	36	11.4
Ultrasound-BI-RADS category		
1	15	4.7
2	10	3.2
3	10	3.2

Table 1. *Cont.*

Variable	No. of Cases	%
4a	82	25.9
4b	72	22.8
4c	75	23.7
5	52	16.5
Image-guided procedure		
Ultrasound-guided	275	87.0
MMG-guided	41	13.0
Needle gauge		
7/10	38	12.0
14/16/18	278	88.0
Operation type		
Mastectomy	191	60.4
BCS	125	39.6
DCIS tumor size (cm), median (IQR)	3.3 (2.6)	
Tumor necrosis area		
None	36	11.4
Focal	178	56.3
Large	102	32.3
DCIS tumor grading		
Low	34	10.7
Intermediate	144	45.6
High	138	43.7
DCIS architecture pattern		
Comedo	122	38.6
Non-comedo	194	61.4
Lymphovascular invasion		
Present	11	3.5
Absent	305	96.5
IDC area		
Multifocal/multicentric	142	44.9
Unifocal	174	55.1
IDC [a]		
T1mi	101	32.0
T1a	92	29.1
T1b	50	15.8
T1c	47	14.9
T2	26	8.2
IDC tumor grading		
1	81	25.6
2	133	42.1
3	44	13.9
Unknown	58	18.4
Estrogen receptor status		
Positive	197	62.3
Negative	119	37.7
Progesterone receptor status		
Positive	176	55.7
Negative	140	44.3
HER2 status		
Positive	110	34.8
Negative	206	65.2
Ki-67		
<20	221	69.9
≥20	70	22.2
Unknown	25	7.9

IQR, interquartile range; MMG, mammography; BI-RADS, Breast Imaging Reporting and Data System; BCS, breast-conserving surgery; DCIS, ductal carcinoma in situ; IDC, invasive ductal carcinoma. Figures are numbers with percentages in parentheses, unless otherwise stated. [a] T stage was defined according to the eighth edition of the American Joint Commission on Cancer TNM staging system for breast cancer.

3.2. Radiologic Features

Regarding the imaging modality for detecting lesions, 236 lesions (74.7%) were ultrasonographically and mammographically detectable, 44 (13.9%) were only ultrasonographically detectable, and 36 (11.4%) were only mammographically detectable. The breasts were predominantly categorized into dense (80.6%) and non-dense (19.4%) categories. The imaging morphology of underestimated IBCs was most commonly a mass with calcifications (164/316, 51.9%) and less commonly a mass without calcifications (85/316, 26.9%) or non-mass (67/316, 21.2%). Forty-nine lesions were categorized as BI-RADS 0 on mammography, and their final assessment was performed after ultrasound examination. The main reason for the difficulty in interpreting mammography was the mass (25/49, 51.0%), followed by focal asymmetry (20/49, 40.8%) and architectural distortion (4/49, 8.2%). Regarding the assessment category of the 316 cases based on ultrasound features, 50 (15.8 %) cases were classified as BI-RASDS 4a, 71 (22.5%) cases as 4b, 78 (24.7%) cases as 4c, and 36 (11.4%) cases as 5.

3.3. Final Pathological Findings

The median tumor size of DCIS on final pathology was 3.3 cm (range, 0.2–14.0 cm). The DCIS grades were documented to be low in 34 (10.7%), intermediate in 144 (45.6%), and high in 138 (43.7%) patients. The architecture growth pattern of DCIS was composed of 38.6% comedo type and 61.4% non-comedo type. Tumor necrosis was absent in 36 (11.4%) patients and was present in 280 (88.6%) patients. LVI was reported to be absent in most cases (305/316, 96.5%). Of the entire cohort, the histological type of all invasive carcinomas was ductal. Regarding the IDC distribution on the final pathology, a total of 174 (55.1%) cases presented with unifocal lesions, and the remaining 142 (44.9%) cases presented with multifocal or multicentric lesions. A total of about 60% of IDC tumors are less than or equal to 0.5 cm in size. Only four (1.3%) tumors were found, and the size of IDC was larger than the DCIS extent. In terms of IDC tumor grading, 81 (25.6%) cases were defined as grade 1, 133 (42.1%) as grade 2, and 44 (13.9%) as grade 3. ER was positive in 197 (62.3%), PR in 176 (55.7%), and HER-2 in 110 (34.8%) cases. Ki67 was finally evaluated in 291 of these 316 patients, and the remaining 25 cases were non-evaluable because the lesions were too small to be stained. Of the 291 patients, a high Ki67 proliferation index ($\geq$20) was observed in 70 (24.1%) and low (<20) in 221 (75.9%) patients.

3.4. Evaluation of Axillary Lymph Node Status

Of the 316 patients, 308 (97.5%) underwent both breast surgery and SLNB simultaneously during the first operation, and the remaining eight (2.5%) underwent SLNB for axillary staging after primary breast surgery. Before 2018, the surgical guidelines for patients with a preoperative diagnosis of DCIS in our institution recommended that a SLNB was indicated in those who underwent mastectomy and should be considered in those with risk factors for an IC component including a palpable mass, high grade DCIS, and large area of mammographic calcifications. A SLNB was also considered in patients who underwent BCS if the tumor location might later interfere with the ability to perform SLNB. The major reason for performing breast surgery and SLNB simultaneously in our population was mastectomy (191/308, 62.0%), followed by a palpable mass (47/308, 15.3%), high grade DCIS (24/49, 7.8%), large area of mammographic calcifications (24/308, 7.8%) and tumor location (22/49, 7.1%). The median number of SLNs removed was 2 (range, 1–8). The SLNs showed macrometastasis in 15 (4.7%), micrometastasis in seven (2.2%), isolated tumor cells in one (0.3%), and no metastasis in 293 (92.7%) patients (Table 2). Among the 23 patients with positive SLNs, 17 underwent completion ALN dissection. In 11 out of 17 patients (64.7%), no additional lymph node metastases were found and, in six, micrometastases were found. Of the six patients, four had only one additional positive lymph node and two had extensive nodal disease, with three and 11 additional positive lymph nodes, respectively. Six patients with positive SLNs did not undergo ALN dissection, four of them had micrometastases, one had macrometastasis, and the remaining one had isolated tumor cells.

Table 2. Clinicopathological findings and radiologic features of patients with sentinel lymph node metastasis.

Age (yrs)	Radiologic Morphology	Surgery Type	Final Pathology							
			LVI	DCIS (mm)	IDC (mm)	Molecular Subtype	No. of SLNs [a]	pN by SLNB [b]	No. of LN by ALND [c]	Final TNM Stage [b]
50	non-mass	Mast.	present	26	9	HER2 positive	1/1	pN1	1/17	pT1bN1aM0
38	mass without calcifications	Mast.	absent	37	9	Luminal A	1/1	pN1mi	0/39	pT1bN1miM0
54	mass without calcifications	BCS	absent	11	7	Luminal A	1/1	pN1	0/20	pT1bN1M0
55	mass with calcifications	Mast.	absent	70	<1	HER2 positive	1/2	pN1	0/12	pT1miN1aM0
42	mass with calcifications	Mast.	present	56	12	Luminal B/HER2 positive	1/2	pN1mi	0/20	pT1cN1miM0
69	mass with calcifications	Mast.	present	10	35	Luminal A	1/2	pN1	0/10	pT2N1aM0
41	mass with calcifications	Mast.	present	42	32	Luminal A	1/1	pN1	1/16	pT2N1aM0
41	mass with calcifications	Mast.	absent	6	8	Triple negative	1/1	pN1mi	NP	pT1bN1miM0
68	mass without calcifications	Mast.	absent	52	<1	Luminal A	1/5	pN0(i+)	NP	pT1miN0(i+)M0
59	mass without calcifications	BCS	absent	47	2.5	Triple negative	1/1	pN1	0/20	pT1aN1aM0
53	mass without calcifications	Mast.	absent	46	12	HER2 positive	1/1	pN1	0/44	pT1cN1aM0
42	mass without calcifications	Mast.	absent	60	19	Luminal A	1/1	pN1	NP	pT1cN1aM0
65	mass without calcifications	Mast.	absent	48	20	Luminal A	2/2	pN1	0/14	pT1cN1aM0
64	mass without calcifications	Mast.	present	25	45	Luminal A	1/2	pN1	1/28	pT2N1aM0
47	non-mass	Mast.	present	109	12	HER2 positive	1/2	pN1	0/20	pT1cN1aM0
74	mass with calcifications	Mast.	present	38	<1	HER2 positive	1/2	pN1	1/18	pT1miN1aM0
57	mass with calcifications	Mast.	absent	50	17	Luminal B HER2 negative	1/2	pN1mi	NP	pT1cN1miM0
37	mass with calcifications	BCS	absent	18	18	Luminal B/HER2 negative	1/2	pN1mi	NP	pT1cN1miM0
39	mass with calcifications	Mast.	present	47	39	Luminal B/HER2 negative	3/3	pN1	3/12	pT2N2aM0
42	mass with calcifications	BCS	absent	40	31	Luminal B/HER2 negative	2/3	pN1	11/27	pT2N3aM0
67	mass without calcifications	Mast.	absent	45	5	Luminal A	1/2	pN1mi	0/11	pT1aN1miM0
44	non-mass	Mast.	absent	47	1.6	Luminal B/HER2 negative	1/2	pN1	0/17	pT1aN1aM0
55	non-mass	BCS	absent	34	32	Luminal A	1/1	pN1mi	NP	pT2N1miM0

LVI, lymphovascular invasion; DCIS, ductal carcinoma in situ; IDC, invasive ductal carcinoma; SLNs, sentinel lymph nodes; SLNB, sentinel lymph node biopsy; ALND, axillary lymph node dissection; Mast., Mastectomy; HER2, human epidermal growth factor receptor 2; BCS, Breast conserving surgery; NP, not performed. [a] Values in table are numbers of sentinel lymph nodes removed (positive/examined). [b] Tumor size and lymph node status were categorized according to the eight edition of the American Joint Commission on Cancer TNM staging system for breast cancer. [c] Values in table are numbers of additional lymph nodes removed by subsequent axillary lymph node dissection (positive/examined).

3.5. Predictors of Sentinel Lymph Node Metastasis

On comparing the clinicopathological findings and radiologic features between patients with negative SLNs and those with positive SLNs, we found significant intergroup differences in IDC tumor size and the presence or absence of LVI. Compared with the patients in the negative SLN group, patients in the positive SLN group were more likely to have an IDC tumor size > 0.5 cm (17/23, 73.9% versus 106/293, 36.2%; $p < 0.001$) and the presence of LVI (8/23, 34.8% versus 3/293, 1.0%; $p < 0.0001$) (Table 3). Among all the clinical variables examined, there were no significant intergroup differences in median patient age, lesion location, and first-degree family history of breast cancer. Although a clinically palpable mass was more common in patients with positive SLNs (17/23, 73.9%) than in those with negative SLNs (157/293, 53.6%), the difference was not statistically significant ($p = 0.059$). Neither radiologic features nor biopsy procedure-associated variables were found to be predictors of SLN metastasis. Mastectomies were performed more frequently in the positive SLN group (78.3%) than in the negative SLN group (59.0%), but the difference was not significant ($p = 0.070$). The two groups were comparable in terms of DCIS tumor grade ($p = 0.797$), DCIS architecture pattern ($p = 0.084$), DCIS tumor size ($p = 0.117$), tumor necrosis area ($p = 0.912$), IDC tumor grade ($p = 0.165$), ER status ($p = 0.458$), PR status ($p = 0.340$), HER2 status ($p = 0.647$), and Ki67 ($p = 0.873$).

Table 3. Univariate analysis of factors influencing the lymph node status in underestimated invasive breast. Carcinoma patients with initial diagnosis of ductal carcinoma in situ by image-guided core needle biopsy.

Variable	Lymph Node		*p* Value
	Negative (n = 293)	Positive (n = 23)	
Age (years), median (IQR)	53.0 (16.0)	53.0 (22.0)	
Lesion location			0.965
Left breast	167 (57.0)	13 (56.5)	
Right breast	126 (43.0)	10 (43.5)	
1st degree family history of breast cancer			0.146
Yes	31 (10.6)	0	
No	262 (89.4)	23 (100.0)	
Palpability			0.059
Palpable	157 (53.6)	17 (73.9)	
Non-palpable	136 (46.4)	6 (26.1)	
Lesion-detecting imaging modality			0.652
Ultrasonography only	42 (14.3)	2 (8.7)	
Mammography only	34 (11.6)	2 (8.7)	
Detected by both ultrasonography and mammography	217 (74.1)	19 (82.6)	
Radiologic morphology			0.389
Mass with calcifications	154 (52.6)	10 (43.5)	
Mass without calcifications	76 (25.9)	9 (39.1)	
Non-mass with calcifications	63 (21.5)	4 (17.4)	
Parenchymal density			0.070
Entirely fatty	8 (2.7)	3 (13.0)	
Scattered fibroglandular	49 (16.7)	3 (13.0)	
Heterogeneously dense	166 (56.7)	13 (56.5)	
Extremely dense	70 (23.9)	4 (17.4)	
MMG-BI-RADS category			0.492
0	43 (14.7)	6 (26.1)	
1	5 (1.7)	1 (4.3)	
2	25 (8.5)	1 (4.3)	
4a	49 (16.7)	1 (4.3)	
4b	65 (22.2)	6 (26.1)	
4c	72 (24.6)	6 (26.1)	
5	34 (11.6)	2 (8.7)	
Ultrasound-BI-RADS category			0.080
1	14 (4.8)	1 (4.3)	
2	10 (3.4)	0	
3	10 (3.4)	0	
4a	80 (27.3)	2 (8.7)	
4b	62 (21.2)	10 (43.5)	

Table 3. *Cont.*

Variable	Lymph Node		*p* Value
	Negative (*n* = 293)	Positive (*n* = 23)	
4c	72 (24.6)	6 (26.1)	
5	34 (11.6)	2 (8.7)	
Ultrasound-BI-RADS category			0.080
1	14 (4.8)	1 (4.3)	
2	10 (3.4)	0	
3	10 (3.4)	0	
4a	80 (27.3)	2 (8.7)	
4b	62 (21.2)	10 (43.5)	
4c	67 (22.9)	8 (34.8)	
5	50 (17.1)	2 (8.7)	
Image-guided procedure			0.751
Ultrasound-guided	254 (86.7)	21 (91.3)	
MMG-guided	39 (13.3)	2 (8.7)	
Needle gauge			>0.999
7/10	36 (12.3)	2 (8.7)	
14/16/18	257 (87.7)	21 (91.3)	
Operation type			0.070
Mastectomy	173 (59.0)	18 (78.3)	
BCS	120 (41.0)	5 (21.7)	
DCIS tumor size (cm), median (IQR)	3.3 (2.6)	4.5 (2.4)	0.117
DCIS tumor grading			0.797
Low	32 (10.9)	2 (8.7)	
Intermediate	132 (45.1)	12 (52.2)	
High	129 (44.0)	9 (39.1)	
DCIS architecture pattern			0.084
Comedo	117 (39.9)	5 (21.7)	
Non-comedo	176 (60.1)	18 (78.3)	
Tumor necrosis area			0.912
None	33 (11.3)	3 (13.0)	
Focal	166 (56.7)	12 (52.2)	
Large	94 (32.1)	8 (34.8)	
IDC area			0.884
Multiple	132 (45.1)	10 (43.5)	
Single	161 (54.9)	13 (56.5)	
IDC tumor size (cm)			<0.001
≦0.5	187 (63.8)	6 (26.1)	
>0.5	106 (36.2)	17 (73.9)	
IDC tumor grading			0.165
1	78 (26.6)	3 (13.0)	
2	119 (40.6)	14 (60.9)	
3	40 (13.7)	4 (17.4)	
Unknown	56 (19.1)	2 (8.7)	
Lymphovascular invasion			<0.0001
Present	3 (1.0)	8 (34.8)	
Absent	290 (99.0)	15 (65.2)	
Estrogen receptor status			0.458
Positive	181 (61.8)	16 (69.6)	
Negative	112 (38.2)	7 (30.4)	
Progesterone receptor status			0.340
Positive	161 (54.9)	15 (65.2)	
Negative	132 (45.1)	8 (34.8)	
HER2 status			0.647
Positive	103 (35.2)	7 (30.4)	
Negative	190 (64.8)	16 (69.6)	
Ki-67			0.873
<20	206 (70.3)	15 (65.2)	
≧20	64 (21.8)	6 (26.1)	
Unknown	23 (7.8)	2 (8.7)	

IQR, interquartile range; MMG, mammography; BI-RADS, Breast Imaging Reporting and Data System; BCS, breast-conserving surgery; DCIS, ductal carcinoma in situ; IDC, invasive ductal carcinoma; HER2, human epidermal growth factor receptor 2. Figures are numbers with percentages in parentheses, unless otherwise stated.

Multivariate analysis demonstrated that an IDC tumor size of >0.5 cm (odds ratio: 3.11; confidence interval: 1.09–8.81; $p = 0.033$) and the presence of LVI (odds ratio: 32.85; confidence interval: 7.56–142.80; $p < 0.0001$) were independent risk predictors of SLN metastasis (Table 4).

Table 4. Multivariate analysis of factors influencing the lymph node status in underestimated invasive breast carcinoma patients with initial diagnosis of ductal carcinoma in situ by image-guided core needle biopsy.

Variable	Odds Ratio	95% Confidence Interval of Odds	*p* Value
IDC tumor size (cm)			
≤0.5	1		
>0.5	3.11	1.09–8.81	0.033
Lymphovascular invasion			
Present	32.85	7.56–142.80	<0.0001
Absent	1		

IDC, invasive ductal carcinoma.

The results of SLNB stratified based on tumor size and LVI are shown in Figure 2. In the current study, the incidence of negative SLNs with tumors that met the features of small IDC tumor size (≤0.5 cm) and absence of LVI was as high as 97.4% (187/192); in contrast, the incidence of tumors that did not meet the above features with negative SLN was only 85.5% (106/124).

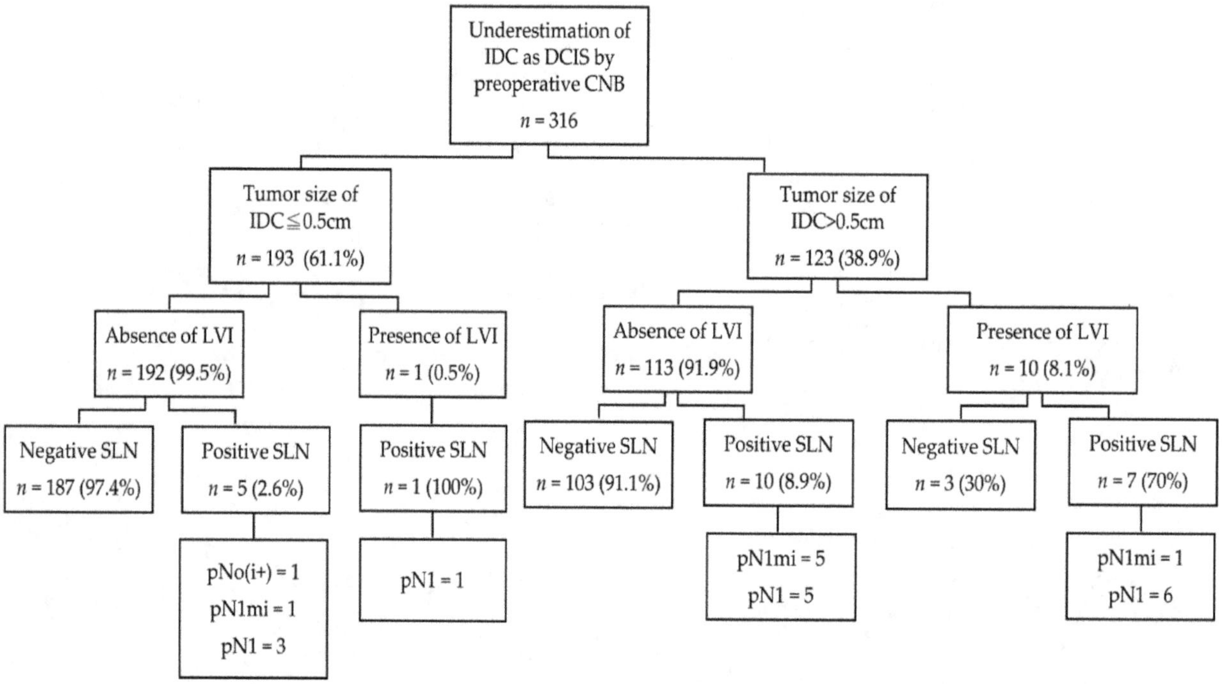

Figure 2. Results of sentinel lymph node biopsy stratified based on tumor size of invasive ductal carcinoma and lymphovascular invasion. IDC, invasive ductal carcinoma; DCIS, ductal carcinoma in situ; CNB, core needle biopsy; LVI, lymphovascular invasion; SLN, sentinel lymph node; pN0(i+), isolated tumor cells; pN1mi, micrometastasis; pN1, 1–3 macrometastasis.

The results of SLNB according to different surgical procedures and the combination of tumor size of IDC (≤0.5 cm) and absence of LVI are shown in Figure 3. In patients undergoing BCS, an extremely low incidence of positive SLNs of 1.3% (1/78) was observed in subgroups without any predictor.

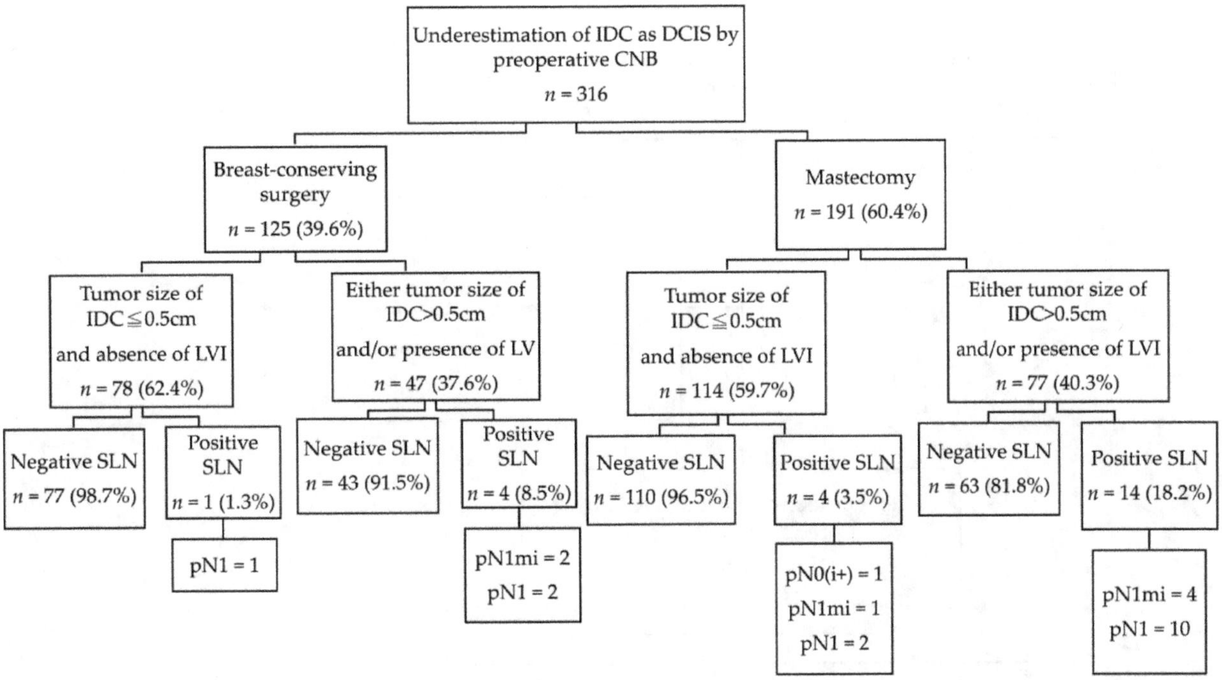

Figure 3. Results of sentinel lymph node biopsy according to different surgical procedures and the combination of tumor size of invasive ductal carcinoma (≦0.5 cm) and absence of lymphovacular invasion. IDC, invasive ductal carcinoma; DCIS, ductal carcinoma in situ; CNB, core needle biopsy; LVI, lymphovascular invasion; SLN, sentinel lymph node; pN0(i+), isolated tumor cells; pN1mi, micrometastasis; pN1, 1–3 macrometastasis.

An incidence of positive SLNs of 4% (2/50) was observed in patients diagnosed with low-risk DCIS, preoperatively in our series (Figure 4). The criteria for defining low-risk DCIS were the same as in the COMET (Comparison of Operative versus Monitoring and Endocrine Therapy) trial, including 40 years of age or older, low/intermediate DCIS without IBC diagnosed on CNB, ER(+) and/or PR(+), HER2(−) and no mass on physical examination or imaging [28].

To investigate whether different predictors existed for aymptomatic (screen-detected) population, we conducted analyses of factors associated with positive SLNs and found a statistically significant correlation of positive SLNs with an IDC tumor size > 0.5 cm (4/5, 80.0% versus 35/115, 30.4%; $p = 0.038$) and the presence of LVI (1/5, 20.0% versus 0/115, 0%; $p = 0.042$) (Table S1). The confirmed predictors associated with positive SLNs in asymptomatic breast cancer patients were the same as those associated with positive SLNs in total population (including asymptomatic and symptomatic breast cancer patients).

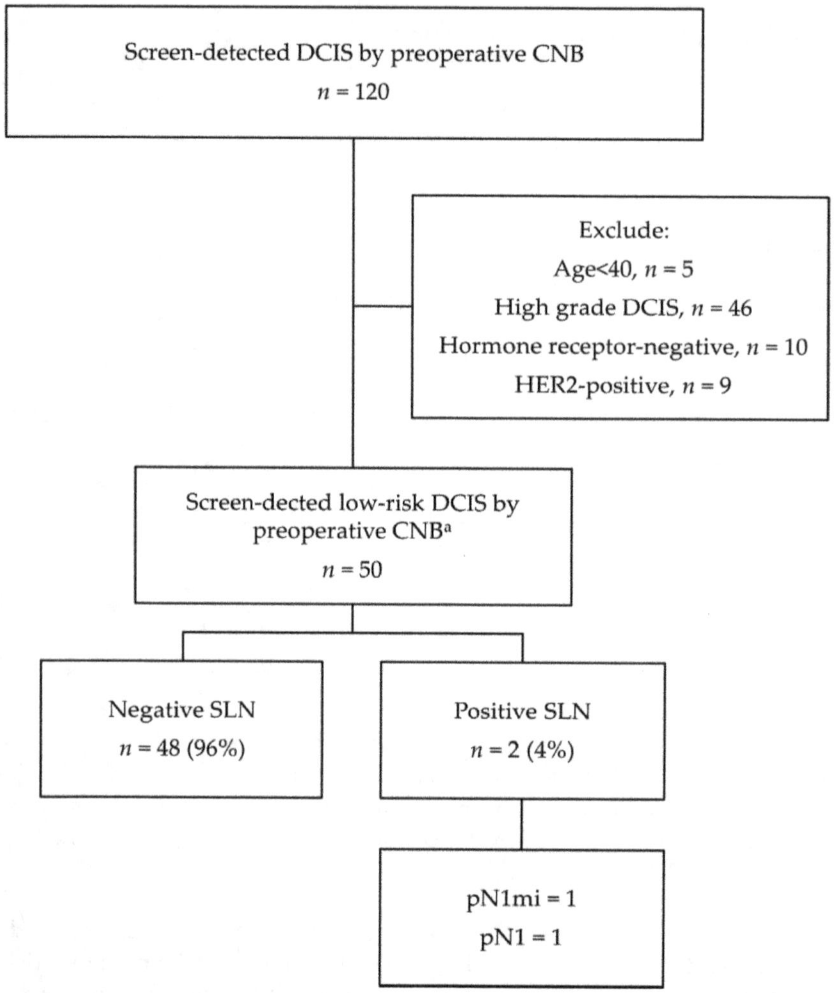

Figure 4. Results of sentinel lymph node biopsy among patients diagnosed with low-risk ductal carcionm in situ preoperatively. DCIS, ductal carcinoma in situ; CNB, core needle biopsy; HER2, human epidermal growth factor receptor 2; SLN, sentinel lymph node; pN1mi, micrometastasis; pN1, 1–3 macrometastasis. [a] The definition of low-risk DCIS is consistent with the inclusion criteria of the COMET(Comparison of Operative versus Monitoring and Endocrine Therapy) trial.

4. Discussion

The overall underestimation rate of DCIS patients by preoperative CNB was 26.5% (329/1240) in our cohort, which was comparable to the 25.9% reported in a previous meta-analysis study containing 7350 cases [3]. In the entire study population of 316 patients with underestimated IBC diagnosed by imaged-guided CNB, the incidence of SLN metastasis was 7.3%, which is within the reported incidence ranging from 0.9–15.6% [7–14] in patients with preoperative DCIS. It is noteworthy that, unlike previous study objects, which were involved in many pure DCIS, our study objects were relatively uniform and only focused on upgrading to IBC postoperatively. We assessed the clinical characteristics, radiologic features, and final pathological findings and identified that an IDC tumor size ≥ 0.5 cm on final pathology and the presence of LVI were independent risk predictors for SLN metastasis findings. To the best of our knowledge, this is the first study to explore the issues arising under the current general treatment guidelines. Moreover, the identified predictive factors in the current study may provide evidence regarding stratification in developing treatment strategies.

Many prior studies have attempted to identify the risk factors for SLN metastasis in patients with preoperative DCIS [7,9,12,14]. Several factors related to clinical characteristics, including young age at diagnosis, palpability, and multifocality, have been demonstrated to be associated with SLN metastasis, but none of them showed a consistent impact on positive SLN among those studies. In our series, unlike previous studies, none of the clinical features were related to SLN metastasis. A possible explanation is that the population composition of the previous studies included most DCIS and a relatively small number of underestimated IBC cases. In fact, the independent factors associated with SLN established by their researches and analyses are highly correlated with the presence of IBC, which has a major influence on SLN metastasis. Therefore, with the composition of our homogeneous study population with IBC, the above factors are relatively unable to achieve clinical significance. In our series, even if the patients who met the inclusion criteria of the COMET trial were classified as low-risk DCIS preoperatively, they still have an incidence of positive SLNs of 4% (2/50) [28], which was even slightly higher than the incidence of positive SLNs of 2.6% (5/192) for those who met the risk predictors of small IDC tumor size ($\leq$0.5 cm) and absence of LVI.

In the present study, all factors related to the radiologic findings or biopsy procedures of breast tumors were also not related to SLN metastasis. Usually, different radiologic features represent distinctions in tissue components, histological type, and histological grade. In our series, according to the fact that the tumor size of DCIS in most lesions (312/316, 98.7%) was larger than that of IDC, it is reasonable to infer that its morphological presentation is still dominated by DCIS. Therefore, the previously identified risk factors associated with radiologic findings for underestimated IBC, such as lesion size and mass formation on mammography or ultrasonography may reflect the aggressiveness of DCIS and thus predict the existence of IBC, but it still lacks effectiveness in predicting SLN metastasis. In our opinion, the determinant factor for the occurrence of SLN metastasis should still be directly related to the nature of the tumor itself, rather than indirectly related to clinical or imaging manifestations.

Regarding the final pathology evaluation, all factors related to the features of DCIS cannot be used to predict the possibility of SLN metastasis. DCIS is a heterogeneous disease in terms of morphology, histology, and biology. In terms of DCIS architecture pattern, compared with non-comedo DCIS, comedo DCIS is recognized as more often associated with the presence of IBC and recurrence after treatment [29–31]. A similar situation can also be observed in tumor grades [22,32]. Although these factors have been recognized as being highly correlated with IBC, there is still no mandatory relationship among them. Once again, similar to clinical features or imaging manifestations, DCIS-related factors still cannot be predictors of SLN metastasis.

In the current study, only the pathologic findings of IDC included tumor size of IDC and LVI, which were confirmed as predictors of SLN metastasis. Moreover, the two identified factors were consistent in predicting SLN metastasis in asymptomatic or symptomatic patients. Many previous studies on underestimated IBC mentioned the positive correlation between the IBC found on final pathology and SLN metastasis, but only a few of them mentioned the impact of the size of IBC on SLN metastasis. Han et al. reported a retrospective analysis of 255 patients with preoperative DCIS and found that the size of IDC was significantly associated with positive SLN [7], which is consistent with our findings. In our study cohort, the T stage for most IDCs (91.8%) was T1. In many studies on predictors of lymph node metastasis for T1 tumors, the size of the tumor always had a determinant influence; however, whether T1a or T1b should be used as the boundary remains controversial [33–35]. In this study, an IDC tumor size of 0.5 cm as the cut-off point is indeed effective in predicting SLN metastasis; however, the optimal cut-off point for IDC tumor size may be revised after the inclusion of more cases.

Theoretically, the process of lymphatic system metastasis is considered to proceed in the order of lymphangiogenesis, then LVI, and finally lymph node metastasis [36]. LVI is a crucial step in breast cancer metastasis [37,38] and is only confirmed by pathological analysis. Numerous studies have previously demonstrated that LVI plays an important role in predicting ALN metastasis in patients with breast cancer [34,39–42]. Ozmen et al.

observed that patients with LVI were more likely to have positive SLNs than those without LVI (51.3% vs. 30.3%, $p = 0.004$) [41]. Similarly, Gajdos et al. demonstrated a significant association between LVI and ALN metastasis in a retrospective study of 850 cases, in which positive lymph nodes were detected in 51% of the patients with LVI than in 19% of those without LVI [42]. In the present study, there was a statistically significant correlation between the presence of LVI and SLN metastasis, being present more frequently in SLN-positive patients than in SLN-negative patients (35.8% vs. 1%, $p < 0.0001$), which is consistent with the research findings mentioned above.

Several studies observed that IDC with accompanying DCIS had a trend to represent a favorable biology in comparison with pure IDC and showed that it was associated with low-grade tumors, smaller tumor size, and less lymph node involvement [43–45]. In a study of 3001 patients with pure IDC (79.4%) and IDC with accompanying DCIS (20.6%) reported by Goh et al., the incidence of LVI in IDC with accompanying DCIS was 7.6% [45]. Furthermore, the incidence of LVI as low as 2.7% (3/112) was documented in a study by Lyson et al. that reported 112 cases of DCIS with microinvasion [46]. These results imply that the smaller the IDCs, the less likely the presence of LVI. Considering that most of the IDCs in the current study were small tumors, 32% (101/316) of the overall cases were categorized as microinvasion ($\leq$1 mm) and 76.9% (243/316) as T1b ($\leq$1 cm); it was not surprising to observe such a low incidence of LVI (3.5%) in our series.

The most important role of SLNB in clinical lymph node-negative breast cancer is to provide information on treatment options, for example, whether a more extensive surgical procedure, such as ALN dissection, or more aggressive systemic drug therapy, such as chemotherapy or target therapy, is required. However, SLNB is never completely free of any side effects, such as bruising, pain, lymphedema, or impairment of upper extremity movement, which are all known possible side effects. Therefore, prospective studies are underway to confirm that certain low-risk groups will have a non-inferior prognosis without receiving SLNB [17–19]. In the current study, the final pathological evaluation of the resected breast specimen showed that, as long as the IDC tumor was > 0.5 cm or had a presence of LVI, the incidence of SLN metastasis would be so high that the omission of SLN was not allowed. In contrast, when no established risk predictor was presented on the final pathology in our series, breast cancer combined with SLN metastasis was as low as 2.6% (5/192), which made us cautiously consider the possibility of omitting SLNB. It is worth nothing that, if no sentinel lymph node biopsy would have been performed for patients without identified risk factors in our series, the administration of systemic therapy would be changed in five patients. The molecular types of the five missed patients were three luminal types, one triple negative type, and the remaining one HER2 positive type. Not surprisingly, the missing information on SLN metastasis would result in no adjuvant chemotherapy for triple negative breast cancer and neither adjuvant chemotherapy nor target therapy for HER2 positive breast cancer, which would be expected to have a greater impact on prognosis than luminal breast cancer with adjuvant hormone therapy. Under such circumstances, for those patients who had not received any adjuvant therapy, adopting more active and short-term follow-up examinations, including axillary lymph nodes as an alternative management, might be able to detect residual disease early, thereby reducing the adverse effects associated with missed diagnosis of nodal metastases.

Since the detection of IDC tumor size and LVI was highly dependent on the pathology of the resected specimen, it was still necessary to perform SLNB at the same time for cases expected to undergo total mastectomy. On the other hand, after BCS, in patients diagnosed with DCIS preoperatively by CNB, with no risk predictors in the final pathological evaluation, omitting SLNB may be an acceptable opinion. This view can be observed in our series of patients undergoing BCS in the absence of any predictor; their SLN metastasis rate was extremely low at 1.3%.

The current study had several limitations. First, since it was a retrospective analysis performed at a single institution, selection bias may have been inevitable. Despite the fact that our research was based on a reliable dataset derived from a relatively homogeneous and large number of cases, the generalization of the findings in our study may not be appropriate for all institutions. Further multi-institutional prospective studies are required. Second, it was difficult to accurately confirm how many cases of patients undergoing mastectomy could actually be replaced by BCS in the current study. In fact, among the patients who underwent mastectomy without any predictive factors in the present study, the four patients with SLN metastasis were accompanied by large DCIS, which made it impossible to perform BCS. This allowed us to reasonably infer that if the objective conditions of the tumor were not added to the patient's preference for surgical procedure selection, more BCS cases without SLN metastasis would be added to the calculation and analysis, resulting in a lower incidence of SLN metastasis than the present value. Third, the overall median follow-up time was not long enough, so we could not assess whether the identified predictor of SLN metastasis in this study is also related to the prognosis of breast cancer.

5. Conclusions

Our study revealed that there were no reliable clinical or imaging features that could be used as a predictor of SLN metastasis in underestimated IDC patients with an initial diagnosis of DCIS by imaged-guided CNB. The current study demonstrated that only the features related to IDC on final pathological assessment, including an IDC tumor size > 0.5 cm and the presence of LVI, could be regarded as predictors of SLN metastasis. Considering the two identified risk factors, the overall incidence of SLN metastasis was very low in the absence of any predictor. Since the predictors established in this study could only be found on resected breast specimens, this study supported the current guidelines for SLNB at the time of mastectomy. For patients diagnosed with DCIS by CNB preoperatively, when invasive cancer is confirmed after BCS, we suggest that SLNB may be omitted for those without any predictors. However, further prospective studies are warranted.

Author Contributions: Conceptualization, C.-C.Y. and S.-C.C.; methodology, C.-C.Y. and Y.-C.C.; software, C.-C.Y.; validation, C.-C.Y., Y.-C.C. and C.H.; formal analysis, C.-C.Y.; investigation, C.-C.Y. and C.H.; resources, C.-C.Y., C.H. and S.-C.C.; data curation, C.-C.Y. and Y.-C.C.; writing—original draft preparation, C.-C.Y.; writing—review and editing, C.-C.Y. and S.-C.C.; visualization, C.H.; supervision, S.-C.C.; project administration, C.-C.Y.; funding acquisition, not available. All authors have read and agreed to the published version of the manuscript.

References

1. Gutwein, L.G.; Ang, D.N.; Liu, H.; Marshall, J.K.; Hochwald, S.N.; Copeland, E.M.; Grobmyer, S.R. Utilization of minimally invasive breast biopsy for the evaluation of suspicious breast lesions. *Am. J. Surg.* **2011**, *202*, 127–132. [CrossRef]
2. Siziopikou, K.P. Ductal carcinoma in situ of the breast: Current concepts and future directions. *Arch. Pathol. Lab. Med.* **2013**, *137*, 462–466. [CrossRef]
3. Brennan, M.E.; Turner, R.M.; Ciatto, S.; Marinovich, M.L.; French, J.R.; Macaskill, P.; Houssami, N. Ductal carcinoma in situ at core-needle biopsy: Meta-analysis of underestimation and predictors of invasive breast cancer. *Radiology* **2011**, *260*, 119–128. [CrossRef]
4. Lyman, G.H.; Somerfield, M.R.; Bosserman, L.D.; Perkins, C.L.; Weaver, D.L.; Giuliano, A.E. Sentinel Lymph Node Biopsy for Patients With Early-Stage Breast Cancer: American Society of Clinical Oncology Clinical Practice Guideline Update. *J. Clin. Oncol.* **2017**, *35*, 561–564. [CrossRef]
5. Veronesi, U.; Paganelli, G.; Viale, G.; Luini, A.; Zurrida, S.; Galimberti, V.; Intra, M.; Veronesi, P.; Robertson, C.; Maisonneuve, P.; et al. A randomized comparison of sentinel-node biopsy with routine axillary dissection in breast cancer. *N. Engl. J. Med.* **2003**, *349*, 546–553. [CrossRef] [PubMed]
6. Crane-Okada, R.; Wascher, R.A.; Elashoff, D.; Giuliano, A.E. Long-term morbidity of sentinel node biopsy versus complete axillary dissection for unilateral breast cancer. *Ann. Surg. Oncol.* **2008**, *15*, 1996–2005. [CrossRef]
7. Han, J.S.; Molberg, K.H.; Sarode, V. Predictors of invasion and axillary lymph node metastasis in patients with a core biopsy diagnosis of ductal carcinoma in situ: An analysis of 255 cases. *Breast J.* **2011**, *17*, 223–229. [CrossRef]

8. Prendeville, S.; Ryan, C.; Feeley, L.; O'Connell, F.; Browne, T.J.; O'Sullivan, M.J.; Bennett, M.W. Sentinel lymph node biopsy is not warranted following a core needle biopsy diagnosis of ductal carcinoma in situ (DCIS) of the breast. *Breast* **2015**, *24*, 197–200. [CrossRef] [PubMed]
9. Francis, A.M.; Haugen, C.E.; Grimes, L.M.; Crow, J.R.; Yi, M.; Mittendorf, E.A.; Bedrosian, I.; Caudle, A.S.; Babiera, G.V.; Krishnamurthy, S.; et al. Is Sentinel Lymph Node Dissection Warranted for Patients with a Diagnosis of Ductal Carcinoma In Situ? *Ann. Surg. Oncol.* **2015**, *22*, 4270–4279. [CrossRef]
10. van Roozendaal, L.M.; Goorts, B.; Klinkert, M.; Keymeulen, K.B.M.I.; De Vries, B.; Strobbe, L.J.A.; Wauters, C.A.P.; van Riet, Y.E.; Degreef, E.; Rutgers, E.J.T.; et al. Sentinel lymph node biopsy can be omitted in DCIS patients treated with breast conserving therapy. *Breast Cancer Res. Treat.* **2016**, *156*, 517–525. [CrossRef] [PubMed]
11. Heymans, C.; van Bastelaar, J.; Visschers, R.G.J.; Vissers, Y.L.J. Sentinel Node Procedure Obsolete in Lumpectomy for Ductal Carcinoma In Situ. *Clin. Breast Cancer* **2017**, *17*, e87–e93. [CrossRef] [PubMed]
12. Sorrentino, L.; Sartani, A.; Bossi, D.; Amadori, R.; Nebuloni, M.; Truffi, M.; Bonzini, M.; Riggio, E.; Foschi, D.; Corsi, F. Sentinel node biopsy in ductal carcinoma in situ of the breast: Never justified? *Breast J.* **2018**, *24*, 325–333. [CrossRef] [PubMed]
13. Watanabe, Y.; Anan, K.; Saimura, M.; Koga, K.; Fujino, M.; Mine, M.; Tamiya, S.; Nishihara, K.; Nakano, T.; Mitsuyama, S. Upstaging to invasive ductal carcinoma after mastectomy for ductal carcinoma in situ: Predictive factors and role of sentinel lymph node biopsy. *Breast Cancer.* **2018**, *25*, 663–670. [CrossRef] [PubMed]
14. Zhang, K.; Qian, L.; Zhu, Q.; Chang, C. Prediction of Sentinel Lymph Node Metastasis in Breast Ductal Carcinoma In Situ Diagnosed by Preoperative Core Needle Biopsy. *Front. Oncol.* **2020**, *10*, 590686. [CrossRef] [PubMed]
15. Giuliano, A.E.; McCall, L.; Beitsch, P.; Whitworth, P.W.; Blumencranz, P.; Leitch, A.M.; Saha, S.; Hunt, K.K.; Morrow, M.; Ballman, K. Locoregional recurrence after sentinel lymph node dissection with or without axillary dissection in patients with sentinel lymph node metastases: The American College of Surgeons Oncology Group Z0011 randomized trial. *Ann. Surg.* **2010**, *252*, 426–432. [CrossRef]
16. Galimberti, V.; Cole, B.F.; Zurrida, S.; Viale, G.; Luini, A.; Veronesi, P.; Baratella, P.; Chifu, C.; Sargenti, M.; Intra, M.; et al. Axillary dissection versus no axillary dissection in patients with sentinel-node micrometastases (IBCSG 23-01): A phase 3 randomised controlled trial. *Lancet Oncol.* **2013**, *14*, 297–305. [CrossRef]
17. Gentilini, O.; Veronesi, U. Abandoning sentinel lymph node biopsy in early breast cancer? A new trial in progress at the European Institute of Oncology of Milan (SOUND: Sentinel node vs Observation after axillary UltraSouND). *Breast* **2012**, *21*, 678–681. [CrossRef]
18. Reimer, T.; Hartmann, S.; Stachs, A.; Gerber, B. Local treatment of the axilla in early breast cancer: Concepts from the national surgical adjuvant breast and bowel project B-04 to the planned intergroup sentinel mamma trial. *Breast Care* **2014**, *9*, 87–95. [CrossRef]
19. Van Roozendaal, L.M.; Vane, M.L.G.; van Dalen, T.; van der Hage, J.A.; Strobbe, L.J.A.; Boersma, L.J.; Linn, S.C.; Lobbes, M.B.I.; Poortmans, P.M.P.; Tjan-Heijnen, V.C.G.; et al. Clinically node negative breast cancer patients undergoing breast conserving therapy, sentinel lymph node procedure versus follow-up: A Dutch randomized controlled multicentre trial (BOOG 2013-08). *BMC Cancer* **2017**, *17*, 459. [CrossRef]
20. American College of Radiology. *Breast Imaging Reporting and Data System*, 5th ed.; American College of Radiology: Reston, VA, USA, 2013.
21. Hoda, S.A.; Brogi, E.; Koerner, F.C.; Rosen, P.P. (Eds.) *Rosen's Breast Pathology*, 5th ed.; Wolters Kluwer: Alphen aan den Rijn, The Netherlands, 2021; p. 478.
22. Silverstein, M.J.; Poller, D.N.; Waisman, J.R.; Colburn, W.J.; Barth, A.; Gierson, E.D.; Lewinsky, B.; Gamagami, P.; Slamon, D.J. Prognostic classification of breast ductal carcinoma-in-situ. *Lancet* **1995**, *345*, 1154–1157.
23. Allred, D.C. Ductal carcinoma in situ: Terminology, classification, and natural history. *J. Natl. Cancer Inst. Monogr.* **2010**, *41*, 134–138. [CrossRef]
24. Harrison, B.T.; Hwang, E.S.; Partridge, A.H.; Thompson, A.M.; Schnitt, S.J. Variability in diagnostic threshold for comedo necrosis among breast pathologists: Implications for patient eligibility for active surveillance trials of ductal carcinoma in situ. *Mod. Pathol.* **2019**, *32*, 1257–1262. [CrossRef]
25. Zhan, H.; Quinn, M.; Tian, W.; Yan, L.; Khoury, T. Significance of Removing Comedonecrosis as an Exclusion Criterion in Mammary Low-Risk Ductal Carcinoma In Situ Managed in an Active Surveillance Clinical Trial. *Am. J. Clin. Pathol.* **2021**, *26*, aqaa276. [CrossRef]
26. Elston, C.W.; Ellis, I.O. Pathological prognostic factors in breast cancer. I. The value of histological grade in breast cancer: Experience from a large study with long-term follow-up. *Histopathology* **1991**, *19*, 403–410. [CrossRef]
27. Hammond, M.E.; Hayes, D.F.; Dowsett, M.; Allred, D.C.; Hagerty, K.L.; Badve, S.; Fitzgibbons,

P.L.; Francis, G.; Goldstein, N.S.; Hayes, M.; et al. American Society of Clinical Oncology/College of American Pathologists guideline recommendations for immunohistochemical testing of estrogen and progesterone receptors in breast cancer (unabridged version). *Arch. Pathol. Lab. Med.* **2010**, *134*, e48–e72. [CrossRef]

28. Hwang, E.S.; Hyslop, T.; Lynch, T.; Frank, E.; Pinto, D.; Basila, D.; Collyar, D.; Bennett, A.; Kaplan, C.; Rosenberg, S.; et al. The COMET (Comparison of Operative versus Monitoring and Endocrine Therapy) trial: A phase III randomised controlled clinical trial for low-risk ductal carcinoma in situ (DCIS). *BMJ Open* **2019**, *12*, e026797. [CrossRef]
29. Schwartz, G.F.; Patchefsky, A.S.; Finklestein, S.D.; Sohn, S.H.; Prestipino, A.; Feig, S.A.; Singer, J.S. Nonpalpable in situ ductal carcinoma of the breast. Predictors of multicentricity and microinvasion and implications for treatment. *Arch. Surg.* **1989**, *124*, 29–32. [CrossRef]
30. Silverstein, M.J.; Waisman, J.R.; Gamagami, P.; Gierson, E.D.; Colburn, W.J.; Rosser, R.J.; Gordon, P.S.; Lewinsky, B.S.; Fingerhut, A. Intraductal carcinoma of the breast (208 cases). Clinical factors influencing treatment choice. *Cancer* **1990**, *66*, 102–108. [CrossRef]
31. Virnig, B.A.; Tuttle, T.M.; Shamliyan, T.; Kane, R.L. Ductal carcinoma in situ of the breast: A systematic review of incidence, treatment, and outcomes. *J. Natl. Cancer Inst.* **2010**, *102*, 170–178. [CrossRef] [PubMed]
32. Boyages, J.; Delaney, G.; Taylor, R. Predictors of local recurrence after treatment of ductal carcinoma in situ: A meta-analysis. *Cancer* **1999**, *85*, 616–628. [CrossRef]
33. Giuliano, A.E.; Barth, A.M.; Spivack, B.; Beitsch, P.D.; Evans, S.W. Incidence and predictors of axillary metastasis in T1 carcinoma of the breast. *J. Am. Coll. Surg.* **1996**, *183*, 185–189.
34. Barth, A.; Craig, P.H.; Silverstein, M.J. Predictors of axillary lymph node metastases in patients with T1 breast carcinoma. *Cancer* **1997**, *79*, 1918–1922. [CrossRef]
35. Markopoulos, C.; Kouskos, E.; Gogas, H.; Mandas, D.; Kakisis, J.; Gogas, J. Factors affecting axillary lymph node metastases in patients with T1 breast carcinoma. *Am. Surg.* **2000**, *66*, 1011–1013. [PubMed]
36. Ran, S.; Volk, L.; Hall, K.; Flister, M.J. Lymphangiogenesis and lymphatic metastasis in breast cancer. *Pathophysiology* **2010**, *17*, 229–251. [CrossRef] [PubMed]
37. Sleeman, J.P.; Thiele, W. Tumor metastasis and the lymphatic vasculature. *Int. J. Cancer* **2009**, *125*, 2747–2756. [CrossRef] [PubMed]
38. Podgrabinska, S.; Skobe, M. Role of lymphatic vasculature in regional and distant metastases. *Microvasc. Res.* **2014**, *95*, 46–52. [CrossRef] [PubMed]
39. Lauria, R.; Perrone, F.; Carlomagno, C.; De Laurentiis, M.; Morabito, A.; Gallo, C.; Varriale, E.; Pettinato, G.; Panico, L.; Petrella, G.; et al. The prognostic value of lymphatic and blood vessel invasion in operable breast cancer. *Cancer* **1995**, *76*, 1772–1778. [CrossRef]
40. Bader, A.A.; Tio, J.; Petru, E.; Bühner, M.; Pfahlberg, A.; Volkholz, H.; Tulusan, A.H. T1 breast cancer: Identification of patients at low risk of axillary lymph node metastases. *Breast Cancer Res. Treat.* **2002**, *76*, 11–17. [CrossRef]
41. Ozmen, V.; Karanlik, H.; Cabioglu, N.; Igci, A.; Kecer, M.; Asoglu, O.; Tuzlali, S.; Mudun, A. Factors predicting the sentinel and non-sentinel lymph node metastases in breast cancer. *Breast Cancer Res. Treat.* **2006**, *95*, 1–6. [CrossRef]
42. Gajdos, C.; Tartter, P.I.; Bleiweiss, I.J. Lymphatic invasion, tumor size, and age are independent predictors of axillary lymph node metastases in women with T1 breast cancers. *Ann. Surg.* **1999**, *230*, 692–696. [CrossRef]
43. Wong, H.; Lau, S.; Yau, T.; Cheung, P.; Epstein, R.J. Presence of an in situ component is associated with reduced biological aggressiveness of size-matched invasive breast cancer. *Br. J. Cancer.* **2010**, *102*, 1391–1396. [CrossRef] [PubMed]
44. Dieterich, M.; Hartwig, F.; Stubert, J.; Klöcking, S.; Kundt, G.; Stengel, B.; Reimer, T.; Gerber, B. Accompanying DCIS in breast cancer patients with invasive ductal carcinoma is predictive of improved local recurrence-free survival. *Breast* **2014**, *23*, 346–351. [CrossRef] [PubMed]
45. Goh, C.W.; Wu, J.; Ding, S.; Lin, C.; Chen, X.; Huang, O.; Chen, W.; Li, Y.; Shen, K.; Zhu, L. Invasive ductal carcinoma with coexisting ductal carcinoma in situ (IDC/DCIS) versus pure invasive ductal carcinoma (IDC): A comparison of clinicopathological characteristics, molecular subtypes, and clinical outcomes. *J. Cancer Res. Clin. Oncol.* **2019**, *145*, 1877–1886. [CrossRef] [PubMed]
46. Lyons, J.M., 3rd; Stempel, M.; Van Zee, K.J.; Cody, H.S., 3rd. Axillary node staging for microinvasive breast cancer: Is it justified? *Ann. Surg. Oncol.* **2012**, *19*, 3416–3421. [CrossRef]

12

Differential Response of MDA-MB-231 and MCF-7 Breast Cancer Cells to In Vitro Inhibition with CTLA-4 and PD-1 through Cancer-Immune Cells Modified Interactions

Kamil Grubczak [1,*], Anna Kretowska-Grunwald [1], Dawid Groth [1], Izabela Poplawska [2], Andrzej Eljaszewicz [1], Lukasz Bolkun [3], Aleksandra Starosz [1], Jordan M. Holl [1], Marta Mysliwiec [4], Joanna Kruszewska [4], Marek Z. Wojtukiewicz [4] and Marcin Moniuszko [1,5,*]

[1] Department of Regenerative Medicine and Immune Regulation, Medical University of Bialystok, Jerzego Waszyngtona 13, 15-269 Bialystok, Poland; annammkretowska@gmail.com (A.K.-G.); dawid.groth@umb.edu.pl (D.G.); andrzej.eljaszewicz@umb.edu.pl (A.E.); aleksandra.starosz@gmail.com (A.S.); jordanmholl@gmail.com (J.M.H.)

[2] Department of Medical Pathomorphology, Medical University of Bialystok, Jerzego Waszyngtona 13, 15-269 Bialystok, Poland; iptaborda@gmail.com

[3] Department of Haematology, Medical University of Bialystok, M. Sklodowskiej-Curie 24A, 15-276 Bialystok, Poland; lbolkun@gmail.com

[4] Department of Oncology, Medical University of Bialystok, Ogrodowa 12, 15-027 Bialystok, Poland; marta.mysl@gmail.com (M.M.); joannak@umb.edu (J.K.); mzwojtukiewicz@gmail.com (M.Z.W.)

[5] Department of Allergology and Internal Medicine, Medical University of Bialystok, M. Sklodowskiej-Curie 24A, 15-276 Bialystok, Poland

* Correspondence: kamil.grubczak@umb.edu.pl (K.G.); marcin.moniuszko@umb.edu.pl (M.M.);

Abstract: Drugs targeting immune checkpoint molecules have been found effective in melanoma, lung cancer, and other malignancies treatment. Recent studies on breast cancer demonstrated the significance of inhibitory anti-CTLA-4 and anti-PD-1 in the regulation of disease progression. However, seemingly the same types of breast cancer do not always respond unambiguously to immunotherapy. Thus, here we set out to analyze the in vitro effects of inhibiting CTLA-4 and PD-1 on interactions between co-cultured lymphocytes and two selected breast adenocarcinoma cell lines. Breast cancer cells were co-cultured with lymphocytes to evaluate the effects of CTLA-4 and PD-1 inhibition. Proliferation, cell cycle, and viability assessment were measured in cancer cells. IFN-gamma, IL-10, perforin, granzyme B production, and CTLA-4 and PD-1 expression were analyzed in lymphocytes. We found that administration of anti-CTLA-4 improved the anti-cancer activity of T cells with reduced proliferation and viability of MDA-MB-231. Lack of response was observed in the context of MCF-7. In addition, differential expression of checkpoint proteins was found between studied cancer cells lines. Inhibition of molecules was followed by IL-10 and IFN-gamma decrease in lymphocytes co-cultured with MDA-MB-231, not demonstrated in reference to MCF-7. Furthermore, CTLA-4 blockage was associated with reduction of CTLA-4+ and PD-1+ lymphocytes in MDA-MB-231, with a significant increase in MCF-7, reduced by anti-PD-1. Altogether, our study revealed that anti-CTLA-4 and anti-PD-1 treatment can improve lymphocytes effects on breast cancer cells. Favorable effects seemed to be related to breast cancer cells features as differential responses were reported. Novel blocking antibodies strategies should be tested for more effective cancer inhibition.

Keywords: immune checkpoint inhibitors; CTLA-4; PD-1; breast cancer; anti-tumor immunity

---

1. Introduction

Breast cancer is the most common cause of cancer-related death in women. Being the most frequently diagnosed cancer in females it accounts for nearly 23% of total cancer cases [1]. Molecular distinction seen in breast tumors engages numerous therapies to be used in the management of this disease. Aside from surgery, chemo- and radiotherapy, which serve as the basis of breast cancer treatment, targeted therapy with agents directed at specific molecule receptors seems to be taking the leading role in several cases [2]. An example of such is endocrine therapy, where a selective estrogen receptor modulator-tamoxifen is used against ER-positive breast cancer cells resulting in inhibition of their growth and apoptosis [3]. On the contrary, the triple-negative breast cancer (TNBC) subtype has the highest likelihood of recurrence and poorest survival prognosis [4]. The efficacy of current therapeutic solutions remains unsatisfactory and therefore there is a great demand for research into this field.

Immunotherapy has become a leading treatment option for patients with melanoma or lung cancer and is soon to be approved for kidney, bladder, and prostate cancer therapy [5,6]. Immune response checkpoint regulators including CTLA-4 and PD-1 have been shown to play a critical role in cancer development through interactions with B7 proteins, particularly CD80 and CD86. According to Xu et al., the B7 protein family was observed to be amplified in breast cancer, which allowed for the introduction of checkpoint protein modulation in breast cancer treatment [7]. In addition to B7 receptors, the upregulation of their ligands CTLA-4 and PD-1was noted [8,9]. In meta-analysis studies, CTLA-4 polymorphisms have been shown to correlate with breast cancer susceptibility, emphasizing the importance of CTLA-4 in regard to tumor development [10]. Recent research from clinical trials has demonstrated that a single dose of anti-CTLA-4 monoclonal antibody (ipilimumab) leads to increased intratumor T cell density [11], which is associated with a lower risk of chemotherapy resistance and higher overall survival in breast cancer patients [12,13]. In the context of the PD-1/PD-L1 axis, recent studies have demonstrated that breast cancer patients with low levels of PD-1+ tumor-infiltrating lymphocytes (TILs) and high expression of PD-L1 within tumors showed the worst survival rate. This fact is likely associated with tumor-induced suppression of the immune response as a consequence of the PD-L1 interaction with lymphocyte-expressed PD-1 [14]. Promising results have also been seen in PD-L1-positive TNBC patients phase Ib clinical trials where a single-agent pembrolizumab showed antitumor activity in 18.5% of subjects, achieving response durations from 15 to more than 47 weeks, with the best standard chemotherapy response duration oscillating within 4 to 12 weeks [15,16]. On the other hand, results of a phase 2 study KEYNOTE-08 evaluating pembrolizumab monotherapy in TNBC treatment proved somewhat modest, with an objective response rate of around 5.7% in the PD-L1-positive population [16].

An increasing number of studies also incorporate CTLA-4 or PD-1 inhibitors to be used as adjuvant therapy, thereby improving anti-cancer agent activity [17]. In experiments studying populations of mice, the application of anti-CTLA-4 antibodies was found to improve the antitumor activity of gemcitabine by leading to sustained, long-term tumor size reduction [18]. Concomitant treatment of tremelimumab (anti-CTLA-4 IgG_1 antibody) with exemestane has been tested in hormone-responsive breast cancer, demonstrating the induction of ICOS+/CD4-/CD8+ lymphocytes, suggesting enhanced activation of conventional T cells in regard to antitumor immunity in addition to immune suppression as a consequence of reduced regulatory T cell numbers [19]. Sagit-Barfi et al. show that despite ineffective blockage of the PD-1/PD-L1 pathway with anti-PD-L1 alone, its combination with ibrutinib (molecule binding to Bruton's tyrosine kinase) significantly enhanced the antitumor activity of T-cells in mice inoculated with breast and colon carcinoma, among others [20]. Similar results were obtained in mice treated with a combination of anti-PD-1 antibody and doxorubicin, which led to reduced metastasis of 4T1 mammary tumor, unlike treatment with anti-PD-1 alone [21]. Despite somewhat promising results of therapeutic immune checkpoint inhibitors, selection of appropriate agents likely depends on the type of treated cancer, as suggested in recent studies, where tumor cells of breast cancer 4T1 cell line demonstrated significantly lower levels of the CTLA-4 ligand (B7-1) compared to colon carcinoma CT26 cell line, despite similar lower level expression of PD-L1 [22]. The number of studies focusing on the assessment of CTLA-4/ PD-1 inhibition on interactions between lymphocytes and different subtypes of breast cancer remains scarce.

Although research into potential novel approaches to treatment in triple-negative breast cancer does not seem to raise any ambiguity due to its dismal prognosis [4], this cannot be said for ER-positive, PR positive, and HER2-negative breast cancer because these patients show a rather favorable outcome [23]. This tendency has however resulted in a limited number of studies focusing on new therapeutic solutions for treatment-resistant luminal A-type breast cancer patients. To date, the assessment of CTLA-4/ PD-1 inhibition on interactions between lymphocytes and different subtypes of breast cancer has not yet been thoroughly analyzed. Several studies have however associated poorer clinical outcomes of breast cancer patients with the expression of CTLA-4 in the tumor microenvironment, justifying the enormous need for further research in this field [24]. Saleh et al. found that MDA-MB-231 (TNBC) cells upregulated CTLA-4 expression in CD4+CD25− T lymphocytes and downregulated PD-1 expression in those CD4+CD25+. On the contrary, the ER-positive breast cancer cells (MCF-7 cell line) greatly upregulated the PD-1 expression in CD4+CD25− T cells, having no significant impact on CD4+CD25+ lymphocytes [25]. The dissimilar impact of both subtypes of breast cancer cells on the expression of immune checkpoints in the co-cultured T cells requires extensive studies in this field to establish relevant immune checkpoint inhibitor-based approaches, which will be highly effective in both mono- and polytherapy of different subtypes of breast cancer.

2. Materials and Methods

2.1. *Preparation of MDA-MB-231 and MCF-7 Breast Cancer Cell Line Cells*

MDA-MB-231 (triple-negative) and MCF-7 (ER-positive) breast cancer cell line cells (both adenocarcinomas obtained from the metastatic site; ATCC, Manassas, VA, USA) were thawed from liquid nitrogen, washed twice, and suspended in DMEM medium enriched with FBS and antibiotics. Cells were maintained in culture, 37 °C 5% CO_2, for the next 4–5 passages to obtain a sufficient number of completely functional cells, thus, cells only from the 4th and 5th passages were used in the study. Prior to the experiment MDA-MB-231 and MCF-7 cells were stained with carboxyfluorescein succinimidyl ester (CFSE, Sigma-Aldrich, Saint Louis, MO, USA) for evaluation of proliferating cells following co-culture. Proliferating cells were analyzed within viable 7AAD- (7-aminoactinomycin D) cells (Supplementary Figure S1a).

2.2. *Isolation of Peripheral Blood Mononuclear Cells (PBMC) from Healthy Blood Donors*

Peripheral blood was obtained by venipuncture from 9 healthy blood donors and subjected to gradient density centrifugation (Histopaque-1077, Sigma-Aldrich) to isolate peripheral blood mononuclear cells (PBMC) (the age of donors was within the range of 26 –35 years; with equal distribution in the context of sex). The obtained PBMC were washed twice in phosphate-buffered saline without calcium and magnesium (PBS, Biomed Lublin) and frozen in cryoprotectant—10% DMSO (DMSO, Sigma-Aldrich) in fetal bovine serum (FBS, Gibco), and stored in liquid nitrogen for the experiments. Prior to co-culture with MDA-MB-231 or MCF-7 cancer cell line cells PBMC were thawed, washed twice, counted, and suspended in DMEM medium enriched with FBS and antibiotic (Gentamicin, Sigma-Aldrich). Due to the use of short co-cultures (up to 24 h) with initially activated PBMC (anti-CD3ε, protocol described in the following subsection), the role of HLA compatibility was excluded in the observed phenomenon, as such mechanisms require longer time intervals, even weeks [26], to develop reactivity in case of lack of histocompatibility. A comparable experimental model is used commonly worldwide and is justified by numerous studies [27,28]. All research was performed in accordance with relevant guidelines/regulations. Informed consent was obtained from all healthy blood donors from whom peripheral blood was collected. The collection of blood was approved by the Local Bioethical Committee at Medical University of Bialystok, approval number R-I-002/61/2015.

2.3. *Co-Cultures of MDA-MB-231 and MCF-7 Breast Cancer Cell Line Cells with PBMC of Healthy Blood Donors*

CFSE-stained MDA-MB-231 or MCF-7 were applied into culture plates (2×10^5 cells/well) and subjected to initial culture to achieve attachment of cells to the surface. Subsequently, PBMC were stimulated with 1 μL/mL of human CD3 epsilon antibody (clone UCHT1) (anti-hCD3ε, R&D Systems, Minneapolis, MN, USA), placed onto MDA-MB-231 or MCF-7 breast cancer cells (2×10^6 of PBMC per well) and incubated for the next 24-h, 37 °C 5% CO_2. Noteworthy, for each repetition with MDA-MB-231 or MCF-7 cell line, separate PBMC material was used from a single donor—there was no pooling of the PBMC prior application on the wells. Additionally, the experimental layout included MDA-MB-231 of MCF-7 co-cultured with PBMC in the presence of 3 μg/mL anti-CTLA-4 (clone AS32; monoclonal IgG1; company provided reactivity to the extracellular domain of the human CTLA-4) (anti-CTLA-4/-CD152, Invitrogen, Waltham, MA, USA) or 3 μg/mL anti-PD-1 (polyclonal IgG; company provided reactivity to the extracellular domain of the human PD-1) (anti-PD-1/-CD279, R&D Systems) antibodies, and wells with cancer cells alone, cancer cells with 25 ng/mL of colcemid (negative control for proliferation) (Colcemid, Biowest, Nuaille, France) and PBMC alone. The ratio of cancer cells to PBMC and culture time was carefully selected in preliminary experiments, thus obtaining inhibition/killing rate allowing us to monitor additional effects caused by the application of anti-CTLA-4/PD-1. In addition, in the course of the preliminary investigation, we also validated the experimental model of lymphocyte blocking with anti-CTLA-4 or anti-PD-1. In accordance with available literature mentioned in the 'Introduction' section, implementation of the CTLA-4 or PD-1 blockage was intended to prevent their inhibitory effects on lymphocytes activation, proliferation, and effector activity (Supplementary Figure S2a—self-made scheme based on information provided in references [29–31]. Noteworthy, we confirmed that selected blocking antibodies exerted expected effects on the action of the lymphocytes, demonstrated as facilitated and increased activation (CD69 early-activation marker) and effective production of inflammatory cytokine (IFN-gamma) where immunosuppressive pathway related to CTLA-4 or PD-1 was restrained (Supplementary Figure S2b).

Following incubation, supernatants containing non-adherent cells were aspirated and centrifuged to obtain cells and supernatants for the next experiments. MDA-MB-231 and MCF-7 breast cancer cells were washed twice with PBS and trypsinized with 0.25% trypsin (2.5% Trypsin, Sigma-Aldrich). Detached cells were suspended in an enriched DMEM medium to inactivate trypsin, washed twice in PBS, and used for flow cytometric analysis.

2.4. *Flow Cytometric Analysis of MDA-MB-231 and MCF-7 Breast Cancer Cell Line Cells Following Co-Cultures*

Analysis of MDA-MB-231 cells proliferation status was conducted with the use of CFSE staining and additional staining with 7AAD to exclude dead cells. Negative control of colcemid-treated MDA-MB-231 cells was used to set the gate and evaluate the frequency of proliferating cells. As the CFSE binds covalently to the cytoplasmic proteins and its amount is constant from the beginning, it is evenly distributed in the daughter cells in the course of proliferation. The use of 7AAD dye allowed for additional analysis of viable cell events within studied cancer models. Cell cycle analysis was performed with the use of NSS reagent containing 50 μg/mL propidium iodide (Propidium iodide, PI, Sigma-Aldrich) and 0.035% nonylphenylpolyethylene (Neonidet P40 Substitute, Sigma-Aldrich), followed by the addition of 10 μg/mL RNase solution (RNase A solution, Sigma-Aldrich). Flow cytometric analysis allowed three cell cycle phases to be distinguished: G1-phase, S-phase, and G2-phase. Proliferation and cell cycle data were acquired with the use of a FACS Calibur flow cytometer (BD Bioscience, Franklin Lakes, NJ, USA) and subsequent analysis was performed using FlowJo software (TreeStar Inc., Ashland, OR, USA). Combination of viability, proliferation, and cell cycle assessment allowed for the complex determination of the function-related events within breast cancer cells in the described co-culture conditions (Supplementary Figure S1b).

2.5. Flow Cytometric Analysis of PBMC after Co-Culture with MDA-MB-231 and MCF-7

Lymphocytes present in supernatants of PBMC and MDA-MB-231 or MCF-7 cells co-culture were stained with fluorochrome-conjugated monoclonal antibodies including: anti-CD3 FITC (clone SK7), anti-CD3 PerCP (clone SK7), anti-CD4 PerCP (clone SK3), anti-CD8 FITC (clone HIT8a), anti-CD152/CTLA-4 APC (clone BNI3), anti-CD279/PD-1 PE (clone MIH4) (BD Bioscience). Moreover, immune checkpoint proteins were studied, both on the surface of lymphocytes and MDA-MB-231/MCF-7 with the use of anti-CTLA-4 APC, anti-PD-1 PE, anti-PD-L1 PE (clone MIH1), anti-CD80 BB515 (clone L307.4), and anti-CD86 PE-Cy5 (clone IT2.2). In addition, following co-culture with MDA-MB-231 or MCF-7, cancer cells supernatants containing non-adherent lymphocytes were subjected to additional 6h stimulation with PMA, ionomycin, and Brefeldin A (Leukocyte Activation Cocktail, BD Bioscience) to evaluate the effects of the presence of breast cancer cells on the production of IFN-gamma and IL-10 by lymphocytes. Cells were stained with the following monoclonal antibodies for staining extracellular markers: anti-CD4 PerCP (clone SK3), anti-CD8 APC (clone SK1), anti-CD3 FITC (clone SK7), and anti-IFN-gamma PE (clone 4S.B3) or anti-IL-10 PE (clone JES3-19F1) after the permeabilization step to assess intracellular cytokines. Intracellular staining procedures were also implemented following co-culture with cancer cells to evaluate perforin (AlexaFluo647-conjugated, clone δG9) and granzyme B (PE-conjugated, clone GB11) production by lymphocytes. Flow cytometric data were acquired with the use of a FACS Calibur flow cytometer (BD Bioscience, USA) and subsequent analysis was performed using FlowJo software (TreeStar Inc., Ashland, USA). Production of IFN-gamma and IL-10 to evaluate inflammatory cytokines crucial in the context of effector function regulation, and perforin and granzyme B to establish lymphocyte-related cytotoxic function were assessed within CD4+, CD8+ and the total pool of lymphocytes (with anti-CD3 PE-Cy7 and anti-CD8 FITC antibodies implemented) (Supplementary Figure S1c,d). Evaluation of CTLA-4 and PD-1 levels within CD4+ and CD8+ lymphocyte subsets included frequencies of CTLA-4- and PD-1-expressing cells and mean fluorescence intensities (MFI) within these populations (Supplementary Figure S1c–e). An in-depth description of the antibodies used, their specificity, and representative dot plots and histograms including FMO controls were presented within supplementary materials. Thus, effective binding to the studied targets and their specific reactivity was confirmed (Supplementary Figure S3).

2.6. Colorimetric Assessment of LDH Activity-Based Cytotoxicity

Supernatants from co-cultures of MDA-MB-231 or MCF-7 cancer cells with PBMC, and inhibition of CTLA-4 or PD-1, were subjected to analysis of LDH activity following 24-h incubation to evaluate the cytotoxicity of the described layouts in reference to breast cancer cells. Analysis was performed with the use of the Pierce LDH Cytotoxicity Assay Kit (Thermo Scientific, Rockford, IL, USA). In accordance with the kit instruction, following 30-min incubation with Reaction Mixture, Stop Solution was added and absorbance was measured at 480 and 680 using the Epoch plate-reader (BioTek Instruments, Winooski, VT, USA) to determine LDH activity. Data were presented as LDH activity-associated absorbance after subtraction of values measured in blank control—enriched cell culture medium used in the experiments. An increase in LDH activity in the tested supernatants indicated its release from cancer cells (as there was no change in the viability of PBMC in flow cytometric data—data not shown), and which presence extracellularly is always associated with disturbances in the membrane-cell damage.

2.7. Statistical Analysis

Due to the non-normal distribution of the data, the non-parametric Wilcoxon signed-rank test was used for statistical analysis of the paired results, and Mann-Whitney for unpaired data. Estimation of the Gaussian distribution of the data was performed with the use of Shapiro–Wilk and D'Agostino Pearson normality tests. Two independent tests were required to confirm the normality of the distribution, otherwise, data were further tested with non-parametric tests. Acquired flow cytometric and colorimetric data were presented on graphs as a relative percentage compared to MDA-MB-231/MCF-7 or PBMC alone defined as initial 100%. Statistics were generated using GraphPad Prism software (GraphPad Software Inc., San Diego, CA, USA). Statistical differences were indicated with asterisks: * $p < 0.05$, ** $p < 0.01$, *** $p < 0.001$, **** $p < 0.0001$, or values for non-significant data but showing tendency and vales close to p-value of 0.05. As described within the figures, statistically significant differences were indicated when the selected group was compared to cells alone (black values/asterisks) or cells co-cultured with PBMC (light grey values/asterisks). Additional brackets above two cell types within certain groups were applied to clearly demonstrate the presence of significant differences in response between MCF-7 and MDA-MB-231 cell lines if present.

3. Results

3.1. Effects of CTLA-4 and PD-1 Blockage on Proliferation Status of MDA-MB-231 and MCF-7 Cells in Presence of PBMC

Despite the lack of changes in the proliferation rate of MDA-MB-231 cancer cells in the presence of anti-CD3-stimulated PBMC alone following 24-h co-culture, we found that inhibition of CTLA-4 on the surface of mononuclear cells allowed for significant reduction of proliferating cancer cells, even when compared to MDA-MB-231 affected by lymphocytes alone. No changes in the proliferation status of breast cancer cells were observed with reference to additional inhibition of PD-1 in co-culture with PBMC. Interestingly, the response of MCF-7 cancer cells to CTLA-4 blockage was significantly different compared to the MDA-MB-231 cell line. In addition, no changes were observed in other studied layouts, both when compared to MCF-7 alone or in co-culture with PBMC (Figure 1a). Assessment of viable cell events related to MCF-7 or MDA-MB-231 cancer cells revealed that only the latter one responded with lower viable cells number compared to co-culture with PBMC when blockage of PD-1 was introduced (Figure 1d).

3.2. Cell Cycle Status of MDA-MB-231 or MCF-7 Cells in Presence of PBMC Alone, and Additional Inhibition of CTLA-4 and PD-1

In accordance with the results observed in the proliferation assay, inhibition of CTLA-4 on the surface of PBMC allowed for the significant arrest of MDA-MB-231 cancer cells in the G1/S-phase of the cell cycle. In addition, despite the lack of significant changes in proliferation status, the presence of PBMC alone and in combination with PD-1-blockage allowed for the significant arrest of breast cancer cells in the G1/S-phase. In accordance with proliferation data, no crucial changes were demonstrated in the context of MCF-7 breast cancer cells with only a slight increase in G1-phase cells when anti-PD-1 was applied (Figure 1b).

3.3. Cytotoxicity of PBMC Alone, and Additional Inhibition of CTLA-4 and PD-1 with Reference to MDA-MB-231 or MCF-7 Cells

Assessment of LDH activity in supernatants of cultured MDA-MB-231 or MCF-7 breast cancer cells revealed significant cytotoxic activity of PBMC on these cells. Importantly, more pronounced effects were observed in the additional application of CTLA-4 inhibition, with approximately 32% higher LDH activity in supernatants compared to MDA-MB-231 treated with PBMC only. We did not find significant differences between MDA-MB-231 cells treated with PBMC alone versus treatment with PBMC and the additional inhibition of PD-1. Furthermore, despite the effective activity of PBMC against MCF cancer cells, it was less pronounced compared to that observed in MDA-MB-231 cells. Moreover, even though cytotoxicity was reported in the MCF-7 cell line in the settings tested, none of the inhibitory antibodies applied-anti-CTLA-4 or anti-PD-1, caused significant effects on the viability of MCF-7 cells co-cultured with PBMC only (Figure 1c).

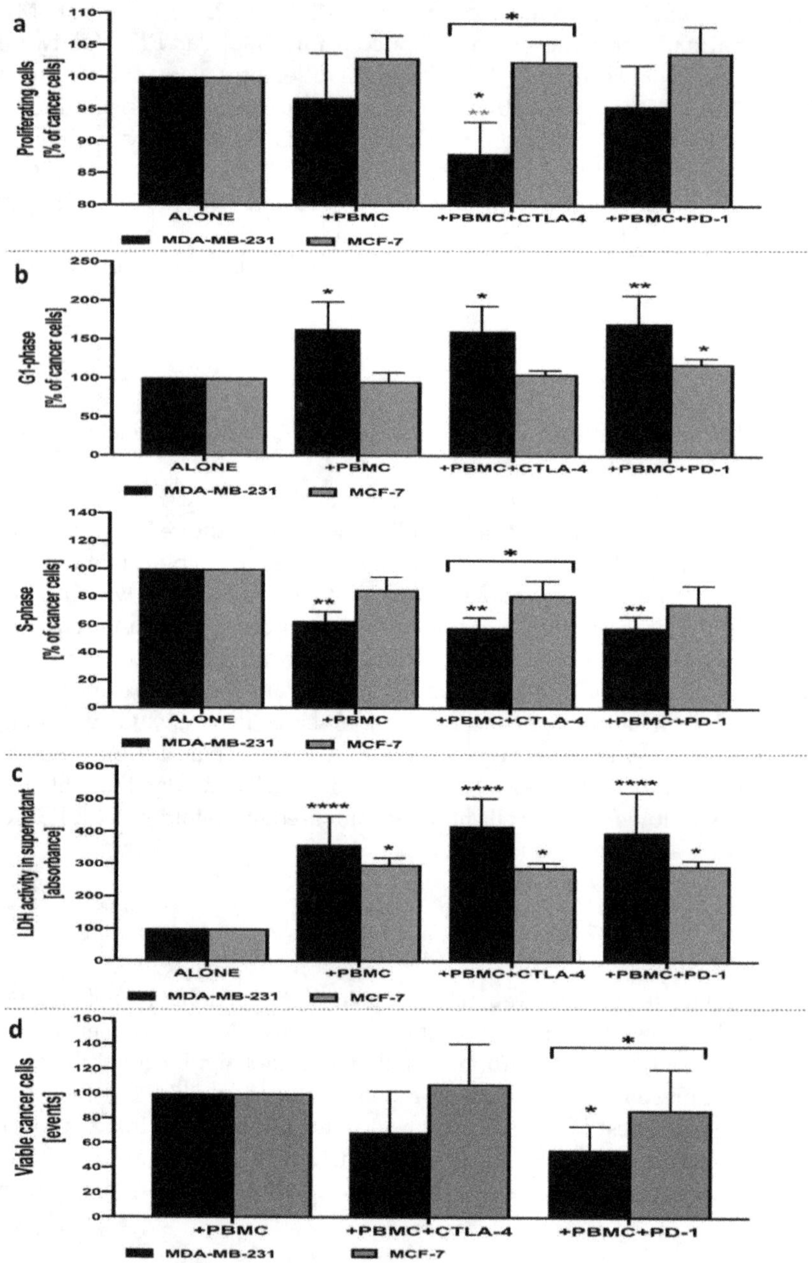

Figure 1. Analysis of MDA-MB-231 and MCF-7 breast cancer-associated parameters. Proliferation status of CFSE-labeled MDA-MB-231/MCF-7 breast cancer cells following 24-h incubation with PBMC alone, and with the addition of CTLA-4 or PD-1 inhibitors (**a**). Cell cycle status of MDA-MB-231/MCF-7 breast cancer cells following 24-h incubation with PBMC alone, and with the addition of CTLA-4 or PD-1 inhibitors, based on the frequency of cancer cells in G1- (upper graph) and S-phase (lower graph) (**b**). Cytotoxic effects of PBMC alone, and with the addition of CTLA-4 or PD-1 inhibitors, on MDA-MB-231/MCF-7 breast cancer cells following 24-h incubation, based on the activity of LDH in supernatants (**c**) ($n = 10$). Evaluation of viable cancer cells based on dead cells exclusion with 7AAD (**d**). Asterisks above individual cancer cell line columns show the level of significance with colors indicating whether the difference is reported when the specific column is compared to cancer cells alone (black) or co-cultured with PBMC (light grey) (* $p < 0.05$, ** $p < 0.01$, *** $p < 0.001$, **** $p < 0.0001$). Moreover, brackets with significance demonstrated are applied when there was a difference in response between MDA-MB-231 and MCF-7 cells.

3.4. Differential Expression of Immune Checkpoint Proteins on the Surface of Tested PBMC and MDA-MB-231/MCF-7 Breast Cancer Cells

Analysis of selected immune checkpoint proteins on the breast cancer cells surface revealed significant differences in the pattern of expressed markers. In reference to MDA-MB-231 cells, PD-L1 expression was found to dominate above all in the context of both the frequency of cells and mean expression on the surface. The frequency of PD-1 was also found to be slightly increased, however, its levels were found to stand out predominantly in MCF-7 cancer cells. A certain percentage of MCF-7 cells was also reported to express CD86, nonetheless, it was PD-1 that dominated in these cells. Noteworthy, PD-1 and PD-L1 levels predominantly were significantly different between MDA-MB-231 and MCF-7 breast cancer cells (Figure 2a).

In the context of immune checkpoint proteins levels within lymphocytes, we found that the PD-1 marker is dominant above all analyzed, with a surprisingly small contribution of CTLA-4 in the context of frequency in studied cell populations. Noteworthy, CD8+ lymphocytes demonstrated significantly higher frequencies when compared to CD4+ T cells or even the total pool of lymphocytes. Interestingly, despite the lack of distinction in the context of frequency, CD80 marker mean expression was different between CD8+ and CD4+ or total lymphocytes, thus, providing a potential target for other further studies (Figure 2b).

3.5. IFN-Gamma and IL-10 Production by Lymphocytes in Response to MDA-MB-231/MCF-7 Presence, and with Additional Inhibition of CTLA-4 or PD-1

First, it is worth noting that significant effects of cancer cells' presence and applied treatment were only reported in reference to co-cultures with MDA-MB-231 breast cancer cells. No changes were demonstrated in cell cultures involving MCF-7 use, with only a slight tendency for higher levels of IL-10-producing CD8+ lymphocytes in co-culture with PBMC and anti-PD-1 presence. In addition, changes in IFN-gamma and IL-10 production reported in MDA-MB-231 were significantly different compared to MCF-7, predominantly through influence on CD8+ T cell population in the context of IL-10 and CD4+ lymphocytes as far as IFN-gamma was concerned. We found that inhibition of CTLA-4 or PD-1 on the surface of PBMC in co-culture with MDA-MB-231 significantly reduced the ability of lymphocytes to produce IFN-gamma in response to additional stimulation with PMA and ionomycin. The decline in IFN-gamma production seems to be associated predominantly with reduced production of that cytokine within CD4+, but not to the same extent in CD8+ lymphocytes. Changes in IFN-gamma apply not only to intracellular production but are also reflected in the decreased number of IFN-gamma-producing CD4+ lymphocytes in the presence of MDA-MB-231 alone, or with additional CTLA-4 or PD-1 inhibition. In addition, despite a lack of changes in intracellular production, the decline was also observed in the frequency of IFN-producing CD8+ lymphocytes when CTLA-4 was blocked. Regarding IL-10 production within lymphocytes, its reduced values were found in lymphocytes cultured in the presence of MDA-MB-231 alone, and additional CTLA-4 or PD-1 inhibition. Interestingly, such decline was shown to be associated with decreased production of IL-10 within CD8+, but not in CD4+ lymphocytes. In addition, effects exerted by PD-1 blockage seem to be more pronounced compared to co-culture with MDA-MB-231 alone or in combination with CTLA-4 inhibition. Furthermore, a significant decline in IL-10 production by CD8+ lymphocytes was accompanied by lower frequencies of IL-10-producing CD8+ lymphocytes (Figure 3a–c).

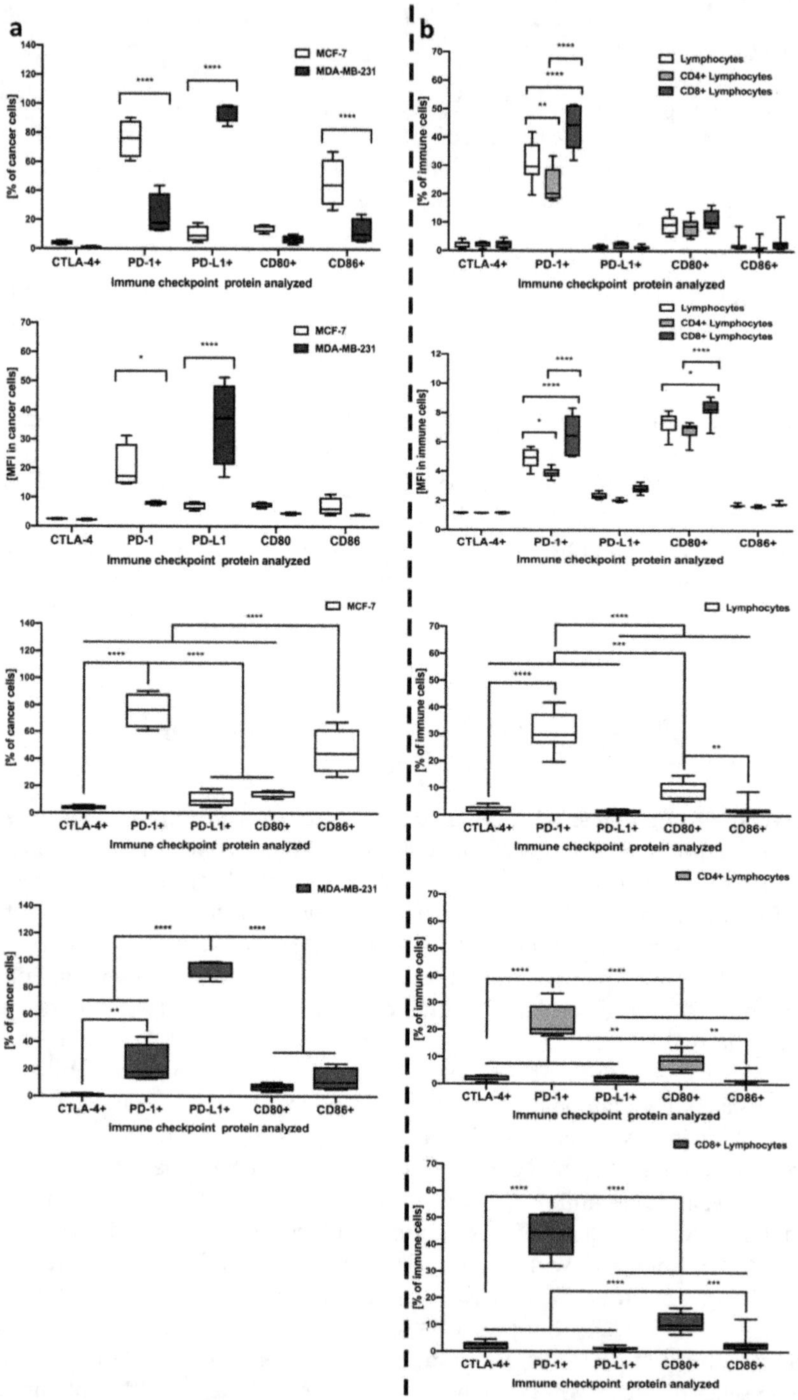

Figure 2. Evaluation of CTLA-4, PD-1, PD-L1, CD80, and CD86 immune checkpoint proteins on the studied cells. Acquired data included frequency of cells expressing selected markers and mean expression (MFI) on single cells, analyzed within MDA-MB-231/MCF-7 cancer cells ($n = 8$) (**a**) and lymphocytes including CD4+, CD8+, and the total pool of lymphocytes ($n = 7$) (**b**). The first two rows demonstrate significant differences between MDA-MB-231/MCF-7 or different lymphocyte subsets within each of the immune checkpoint proteins tested. Left column, rows 3–4, demonstrate the profile of immune checkpoint proteins within MCF-7 and MDA-MB-231, respectively. In the right column, rows 3–5, differences between studied checkpoint proteins are indicated for all studied lymphocyte subsets separately (statistically significant differences are indicated with asterisks) (* $p < 0.05$, ** $p < 0.01$, *** $p < 0.001$, **** $p < 0.0001$).

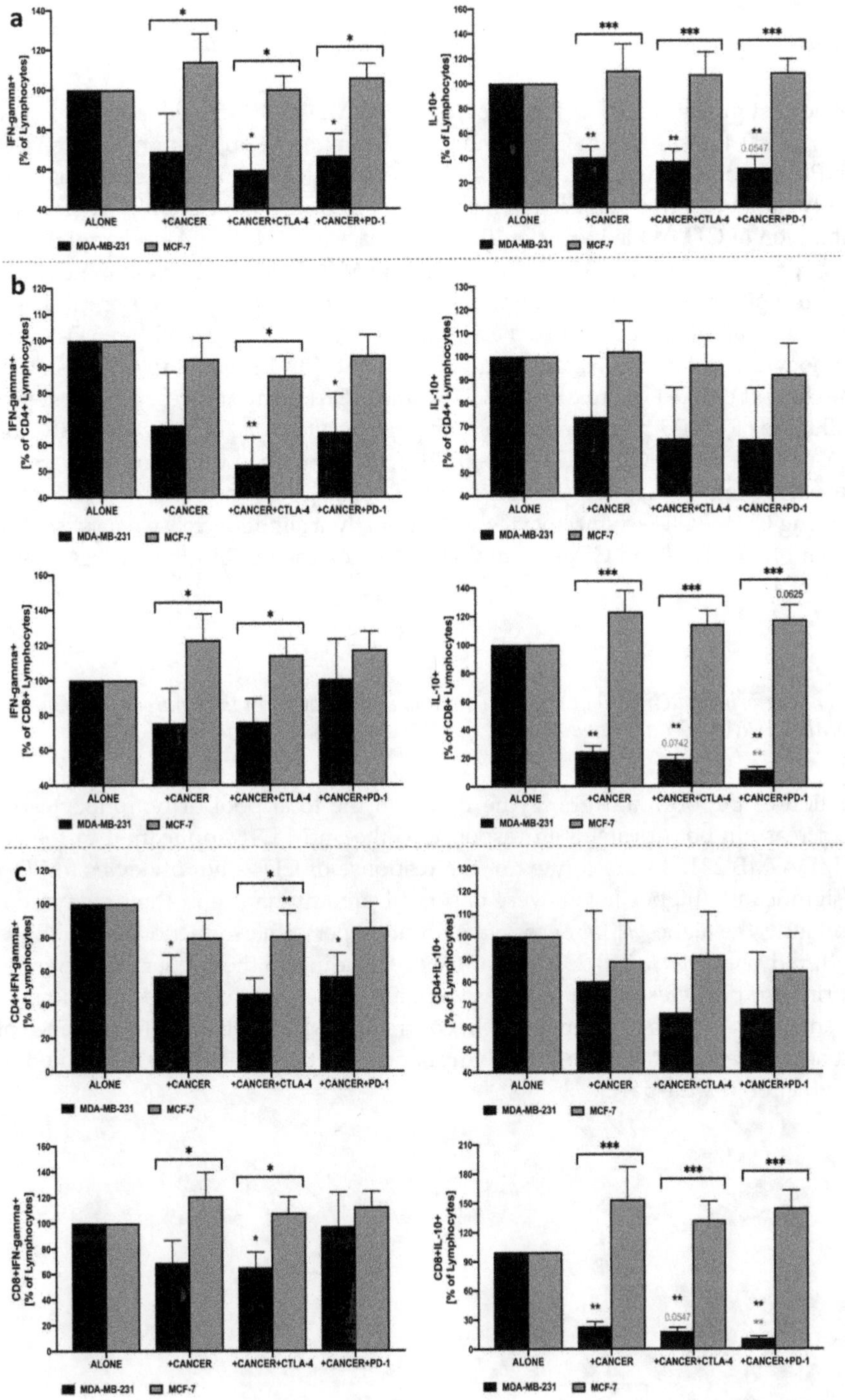

Figure 3. Analysis of IFN-gamma and IL-10 production within lymphocytes co-cultured with MDA-MB-231/MCF-7. Production of IFN-gamma and IL-10 in the total pool of lymphocytes (**a**), within CD4+ and CD8+ lymphocyte subsets (**b**), and frequencies of IFN-gamma- and IL-10-producing CD4+ and CD8+ lymphocytes (**c**) ($n = 8$). Asterisks above individual cancer cell line columns show the level of significance with colors indicating whether a difference is reported when the specific column is compared to cancer cells alone (black) or co-cultured with PBMC (light grey) (* $p < 0.05$, ** $p < 0.01$, *** $p < 0.001$, **** $p < 0.0001$). Moreover, brackets with significance demonstrated are applied when there was a difference in response between MDA-MB-231 and MCF-7 cells.

3.6. Alterations in CTLA-4 and PD-1 on the Surface of Lymphocytes in Co-Culture with MDA-MB-231/MCF-7 and Additional Presence of CTLA-4 or PD-1 Inhibition

We found that inhibition of PD-1 in co-culture with MDA-MB-231 led to a decrease in the frequency of PD-1+ cells within CD4+ and CD8+ lymphocyte populations, as well as a decrease in PD-1 expression in both subsets. Furthermore, a decline in the frequency of CD8+PD-1+ lymphocytes was observed in the presence of CTLA-4 or PD-1 blockage. Additionally, inhibition of CTLA-4 led to a significant decrease in CD4+CTLA-4+ lymphocytes. Interestingly, contrary to MDA-MB-231, the presence of MCF-7 was mostly associated with completely different effects exerted on lymphocyte's expression of CTLA-4 or PD-1. We found, inter alia, that MCF-7 cells caused an increase in CTLA-4 levels within CD4+ and CD8+ lymphocytes. Noteworthy, implementation of anti-PD-1 seemed to diminish that effect in the context of PD-1 expression on CD4+ and CD8+ lymphocytes. The most pronounced influence of MCF-7 breast cancer cells on lymphocytes was found when analyzing CD4+CTLA-4+/PD-1+ and CD8+CTLA-4+/PD-1+ frequencies in total lymphocytes. In accordance with general PD-1 expression, here, PD-1 blockage also reduced the fraction of PD-1-expressing CD4+/CD8+ lymphocytes. Additionally, a slight decrease was observed in the population of CD4+ and CD8+ with CTLA-4 when the inhibition of CTLA-4 was applied (Figure 4a–c).

3.7. Changes in Perforin and Granzyme B Production by Lymphocytes in the Course of Co-Culture with MDA-MB-231/MCF-7 and Implementation of CTLA-4 and PD-1 Inhibition

Evaluation of perforin and granzyme B within the total pool of lymphocytes revealed an increase in both proteins in response to the anti-PD-1 application in the co-culture of MDA-MB-231. In the context of the response of CD4+ lymphocytes to PD-1 blockage, significantly higher levels were observed predominantly in the granzyme B level. Importantly, the highest differences were found in perforin production when PBMC were co-cultured with MDA-MB-231 and anti-PD-1 leading to the higher frequency of CD8+Perforin+lymphocytes. Slight changes were also observed in these populations of cells when anti-CTLA-4 was implemented. In contrary to MDA-MB-231, the presence of MCF-7 did not cause essential changes in lymphocytes in the context of granzyme B or perforin production (Figure 5a–c).

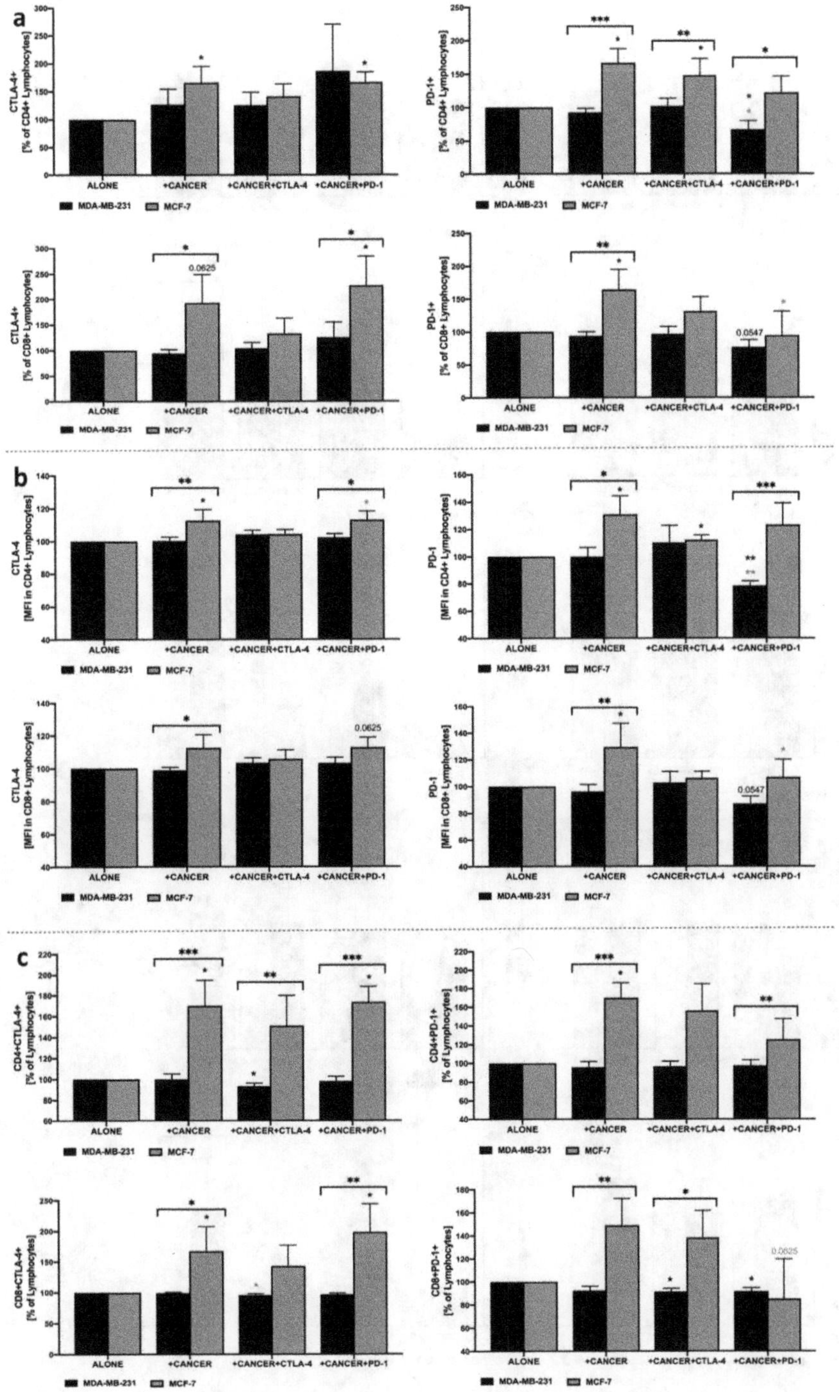

Figure 4. Evaluation of CTLA-4 and PD-1 levels in lymphocytes in response to co-culture with MDA-MB-231/MCF-7. Changes in frequency of CTLA-4+ and PD-1+ cells within CD4+ and CD8+ lymphocytes (**a**), expression of these markers presented as mean fluorescence intensity (MFI) (**b**), and percentage of CTLA-4+ or PD-1+ CD4+ and CD8+ cells within total pool of lymphocytes (**c**) ($n = 8$). Asterisks above individual cancer cell line columns show the level of significance with colors indicating whether a difference is reported when the specific column is compared to cancer cells alone (black) or co-cultured with PBMC (light grey) (* $p < 0.05$, ** $p < 0.01$, *** $p < 0.001$, **** $p < 0.0001$). Moreover, brackets with significance demonstrated are applied when there was a difference in response between MDA-MB-231 and MCF-7 cells.

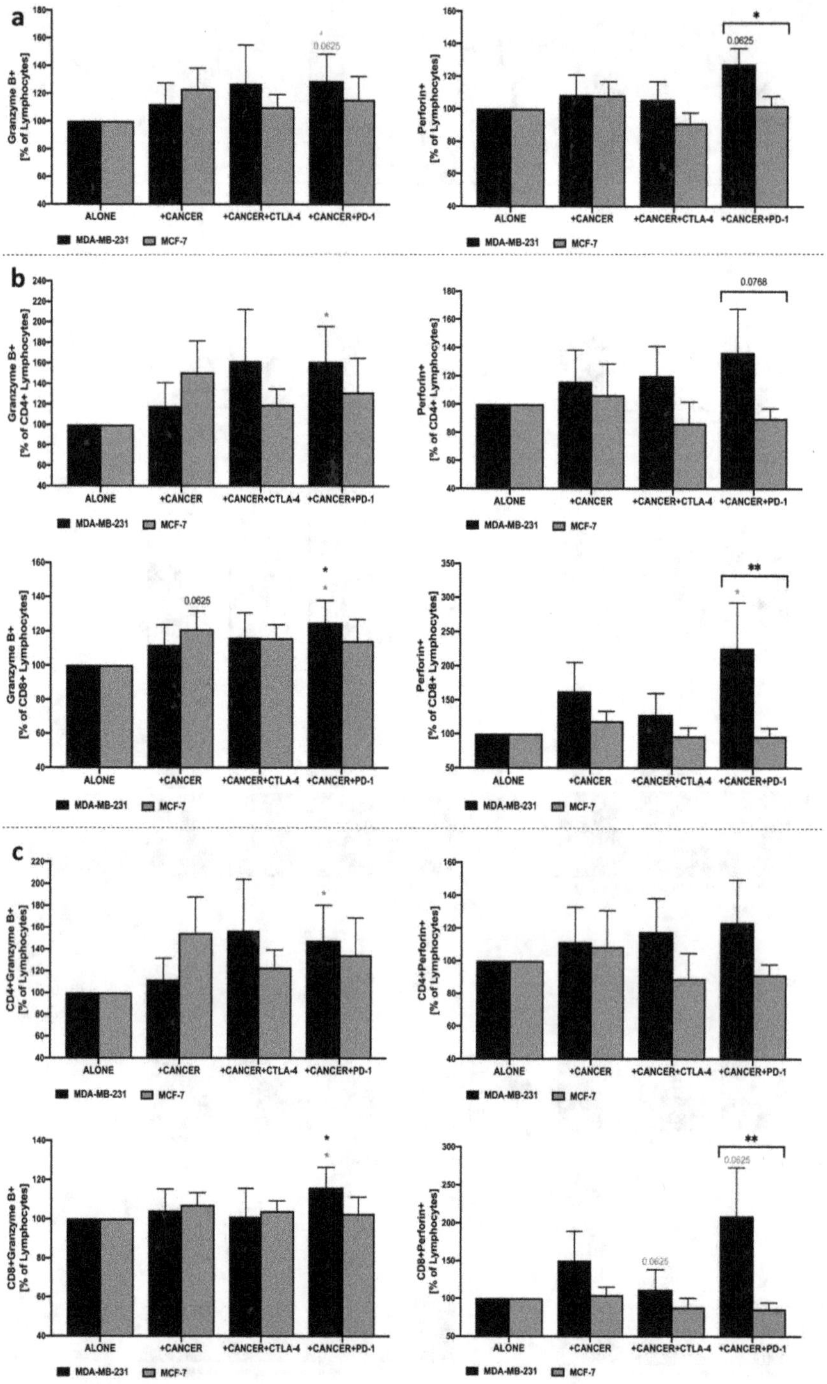

Figure 5. Granzyme B and perforin production in PBMC following co-culture with MDA-MB-231/MCF-7 and CTLA-4/PD-1 blockage. Changes in frequency of granzyme B+ and perforin+ cells were presented as the frequency within total lymphocytes (**a**), CD4+ and CD8+ lymphocytes (**b**), and percentage of granzyme B+ or perforin+ CD4+/CD8+ cells within the total pool of lymphocytes (**c**) ($n = 6$). Asterisks above individual cancer cell line columns show the level of significance with colors indicating whether the difference is reported when the specific column is compared to cancer cells alone (black) or co-cultured with PBMC (light grey) (* $p < 0.05$, ** $p < 0.01$, *** $p < 0.001$, **** $p < 0.0001$). Moreover, brackets with significance demonstrated are applied when there was a difference in response between MDA-MB-231 and MCF-7 cells.

4. Discussion

Cytotoxic T lymphocyte-associated antigen 4 (CTLA-4) and programmed cell death protein 1 (PD-1), both representing the immune checkpoint receptor family, are essential factors in maintaining homeostasis of the immune system through negatively regulating immune responses, providing self-tolerance [29]. This phenomenon can be also observed in the tumor microenvironment, where the overexpression of inhibitory immune checkpoints causes the depletion in anti-tumor activity resulting in tumor cells' proliferation and metastasis [30]. Therefore, inhibiting the axis between cancer and immune cells through antibodies directed at CTLA-4/PD-1 leads to the invaluable improvement in treatment efficacy of numerous malignant tumors especially melanoma, lung cancer, and breast cancer [6,31]. The effectiveness of CTLA-4 blocking is supported by studies demonstrating prolonged cells activation and sustained inflammation [32]. Here we implemented in vitro model involving breast cancer cell lines (MDA-MB-231 and MCF-7) and healthy PBMC (Supplementary Figure S2; model justified by numerous studies [27,28] to reveal how blocking of CTLA-4 or PD-1 might contribute to anti-cancer effects, and whether its support initially presumed hypothesis.

In accordance with previous results suggesting the favorable role of anti-CTLA-4 antibodies in supporting gemcitabine-based suppression of tumor growth in mice (with anti-CTLA-4 alone exhibiting a slight hampering effect) [17], we found that CTLA-4 blockage effectively supports the response of immune cells against cancer cells. However, here we demonstrated that not only type of breast cancer is essential to obtain the same response but also individual features of cancer cells. The triple-negative model of breast cancer was the one responding with growth inhibition to additional implementation with anti-CTLA-4. Such changes were not found when MCF-7 cells (ER-positive) were used, thus suggesting the need for careful consideration of immunotherapy application in breast cancers. In the study of Peng et al., the molecular analysis of CTLA-4 expression on different subtypes of breast cancer cells showed the highest CTLA-4 level in TNBC, which seems to be a direct confirmation of our results [33].

Analysis of immune checkpoint proteins on tested breast cancer cells revealed the difference between them also in the context of these molecules apart from hormone receptors. The obtained data demonstrated the dominance of PD-L1 in MDA-MB-231 and PD-1 in breast cancer cells. In addition, PD-1 seemed to be the predominant checkpoint protein. Despite low levels of CTLA-4 on the surface of the lymphocytes, its inhibition was still more effective in reducing MDA-MB-231 cell proliferation than PD-1 blockage. These data suggest the need for future mechanistic research to comprehensively study mutual interactions between immune checkpoints and breast cancer cells modulation in the immunotherapeutic application.

In experiments with dendritic cells transfected with anti-CTLA-4 antibody mRNA, the activity of this immune modulator was associated with the enhancement of antigen-specific cytotoxic T lymphocytes (CTL) responses against breast cancer cells, including MCF-7, MDA-MB-231, and T4D7 cell lines [34]. On the contrary, we observed that application of anti-CTLA-4 (and PD-1 partially) antibodies into the tumor micro-environment inhibits CD4+ and CD8+ cell activity affecting their interaction with breast cancer cells. Here, however, changes were only observed in MDA-MB-231 and not MCF-7 breast cancer cells. In the context of PD-1 inhibition, lack of changes in MDA-MB-231 breast cancer cell proliferation would appear to be in accordance with previous data indicating no effects on survival and metastasis of tumors treated only with anti-PD-1 antibodies [20]. Interestingly, blockage of PD-1 was still found to affect cancer cells viability compared to the co-culture with PBMC alone. Additionally, MCF-7, as in the case of proliferation, did not demonstrate an unambiguous response to selected immunotherapeutic in the context of viability.

The results of our study on the effects of breast cancer cells on the cytokine production profile of CD4+ and CD8+ lymphocytes are reflected in research conducted recently in animal models by da Cunha et al. Both research teams demonstrated that the presence of breast cancer cells did not affect the frequency of IL-10-producing CD4+ T cells, but instead significantly reduced IL-10-positive CD8+ T cells. Furthermore, in both CD4+ and CD8+ T cells, interaction with tumor cells did not influence the production of IFN-gamma [35]. Interestingly, we found that ER-positive MCF-7 cancer cells unlike MDA-MB-231 did not respond with a decline in IFN-gamma or IL-10 production in lymphocytes. Furthermore, previously obtained data from other research teams has indicated that failure of NAC treatment and lack of complete response was significantly associated with the immunosuppressive activity of IL-10 [36] Interestingly, we found that the application of CTLA-4 blocking antibodies effectively reduced the production of IL-10 within lymphocytes, predominantly through a decline in IL-10+ CD8+ cell frequency. Therefore, blockage of CTLA-4 on lymphocytes might allow for overriding adverse suppression of the anti-tumor immune response through reduction of cells bearing suppressive potential, including IL-10-producing Th2 cells, or possibly even Foxp3+ regulatory T cells or IL-10-producing regulatory B cells. Such a favorable role of immunosuppressive Foxp3+ T cell depletion was demonstrated previously in a mouse model of mammary carcinoma where reduced immunosuppressive activity significantly affected tumor progression through increased cancer cell death and improved overall survival [37]. In line with this, Pruitt et al. showed that the presence of immune checkpoint modulators inhibits induction of regulatory T cells and related immunosuppressive effects [34]. In addition to changes in IFN-gamma or IL-10, granzyme B/perforin-related cytotoxic effects were clearly detected when anti-PD-1 (partially anti-CTLA-4) was implemented in co-culture of PBMC with MDA-MB-231. Importantly, no changes were found when the ER-positive MCF-7 model was tested. In general, however, features of breast cancer must be carefully monitored before any therapeutic approach will be implemented as these might affect the effectiveness of the response to the immunotherapy.

Experiments conducted by Chen et al. showed that inhibition of anti-tumor response might not only occur through the interaction of tumor receptors with T cell-expressed CTLA-4, but also via suppression of dendritic cell function as a consequence of their interaction with CTLA-4+ breast cancer cells. Furthermore, blockage of CTLA-4 on breast cancer cells led to the restoration of dendritic and T cells activity with concomitant inhibition of cancer cell proliferation [38]. These data are in accordance with the results obtained in our study where CTLA-4 inhibition led to a significant reduction of breast cancer cell proliferation. However, we consider the blocking of anti-tumor activity is associated with cancer cell interaction with CTLA-4+ lymphocytes, thus, making the T cells of crucial importance, as far as MDA-MB-231 cells are considered. In the study by Kaewkangsadan et al., it has been demonstrated that unlike intratumoral infiltration by CD4+ and CD8+ T cells, tumor-infiltrating CTLA-4+ and PD-1+ T cell levels were not associated with pathological complete response (pCR) following neoadjuvant chemotherapy (NAC) in large and locally advanced breast cancers (LLABC) [36]. In the present study, we have shown that blockage of CTLA-4 receptor on lymphocytes and concomitant reduction of CD4+CTLA-4+ and CD8+PD-1+ cells seem to be a crucial element in inhibition of MDA-MB-231 breast cancer cell proliferation and their arrest in the G1-phase.

Additionally, our results, in combination with data from Page et al. indicate that application of anti-CTLA-4 antibodies is likely not only to increase the number of infiltrating T cells in the tumor environment showed by their team, but also to reduce the proportion of unfavorable immunosuppressive populations of CTLA-4+ lymphocytes as demonstrated by change of lymphocytes phenotype in our study [11]. In contrast, PD-1 blocking did not affect the proliferation status of MDA-MB-231 cells, even though it effectively reduced the frequency of PD-1+ CD4+ and CD8+ lymphocytes. It is worth noting that the reduced frequency of PD-1-expressing lymphocytes might have favorable effects on avoiding tumor-induced PD-L1-driven suppression of the immune response which has been previously suggested to be responsible for the reduced survival of breast cancer patients [18]. Other research teams have indicated the possible association between the number of PD-1-positive T lymphocytes infiltrating the tumor environment with worse overall survival rate in breast cancer patients [39,40]. With reference to PD-1 expression within lymphocyte subsets, slight differences in response to anti-PD-1 blockage seem to be associated with differential expression of PD-1 in tumor-associated lymphocytes, predominantly in CD4+ T cells [41]. In fact, PD-1 expression is different between CD4+ and CD8+ lymphocytes but here we demonstrated that the latter population exhibit the highest levels of PD-1, with relatively lower levels of CTLA-4 in both cell types simultaneously. Noteworthy, the presence of MCF-7 cells led to completely different changes compared to MDA-MB-231 in reference to CTLA-4 or PD-1 expression. Co-culture of PBMC with MCF-7 breast cancer cells is causing an increase in CTLA-4 and PD-1 expression within lymphocytes. In the study of Saleh et al., the MCF-7 breast cancer cells greatly upregulated the PD-1 expression in CD4+CD25− T cells, having no significant impact on CD4+CD25+ lymphocytes [25]. Furthermore, we reported that anti-PD-1 application predominantly diminished these effects. Cumulatively, such an increase in selected immune checkpoint proteins might be a possible explanation of the different responses of MCF-7 cancer cells when compared to MDA-MB-231.

Unlike Sagiv-Barfi et al. who demonstrated the effects of a lack of PD-L1-blockage IFN-gamma production in CD44+ central memory T cells(19), here we have shown a significant reduction of IFN-gamma-producing T cells (exclusively CD4+ lymphocytes) in response to anti-PD-1 and anti-CTLA-4 inhibition. Such phenomenon, however, was only observed in triple-negative MDA-MB-231 cancer cells, not MCF-7. Another research group showed that the supportive potential of CTLA-4 blockage in HER2/Neu antibody and triciribine combination treatment of mouse mammary tumors was associated with increased concentrations of IFN-gamma in tumor lysates and plasma [42]. Interestingly, Sagiv-Barfi et al. reported that PD-L1 inhibition combined with ibrutinib treatment (in A20 lymphoma cell line) led to increased frequency of IFN-gamma-producing CD44+ central memory T cells [19]. Likewise, the application of anti-PD-1 with anti-GITR antibodies synergistically induced the production of IFN-gamma in tumor-associated lymphocytes. However, in accordance with our data, PD-1 monotherapy did not affect the frequencies of IFN-gamma-producing CD8+ T cells [43]. Moreover, we found that cytotoxicity against MDA-MB-231 breast cancer cells was associated with an increase in granzyme B and perforin B. As indicated above, such effect was not obtained in the MCF-7 cancer cell line co-cultured with PBMC. To summarize, we assume that the observed reduction in the number of IFN-gamma-producing CD4+ T cells might be simultaneously associated with an increased release of IFN-gamma into the cancer cell micro-environment in triple-negative MDA-MB-231 cancer cells. It was followed additionally by an increase in cytotoxicity-related perforin/granzyme B within lymphocytes. It is worth noting that previous studies in mouse models of breast cancer demonstrated that repetitive administration of PD-1/PD-L1 axis-blocking antibodies can cause fatal hypersensitivity reactions [44]. Based on the obtained results, we presume that such phenomenon might be associated with IFN-gamma reduction within lymphocytes following anti-PD-1 administration, which in fact has been shown in numerous studies to play a protective role in the context of excessive immune responses [45,46]. Considering observed differences in immune checkpoint proteins in tested breast cancer cell lines, appropriate selection of these molecules' inhibitors might decrease these adverse effects, maintaining anti-cancer effects adjusted to cancer type.

5. Conclusions

The obtained results indicate the advantageous properties of CTLA-4 blockage within lymphocytes in the suppression of breast cancer cell proliferation. However, our data revealed that responses of cancer cells might be different depending on surface expression of hormone receptors, or as indicated in here, variations in immune checkpoint molecules. Thus, further experiments would be crucial to carefully consider the therapeutic anti-tumor potential of CTLA-4 modulation in the context of breast cancer treatment. In addition, combining immune checkpoint inhibitors with factors amplifying their effects is another issue of current investigation. One of them is demonstrated in an animal model blockage of CD73 leading to improved efficiency of anti-CTLA-4- or anti-PD1-induced antitumor activity in colon, prostate, and breast cancer subjects [47]. Here demonstrated the contribution of other checkpoint molecules such as CD80 suggest that studies on the combinatory application of these protein inhibitors might be of great importance, especially considering different features of only seemingly the same types of breast cancers. Furthermore, recent data has been shown to be promising regarding anti-SEMA4D antibody (semaphorin 4D, CD100) and its enhancing properties in relation to immunomodulation of the anticancer ability of anti-CTLA4/PD-1 antibody activity [48]. This data has been crucial in shedding new light on novel therapeutic approaches involving a combination of CD100 and immune checkpoint blocking antibodies.

Author Contributions: K.G., M.Z.W., and M.M. (Marcin Moniuszko) have made a substantial contribution to the project concept. K.G., M.M. (Marcin Moniuszko) have designed the work and supervised project implementation. K.G., A.K.-G., D.G., I.P., A.E., L.B., A.S., M.M. (Marta Mysliwiec), J.K. and J.M.H. have performed the experiments, acquired and analyzed data. K.G., A.K.-G. and M.M. (Marcin Moniuszko) summarized the data and prepared the manuscript. All authors read and approved the final manuscript.

References

1. Coms¸a, S¸.; Cîmpean, A.M.; Raica, M. The Story of MCF-7 Breast Cancer Cell Line: 40 years of Experience in Research. *Anticancer Res.* **2015**, *35*, 3147–3154.
2. McDonald, E.S.; Clark, A.S.; Tchou, J.; Zhang, P.; Freedman, G.M. Clinical Diagnosis and Management of Breast Cancer. *J. Nucl. Med.* **2016**, *57* (Suppl. 1), 9S–16S. [CrossRef]
3. Li, W.; Shi, X.; Xu, Y.; Wan, J.; Wei, S.; Zhu, R. Tamoxifen promotes apoptosis and inhibits invasion in estrogen-positive breast cancer MCF-7 cells. *Mol. Med. Rep.* **2017**, *16*, 478–484. [CrossRef]
4. Dent, R.; Trudeau, M.; Pritchard, K.I.; Hanna, W.M.; Kahn, H.K.; Sawka, C.A.; Lickley, L.A.; Rawlinson, E.; Sun, P.; Narod, S.A. Triple-negative breast cancer: Clinical features and patterns of recurrence. *Clin. Cancer Res.* **2007**, *13*, 4429–4434. [CrossRef]
5. Sharma, P.; Allison, J.P. The future of immune checkpoint therapy. *Science* **2015**, *348*, 56–61. [CrossRef]
6. Ishida, Y. PD-1: Its Discovery, Involvement in Cancer Immunotherapy, and Beyond. *Cells* **2020**, *9*, 1376. [CrossRef] [PubMed]
7. Xu, Z.; Shen, J.; Wang, M.H.; Yi, T.; Yu, Y.; Zhu, Y.; Chen, B.; Chen, J.; Li, L.; Li, M.; et al. Comprehensive molecular profiling of the B7 family of immune-regulatory ligands in breast cancer. *Oncoimmunology* **2016**, *5*, e1207841. [CrossRef]
8. Jaberipour, M.; Habibagahi, M.; Hosseini, A.; Habibabad, S.R.; Talei, A.; Ghaderi, A. Increased CTLA-4 and FOXP3 transcripts in peripheral blood mononuclear cells of patients with breast cancer. *Pathol. Oncol. Res.* **2010**, *16*, 547–551. [CrossRef] [PubMed]
9. Kolacinska, A.; Cebula-Obrzut, B.; Pakula, L.; Chalubinska-Fendler, J.; Morawiec-Sztandera, A.; Pawlowska, Z.; Zawlik, I.; Morawiec, Z.; Jesionek-Kupnicka, D.; Smolewski, P. Immune checkpoints: Cytotoxic T-lymphocyte antigen 4 and programmed cell death protein 1 in breast cancer surgery. *Oncol. Lett.* **2015**, *10*, 1079–1086. [CrossRef] [PubMed]
10. Dai, Z.; Tian, T.; Wang, M.; Liu, X.; Lin, S.; Yang, P.; Liu, K.; Zheng, Y.; Xu, P.; Liu, M.; et al. CTLA-4 polymorphisms associate with breast cancer susceptibility in Asians: A meta-analysis. *PeerJ* **2017**, *5*, e2815. [CrossRef]
11. Page, D.B.; Yuan, J.; Redmond, D.; Wen, Y.H.; Durack, J.C.; Emerson, R.; Solomon, S.; Dong, Z.; Wong, P.; Comstock, C.; et al. Deep Sequencing of T-cell Receptor DNA as a Biomarker of Clonally Expanded TILs in Breast Cancer after Immunotherapy. *Cancer Immunol. Res.* **2016**, *4*, 835–844.12. [CrossRef] [PubMed]
12. Gajewski, T.F. Cancer immunotherapy. *Mol. Oncol.* **2012**, *6*, 242–250. [CrossRef]
13. Denkert, C.; Loibl, S.; Noske, A.; Roller, M.; Müller, B.M.; Komor, M.; Budczies, J.; Darb-Esfahani, S.; Kronenwett, R.; Hanusch, C.; et al. Tumor-associated lymphocytes as an independent predictor of response to neoadjuvant chemotherapy in breast cancer. *J. Clin. Oncol.* **2010**, *28*, 105–113. [CrossRef] [PubMed]
14. Tsang, J.Y.; Au, W.L.; Lo, K.Y.; Ni, Y.B.; Hlaing, T.; Hu, J.; Chan, S.K.; Chan, K.F.; Cheung, S.Y.; Tse, G.M. PD-L1 expression and tumor infiltrating PD-1+ lymphocytes associated with outcome in HER2+ breast cancer patients. *Breast Cancer Res. Treat.* **2017**, *162*, 19–30. [CrossRef] [PubMed]
15. Nanda, R.; Chow, L.Q.; Dees, E.C.; Berger, R.; Gupta, S.; Geva, R.; Pusztai, L.; Pathiraja, K.; Aktan, G.; Cheng, J.D.; et al. Pembrolizumab in Patients with Advanced Triple-Negative Breast Cancer: Phase Ib KEYNOTE-012 Study. *J. Clin. Oncol.* **2016**, *34*, 2460–2467. [CrossRef]
16. Adams, S.; Schmid, P.; Rugo, H.S.; Winer, E.P.; Loirat, D.; Awada, A.; Cescon, D.W.; Iwata, H.; Campone, M.; Nanda, R.; et al. Pembrolizumab monotherapy for previously treated metastatic triple-negative breast cancer: Cohort A of the phase II KEYNOTE- 086 study. *Ann. Oncol.* **2019**, *30*, 397–404. [CrossRef] [PubMed]
17. American Association for Cancer Research, Checkpoint Inhibitors Boost Power of Antibody-Drug Conjugate. *Cancer Discov.* **2016**, *6*, e61895.

18. Lesterhuis, W.J.; Salmons, J.; Nowak, A.K.; Rozali, E.N.; Khong, A.; Dick, I.M.; Harken, J.A.; Robinson, B.W.; Lake, R.A. Synergistic effect of CTLA-4 blockade and cancer chemotherapy in the induction of anti-tumor immunity. *PLoS ONE* **2013**, *8*, e61895. [CrossRef]
19. Vonderheide, R.H.; LoRusso, P.M.; Khalil, M.; Gartner, E.M.; Khaira, D.; Soulieres, D.; Dorazio, P.; Trosko, J.A.; Rüter, J.; Mariani, G.L.; et al. Tremelimumab in combination with exemestane in patients with advanced breast cancer and treatment-associated modulation of inducible costimulator expression on patient T cells. *Clin. Cancer Res.* **2010**, *16*, 3485–3494. [CrossRef]
20. Sagiv-Barfi, I.; Kohrt, H.E.; Czerwinski, D.K.; Ng, P.P.; Chang, B.Y.; Levy, R. Therapeutic antitumor immunity by checkpoint blockade is enhanced by ibrutinib, an inhibitor of both BTK and ITK. *Proc. Natl. Acad. Sci. USA* **2015**, *112*, E966–E972. [CrossRef]
21. Black, M.; Barsoum, I.B.; Truesdell, P.; Cotechini, T.; Macdonald-Goodfellow, S.K.; Petroff, M.; Siemens, D.R.; Koti, M.; Craig, A.W.; Graham, C.H. Activation of the PD-1/PD-L1 immune checkpoint confers tumor cell chemoresistance associated with increased metastasis. *Oncotarget* **2016**, *7*, 10557–10567. [CrossRef]
22. Kim, P.S.; Kwilas, A.R.; Xu, W.; Alter, S.; Jeng, E.K.; Wong, H.C.; Schlom, J.; Hodge, J.W. IL-15 superagonist/IL-15RαSushi-Fc fusion complex (IL-15SA/IL-15RαSu-Fc; ALT-803) markedly enhances specific subpopulations of NK and memory CD8+ T cells, and mediates potent anti-tumor activity against murine breast and colon carcinomas. *Oncotarget* **2016**, *7*, 16130–16145. [CrossRef] [PubMed]
23. Gao, J.J.; Swain, S.M. Luminal A Breast Cancer and Molecular Assays: A Review. *Oncologist* **2018**, *23*, 556–565. [CrossRef]
24. Kern, R.; Panis, C. CTLA-4 Expression and Its Clinical Significance in Breast Cancer. *Arch. Immunol. Ther. Exp.* **2021**, *69*, 16. [CrossRef] [PubMed]
25. Saleh, R.; Toor, S.M.; Khalaf, S.; Elkord, E. Breast Cancer Cells and PD-1/PD-L1 Blockade Upregulate the Expression of PD-1, CTLA-4, TIM-3 and LAG-3 Immune Checkpoints in $CD4^+$ T Cells. *Vaccines* **2019**, *7*, 149. [CrossRef] [PubMed]
26. Janeway, C.A., Jr.; Travers, P.; Walport, M.; Shlomchik, M.J. Immunobiology: The Immune System in Health and Disease. In *Principles of Innate and Adaptive Immunity*, 5th ed.; Garland Science: New York, NY, USA, 2001.
27. Courau, T.; Bonnereau, J.; Chicoteau, J.; Bottois, H.; Remark, R.; Miranda, L.A.; Toubert, A.; Blery, M.; Aparicio, T.; Allez, M.; et al. Cocultures of human colorectal tumor spheroids with immune cells reveal the therapeutic potential of MICA/B and NKG2A targeting for cancer treatment. *J. Immunother. Cancer* **2019**, *7*, 74. [CrossRef]
28. Saraiva, D.P.; Matias, A.T.; Braga, S.; Jacinto, A.; Cabral, M.G. Establishment of a 3D Co-culture With MDA-MB-231 Breast Cancer Cell Line and Patient-Derived Immune Cells for Application in the Development of Immunotherapies. *Front. Oncol.* **2020**, *10*, 1543. [CrossRef] [PubMed]
29. Shadbad, M.A.; Hajiasgharzadeh, K.; Baghbanzadeh, A.; Safarpour, H.; Mokhtarzadeh, A.; Brunetti, O.; Yue, S.C.; Silvestris, N.; Baradaran, B. Immune Checkpoints and CAR-T Cells: The Pioneers in Future Cancer Therapies? *Int. J. Mol. Sci.* **2020**, *21*, 8305.
30. Derakhshani, A.; Hashemzadeh, S.; Asadzadeh, Z.; Shadbad, M.A.; Rasibonab, F.; Safarpour, H.; Jafarlou, V.; Solimando, A.G.; Racanelli, V.; Singh, P.K.; et al. Cytotoxic T-Lymphocyte Antigen-4 in Colorectal Cancer: Another Therapeutic Side of Capecitabine. *Cancers* **2021**, *13*, 2414. [CrossRef]
31. Rotte, A. Combination of CTLA-4 and PD-1 blockers for treatment of cancer. *J. Exp. Clin. Cancer Res.* **2019**, *38*, 255. [CrossRef] [PubMed]
32. Abramiuk, M.; Be̜bnowska, D.; Hrynkiewicz, R.; Polak, P.N.G.; Kotarski, J.; Rolin′ ski, J.; Grywalska, E. CLTA-4 Expression is Associated with the Maintenance of Chronic Inflammation in Endometriosis and Infertility. *Cells* **2021**, *10*, 487. [CrossRef]
33. Peng, Z.; Su, P.; Yang, Y.; Yao, X.; Zhang, Y.; Jin, F.; Yang, B. Identification of CTLA-4 associated with tumor microenvironment and competing interactions in triple negative breast cancer by co-expression network analysis. *J. Cancer* **2020**, *11*, 6365–6375. [CrossRef]
34. Pruitt, S.K.; Boczkowski, D.; de Rosa, N.; Haley, N.R.; Morse, M.A.; Tyler, D.S.; Dannull, J.; Nair, S. Enhancement of anti-tumor immunity through local modulation of CTLA-4 and GITR by dendritic cells. *Eur. J. Immunol.* **2011**, *41*, 3553–3563. [CrossRef] [PubMed]
35. da Cunha, A.; Michelin, M.A.; Murta, E.F.C. Phenotypic profile of dendritic and T cells in the lymph node of Balb/C mice with breast cancer submitted to dendritic cells immunotherapy. *Immunol. Lett.* **2016**, *177*, 25–37. [CrossRef]
36. Kaewkangsadan, V.; Verma, C.; Eremin, J.M.; Cowley, G.; Ilyas, M.; Eremin, O. Crucial Contributions by T Lymphocytes (Effector, Regulatory, and Checkpoint Inhibitor) and Cytokines (TH1, TH2, and TH17) to a Pathological Complete Response Induced by Neoadjuvant Chemotherapy in Women with Breast Cancer. *J. Immunol. Res.* **2016**, *2016*, 4757405. [CrossRef] [PubMed]
37. Bos, P.D.; Plitas, G.; Rudra, D.; Lee, S.Y.; Rudensky, A.Y. Transient regulatory T cell ablation deters oncogene-driven breast cancer and enhances radiotherapy. *J. Exp. Med.* **2013**, *210*, 2435–2466. [CrossRef]
38. Chen, X.; Shao, Q.; Hao, S.; Zhao, Z.; Wang, Y.; Guo, X.; He, Y.; Gao, W.; Mao, H. CTLA-4 positive breast cancer cells suppress dendritic cells maturation and function. *Oncotarget* **2017**, *8*, 13703–13715. [CrossRef]

39. Mao, Y.; Qu, Q.; Chen, X.; Huang, O.; Wu, J.; Shen, K. The Prognostic Value of Tumor-Infiltrating Lymphocytes in Breast Cancer: A Systematic Review and Meta-Analysis. *PLoS ONE* **2016**, *11*, e0152500. [CrossRef] [PubMed]
40. Sun, S.; Fei, X.; Mao, Y.; Wang, X.; Garfield, D.H.; Huang, O.; Wang, J.; Yuan, F.; Sun, L.; Yu, Q.; et al. PD-1(+) immune cell infiltration inversely correlates with survival of operable breast cancer patients. *Cancer Immunol. Immunother.* **2014**, *63*, 395–406. [CrossRef]
41. Muenst, S.; Soysal, S.D.; Gao, F.; Obermann, E.C.; Oertli, D.; Gillanders, W.E. The presence of programmed death 1 (PD-1)-positive tumor-infiltrating lymphocytes is associated with poor prognosis in human breast cancer. *Breast Cancer Res. Treat.* **2013**, *139*, 667–676. [CrossRef] [PubMed]
42. Wang, Q.; Li, S.H.; Wang, H.; Xiao, Y.; Sahin, O.; Brady, S.W.; Li, P.; Ge, H.; Jaffee, E.M.; Muller, W.J.; et al. Concomitant targeting of tumor cells and induction of T-cell response synergizes to effectively inhibit trastuzumab-resistant breast cancer. *Cancer Res.* **2012**, *72*, 4417–4428. [CrossRef] [PubMed]
43. Lu, L.; Xu, X.; Zhang, B.; Zhang, R.; Ji, H.; Wang, X. Combined PD-1 blockade and GITR triggering induce a potent antitumor immunity in murine cancer models and synergizes with chemotherapeutic drugs. *J. Transl. Med.* **2014**, *12*, 36. [CrossRef]
44. Mall, C.; Sckisel, G.D.; Proia, D.A.; Mirsoian, A.; Grossenbacher, S.K.; Pai, C.S.; Chen, M.; Monjazeb, A.M.; Kelly, K.; Blazar, B.R.; et al. Repeated PD-1/PD-L1 monoclonal antibody administration induces fatal xenogeneic hypersensitivity reactions in a murine model of breast cancer. *Oncoimmunology* **2015**, *5*, e1075114. [CrossRef] [PubMed]
45. Meissner, N.; Swain, S.; McInnerney, K.; Han, S.; Harmsen, A.G. Type-I IFN signaling suppresses an excessive IFN-gamma response and thus prevents lung damage and chronic inflammation during Pneumocystis (PC) clearance in CD4 T cell-competent mice. *Am. J. Pathol.* **2010**, *176*, 2806–2818. [CrossRef]
46. Chang, E.Y.; Guo, B.; Doyle, S.E.; Cheng, G. Cutting edge: Involvement of the type I IFN production and signaling pathway in lipopolysaccharide-induced IL-10 production. *J. Immunol.* **2007**, *178*, 6705–6709. [CrossRef] [PubMed]
47. Allard, B.; Pommey, S.; Smyth, M.J.; Stagg, J. Targeting CD73 enhances the antitumor activity of anti-PD-1 and anti-CTLA-4 mAbs. Clin. *Cancer Res.* **2013**, *19*, 5626–5635.
48. Evans, E.E.; Jonason, A.S., Jr.; Bussler, H.; Torno, S.; Veeraraghavan, J.; Reilly, C.; Doherty, M.A.; Seils, J.; Winter, L.A.; Mallow, C.; et al. Antibody Blockade of Semaphorin 4D Promotes Immune Infiltration into Tumor and Enhances Response to Other Immunomodulatory Therapies. *Cancer Immunol. Res.* **2015**, *3*, 689–701. [CrossRef]

13

Prognostic Significance of *O*-GlcNAc and PKM2 in Hormone Receptor-Positive and HER2-Nonenriched Breast Cancer

Wen-Ling Kuo [1,†], Lin-Lu Tseng [2,†], Che-Chang Chang [3,†], Chih-Jung Chen [4,5,†], Mei-Ling Cheng [6,7,†], Hsin-Hung Cheng [2], Meng-Jen Wu [2], Yu-Lun Chen [2], Ruei-Ting Chang [3], Hsiang-Yu Tang [7], Yong-Chen Hsu [4], Wen-Jye Lin [8], Cheng-Yuan Kao [8], Wen-Ping Hsieh [9], Hsing-Jien Kung [10,11] and Wen-Ching Wang [2,*]

1 Division of Breast Surgery, General Surgery, Department of Surgery, Chang Gung Memorial Hospital Linkou Medical Center, Taoyuan City 33305, Taiwan; sylvie5285@gmail.com
2 Institute of Molecular and Cellular Biology and Department of Life Sciences, National Tsing-Hua University, Hsinchu City 30013, Taiwan; linlutseng@gapp.nthu.edu.tw (L.-L.T.); fabiencheng@gmail.com (H.-H.C.); mengjhen@gmail.com (M.-J.W.); utopia_peter@hotmail.com.tw (Y.-L.C.)
3 The Ph.D. Program for Translational Medicine, College of Medical Science and Technology, Taipei Medical University, Taipei City 11031, Taiwan; ccchang168@tmu.edu.tw (C.-C.C.); bulesky7879@hotmail.com (R.-T.C.)
4 Department of Pathology and Laboratory Medicine, Taichung Veterans General Hospital, Taichung City 40705, Taiwan; cjchen1016@gmail.com (C.-J.C.); shuyongjen@hotmail.com (Y.-C.H.)
5 School of Medicine, Chung Shan Medical University, Taichung City 40201, Taiwan
6 Department of Biomedical Sciences, College of Medicine, Chang Gung University, Taoyuan City 33302, Taiwan; chengm@gap.cgu.edu.tw
7 Metabolomics Core Laboratory, Healthy Aging Research Center, Chang Gung University, Taoyuan City 33302, Taiwan; tangshyu@gmail.com
8 Immunology Research Center, National Health Research Institutes, Miaoli County 35053, Taiwan; wjlin@nhri.edu.tw (W.-J.L.); chengyuankao@nhri.edu.tw (C.-Y.K.)
9 Institute of Statistics, National Tsing Hua University, Hsinchu City 30013, Taiwan; wphsieh@stat.nthu.edu.tw
10 Graduate Institute of Cancer Biology and Drug Discovery, Taipei Medical University, Taipei City 11031, Taiwan; hkung@tmu.edu.tw
11 Department of Biochemistry and Molecular Medicine, University of California Davis School of Medicine, University of California Davis Cancer Centre, Sacramento, CA 95817, USA
* Correspondence: wcwang@mx.nthu.edu.tw;
† These authors contributed equally to this work.

Abstract: Predictive metabolic biomarkers for the recurrent luminal breast cancer (BC) with hormone receptor (HR)-positive and human epidermal growth factor receptor type 2 (HER2)-negative are lacking. High levels of *O*-GlcNAcylation (*O*-GlcNAc) and pyruvate kinase isoenzyme M2 (PKM2) are associated with malignancy in BC; however, the association with the recurrence risk remains unclear. We first conduct survival analysis by using the METABRIC dataset to assess the correlation of PKM2 expression with BC clinical outcomes. Next, patients with HR$^+$/HER2- luminal BC were recruited for PKM2/*O*-GlcNAc testing. Logistic regression and receiver operating characteristic curve analysis were performed to evaluate the 10-year DFS predicted outcome. Survival analysis of the METABRIC dataset revealed that high expression of PKM2 was significantly associated with worse overall survival in luminal BC. The high expression of *O*-GlcNAc or PKM2 was a significant independent marker for poor 10-year DFS using immunohistochemical analysis. The PKM2 or *O*-GlcNAc status was a significant predictor of DFS, with the combination of PKM2–*O*-GlcNAc status and T stage greatly enhancing the predictive outcome potential. In summary, *O*-GlcNAc, PKM2, and T stage serve as good prognostic discriminators in HR$^+$/HER2$^-$ luminal BC.

Keywords: *O*-GlcNAc; PKM2; HR$^+$/HER2$^-$ luminal breast cancer; metabolism; prognosis

---

1. Introduction

The incidence of breast cancer (BC), a common malignancy in women, is rising sharply in East Asia, particularly in relatively young or premenopausal women, possibly due to a Westernized lifestyle and environmental factors [1]. BC is a highly heterogeneous disease and is molecularly classified into five intrinsic subgroups based on gene expression signatures, which was modified for clinical utility using pathologic parameters and receptor status by immunohistochemistry (IHC) in paraffin-embedded sections [2]: (1) luminal A (human epidermal growth factor receptor type 2 $(HER2)^-$, estrogen receptor (ER) and/or progesterone receptor $(PR)^+$, with Ki-67 < 20%), (2) luminal B ($HER2^-$, ER, and/or PR^+, with Ki-67 > 20% or grade (3)), (3) luminal HER2 ($HER2^+$, ER, and/or PR^+), (4) HER2 ($HER2^+$, ER^-, and PR^-), and (5) triple-negative BC (TNBC; ER^-, PR^-, and $HER2^-$).

The risk of relapse in the Luminal B subtype, which is characterized by positive hormonal receptors (HRs), non-amplified *HER2*, a higher tumor grade, a higher Ki-67 level, and more aggressive tumor behavior, is high and increases at a constant rate up to 10 years after diagnosis [3]. The incidence of the luminal subtype is also higher (i.e., 67%) among cases of premenopausal BC, 72% of which are luminal B with a high tumor grade (grade 2–3) and are associated with worse prognoses than that of luminal A [4–6]. Although luminal A and B harbor overlapping intrinsic markers and distinct clinical and molecular features, genomic analyses have revealed higher frequencies of DNA amplification and chromosomal alterations, as well as a higher tumor mutational burden in luminal B than in luminal A, which offers growth advantage independent of estrogen stimulation [7].

Clinicopathological parameters, such as tumor diameter and nodal status (TN) as well as tumor grade, are strongly associated with long-term disease-free survival (DFS) in $HR^+/HER2^-$ BC [8]. The Nottingham prognostic index (NPI) is the earliest tool combining nodal status, tumor size, and histological grade to predict outcomes in early BC [9,10]. The clinical treatment score post-5 years (CTS5) integrates tumor size, tumor grade, patient age, and the number of nodes (https://www.cts5-calculator.com (accessed on 7 April 2020)), and provides another useful web-based tool to estimate the risk of late recurrences [11,12]. As a continuous variable, the CTS5 score can be used to categorize patients into low, intermediate, and high-risk groups (<5%, 5–10%, and >10% distant recurrence risk, respectively) after 5 years of endocrine therapy for postmenopausal women. A recent validation study of a large sample of patients with BC using SEER (Surveillance, Epidemiology, and End Results) data has revealed a comparable prognostic power in both premenopausal and postmenopausal patients with BC [13]. In contrast, Sestak et al. recently evaluated CTS5 in the TAILORx trial and reported that the prognostic value is lower in patients aged 50 years or younger than in older patients [14].

Multigene expression signature is clinically useful to predict the relapse risk in $HR^+/HER2^-$ BCs [15]. For instance, OncotypeDx (a 21-gene assay) [16–18] and MammaPrint (a 70-gene assay) [19] offer recurrence scores to determine the benefit of adjuvant chemotherapy. EPclin score by EndoPredict [20], ROR score by Prosigna [21], and a two-gene ratio (*HOXB13/IL17BR*) by Breast Cancer Index [22] are also commercial risk-predicting panels. These gene-expression-based assays are primarily based on the analysis of marker genes, which may offer some clues for understanding complex mechanisms underlying BC progression.

An emerging approach for the prediction of recurrence and risk stratification involves metabolic panels, as cancer cell proliferation and progression are fueled by metabolic reprogramming [23–26]. Warburg metabolism, which diverts glycolytic flux into aerobic glycolysis, is observed in proliferating tumors [25]. In addition, increasing evidence suggests that upregulated *O*-GlcNAcylation of key factors contributes to cancer progression [27,28]. The sugar substrate UDP-*N*-acetylglucosamine (UDP-GlcNAc) generated from the hexosamine biosynthetic pathway (HBP) is utilized for the *O*-GlcNAc modification [27,28]. HBP integrates nutrient status from the metabolism of glucose, amino acids, and fatty acids and is involved in the regulation of signal transduction and metabolic reprogramming [29]. Notably, enhanced *O*-GlcNAcylation is important for BC malignancy, metastasis, and endocrine resistance [30–33].

PKM2, a glycolytic enzyme (conversion of phosphoenolpyruvate into pyruvate), serves as a control point in the metabolic network of cancer cells [34,35]. Metabolites (such as fructose-1,6-bisphosphate, serine, phenylalanine) and post-translational modifications regulate PKM2's pyruvate kinase activity and hence the carbon flow to regulate the Warburg metabolism [34,35]. PKM2 exhibits non-metabolic functions, acting as a coactivator of HIF-1α, Stat3, and β-catenin pathways in the nucleus [36,37] and exhibiting protein kinase activity toward H3 and Stat3 [38–40]. PKM2 also partners with the oncogenic demethylase KDM8, which promotes the nuclear translocation of PKM2 and hence Warburg metabolism [41,42]. Notably, PKM2 is overexpressed in BC and is associated with poor clinical outcomes in a large-scale analysis [42] and in a meta-analysis of breast tumors [42,43]. Furthermore, an elevated degree of *O*-GlcNAcylated PKM2 is found in breast tumors [31]. *O*-GlcNAcylation of PKM2 at threonine 405 and serine 406 promotes tumor growth using a BC xenograft model [44]. Overexpression of PKM2 [45,46] and *O*-GlcNAcylation [30] have been indicated to confer a selection progression advantage to breast cancer. However, whether the expression of *O*-GlcNAc and/or PKM2 is associated with clinical outcomes in different BC subtypes remains unclear. In this study, we evaluated the clinical relevance of PKM2 expression in luminal tumors using the Metabric dataset. We also investigated the association between the expression of PKM2, *O*-GlcNAc, histological grade, and clinical outcomes in a retrospective cohort of endocrine-treated $HR^+/HER2^-$ patients by IHC and survival analysis, with a focus on the risk of recurrence.

2. Materials and Methods

2.1. Dataset Analysis

The METABRIC dataset [47] retrieved from (https://www.cbioportal.org (accessed on 25 March 2021)) was used to evaluate the correlation between PKM2 expression and clinical outcome in luminal tumors. The gene mRNA expression levels were divided into quartiles. A survival analysis was performed between the lowest group (bottom 25%) and the highest group (top 25%) using a log-rank test.

2.2. Study Subjects

A total of 3166 $HR^+/HER2^-$ luminal BC patients who had received therapy at Chang-Gung Memorial Hospital (CGMH), Linkou, Taiwan (2005–2013) were reviewed based on the pathological and clinical properties. The diagnostic criteria for $HR^+/HER2^-$ luminal BC was based on the receptor status (ER, PR, and HER2) by IHC and *HER2* amplification by fluorescence in situ hybridization (FISH) in invasive cancer as the following: HR^+, more than 1% positive for ER or PR; $HER2^-$, an IHC score of 0 to 1+, or 2+ with non-amplified *HER2* by FISH. One hundred and sixty-nine $HR^+/HER2^-$ patients who had concluding pathologic reports and no other malignancies were firstly selected. Seven patients were excluded for the following reasons: 4 cases with incomplete initial diagnostic information, 2 with mucinous carcinoma, and 1 with no available formalin-fixed paraffin-embedded block of the primary tumor. The final number of enrollments was 162, including 50 patients with documented recurrence and 112 patients without any recurrence over 10 years (Figure 1 and Table 1). Demographic factors of this retrospective cohort included age, history of diabetes, ER and PR status, tumor size, grade, TN stage, surgical treatment, chemotherapy use, endocrine therapy, and radiotherapy. The time and location of recurrence were documented. The study protocols have been approved by the Institutional Review Board of CGMH (IRB#201700716A3).

2.3. IHC Assessment

Consecutive paraffin-embedded serial sections of specimens (n = 162) were obtained from CGMH for single IHC staining of PKM2 and *O*-GlcNAc. The specimens were deparaffinized and rehydrated with xylene (Sigma-Aldrich) and ethanol (100% ethanol for 10 min, 95% ethanol for 5 min, 80% ethanol for 3 min, 70% ethanol for 3 min, 50% ethanol for 2 min, and then deionized water for 5 min). For antigen retrieval, specimens were incubated with citrate buffer at pH 6.0 (10 mM citrate, 0.05% Tween 20) and autoclaved at 121 °C for 20 min. The immunostaining procedures were performed using Novolink Polymer

Detection System (Leica) according to the manufacturer's manual. In brief, tissues were stained with anti-*O*-GlcNAc or anti-PKM2 for 60 min at room temperature. The working dilution of the primary antibody was 1:50 for anti-*O*-GlcNAc (838004, Biolegend, San Diego, CA, USA) and 1:100 for anti-PKM2 (D78A4, Cell Signaling Technology, Danvers, MA, USA). The IHC results were reviewed blindly by two pathologists (CJ Chen and YC Hsu) based on two parameters: the staining intensity score (0 = negative; 1 = weak; 2 = moderate; and 3 = strong), and the percentage of immunopositive cells (0–100) [48,49]. The Q score (0–300) was calculated by multiplying these two parameters. Two groups were stratified based on the Q score: low expression ($Q \leq$ mean) and high expression ($Q >$ mean). Kaplan–Meier analysis was conducted to evaluate the clinical relevance.

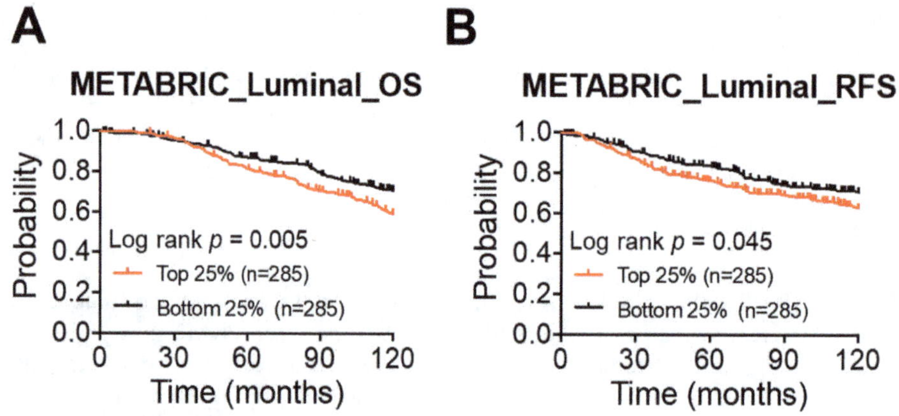

Figure 1. High expression of PKM2 is significantly associated with worse overall survival in luminal tumors. (**A**,**B**) A 10-year overall survival (**A**) and relapse-free survival (**B**) analysis based on the expression level of PKM2 in luminal tumors. Data were obtained from the METABRIC online dataset. The mRNA expression levels of PKM2 were divided into quartiles. An analysis between the top quartile group (top 25%) and the bottom one (bottom 25%) was then compared by a log-rank test.

2.4. Statistical Analysis

A Chi-square test was performed to compare clinicopathological properties of the patients with categorical variables. Kaplan–Meier analysis was conducted to assess overall patient survival, which was estimated as the time from diagnosis until death or until last follow-up. The log-rank test was used to determine the statistical significance between groups. Spearman's correlation was performed to evaluate the status of *O*-GlcNAc, PKM2, or CTS5 with each of the clinical parameters. Differences were considered significant at $p < 0.05$. All *p*-values were obtained from 2-sided tests.

Logistic regression analysis was used to assess the contribution of the expression of *O*-GlcNAc and PKM2 and/or the CTS5 score in prognosis. A *p*-value of less than 0.05 was considered significant. The receiver operating characteristic (ROC) curve was plotted based on the set of sensitivity and specificity. The area under the curve (AUC) was computed using numerical integration of the ROC curves. Cox regression analysis was conducted to characterize the effect of one (*O*-GlcNAc, PKM2, invasive tumor size, T stage, or CTS5) or multiple variables (*O*-GlcNAc, PKM2, and/or a clinical parameter) upon the time of a DFS event takes to happen. Univariate and multivariate Cox regression, as well as logistic regression analyses, were performed using IBM SPSS, version 25 (IBM Corp. New York, NY, USA).

Table 1. Clinical properties of patients.

Factors		Non-Recurrent No. (%), n = 112	Recurrent No. (%), n = 50	p-Value
Molecular subtype	Luminal A Luminal B	73 (65.2) 39 (34.8)	35 (70.0) 15 (30.0)	0.548
Age (years)	Median (IQR)	51.0 (16.0)	53.0 (22.0)	0.517
Age (years)	≤ 50 > 50	51 (45.5) 61 (54.5)	20 (40.0) 30 (60.0)	0.512
Diabetes mellitus	No Yes	104 (92.9) 8 (7.1)	45 (90.0) 5 (10.0)	0.542
Operation type	Mastectomy Breast conservation	62 (55.4) 50 (44.6)	27 (54.0) 23 (46.0)	0.873
Invasive tumor size (cm)	Median (IQR)	1.9 (1.4)	2.4 (1.7)	0.019
SBR grade	1 2 3	13 (11.6) 61 (54.5) 38 (33.9)	5 (10.0) 30 (60.0) 15 (30.0)	0.806
Estrogen receptor	Negative Positive	4 (3.6) 108 (96.4)	0 50 (100.0)	0.312
Progesterone receptor	Negative Positive	11 (9.8) 101 (90.2)	3 (6.0) 47 (94.0)	0.553
Ki67 index (%)	< 25% ≥ 25%	30 (26.8) 16 (14.3)	17 (34.0) 16 (32.0)	0.006
	Missing	66 (58.9)	17 (34.0)	
T stage	T1a T1b T1c T2 T3 T4	0 8 (7.1) 54 (48.2) 45 (40.2) 5 (4.5) 0	1 (2.0) 1 (2.0) 14 (28.0) 30 (60.0) 3 (6.0) 1 (2.0)	0.014
N stage	N0 N1 N2 N3	56 (50.0) 40 (35.7) 12 (10.7) 4 (3.6)	21 (42.0) 22 (44.0) 3 (6.0) 4 (8.0)	0.353
Stage	I II III	40 (35.7) 55 (49.1) 17 (15.2)	9 (18.0) 33 (66.0) 8 (16.0)	0.067
Chemotherapy	No Yes	19 (17.0) 93 (83.0)	7 (14.0) 43 (86.0)	0.635
Hormone therapy	No Yes	3 (2.7) 109 (97.3)	2 (4.0) 48 (96.0)	0.645
Radiotherapy	No Yes	57 (50.9) 55 (49.1)	23 (46.0) 27 (54.0)	0.565

3. Results

3.1. Clinical Relevance of PKM2 Expression in Luminal Tumors

PKM2 is overexpressed in the breast tumors [42] and associated with poor BC prognosis in a meta-analysis [43]. We sought to further evaluate the clinical relevance of *PKM2* expression in the luminal tumors using the METABRIC cohort defined by PAM50 [47]. Figure 1A shows that patients with high PKM2 expression exhibited a significantly worse 10-year survival than did those with low PKM2 expression (top 25% vs. bottom 25%,

$p = 0.005$). A significantly worse relapse-free survival was also found for the top-quartile group as compared with the bottom-quartile one (top 25% vs. bottom 25%, $p = 0.045$) (Figure 1B). We also evaluated the clinical relevance of *PKM2* expression in the basal and HER2 subtypes of BC tumors using the METABRIC cohort. Figure S1A shows that the basal subtype exhibited a significantly worse 10-year relapse-free-survival (RFS) (top 25% vs. bottom 25%, $p = 0.046$) but no significant difference in a 10-year overall survival (OS) outcome for the PKM2-high expression group. There was no significance for the HER2 subtype (Figure S1B).

These results suggested that high expression of PKM2 is associated with a worse clinical outcome in luminal tumors.

3.2. *High PKM2 and High O-GlcNAc and Predicts Poor Prognosis in $HR^+/HER2^-$ BC*

Patients with $HR^+/HER2^-$ luminal BC ($n = 3166$, 2005–2013 at Chang Gung Memorial Hospital) were classified into two groups based on pathological and IHC features: luminal A (ER and/or PR^+, Ki67 $\leq$ 20%, or grade 1) and luminal B (ER and/or PR^+, Ki67 > 20%, or grade 2 or 3). The luminal B group exhibited a significantly lower survival rate than that of the luminal A group (10-year overall survival (OS), $p < 0.001$; 10-year DFS, $p < 0.001$) (Figure 2A,B), revealing the substantial outcome difference between the two subtypes in our hospital-based population.

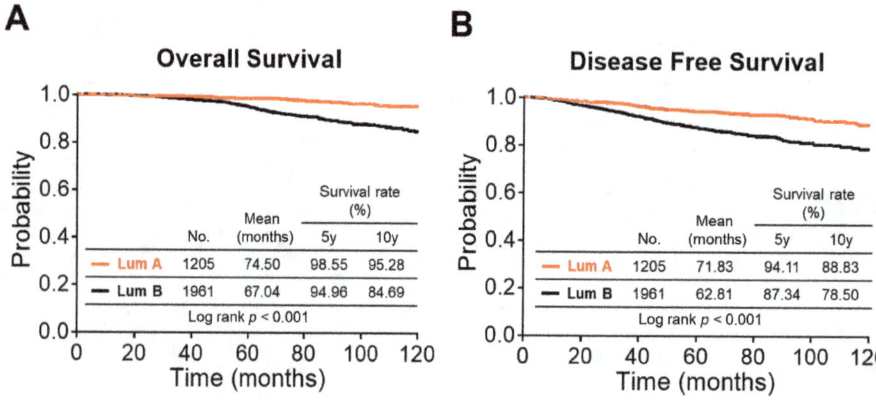

Figure 2. Survival analysis for HR^+ luminal BC at Chang Gung Memorial Hospital (2005–2013). (**A**,**B**) Overall survival (**A**) and DFS (**B**) curves for HR^+ luminal BC at Chang Gung Memorial Hospital (2005–2013). Lum A, luminal A ($n = 1205$); Lum B, luminal B ($n = 1961$). For group comparisons, p-values were determined by a log-rank test.

We next evaluated the clinical relevance of PKM2 abundance in *$HR^+/HER2^-$* luminal BC using IHC analysis. Additionally, we evaluated the clinical association with respect to *O*-GlcNAc expression because of its implication in BC progression and endocrine resistance [30–33]. A retrospective cohort study was conducted on 162 subjects (non-recurrent, $n = 112$, median (interquartile range (IQR)) age, 51.0 (16.0) years; recurrent, $n = 50$, median (IQR) age, 53.0 (22.0) years) who had received BC therapy and were followed up until December, 2018 (median period, 123.4 months, IQR, 107.4–134.1 months) (Figure 3 and Table 1).

O-GlcNAc and PKM2 were characterized by IHC staining for each of the samples (Figure 4). We first conducted Spearman's correlation analyses of the status of *O*-GlcNAc, PKM2, or CTS5 with each of the clinical parameters. We were nonetheless not able to perform analysis for the Ki67 index because of 83 missing values. As shown in Table S1, the Spearman's rank correlation coefficient of *O*-GlcNAc with each of the clinical parameters was low (correlation coefficient = −0.12–0.14), indicating low or no correlation. Similar results were also obtained for the Spearman's rank correlation of PKM2 with each of the clinical parameters (Table S2; correlation coefficient = −0.293-0.149). On the other hand, CTS5 includes the information of tumor size, tumor grade, and the number of nodes, exhibited a strong correlation with invasive tumor size, SBR Grade, T stage, N stage, or Stage (Table S3, correlation coefficient $\geq$0.679). These results together suggest that there was no or low correlation of PKM2 or *O*-GlcNAc expression with each of the clinical parameters in this retrospective cohort. Univariate Cox regression analysis revealed that invasive tumor size ($p = 0.020$), T stage ($p = 0.004$), *O*-GlcNAc expression ($p < 0.001$), or PKM2 expression ($p = 0.048$) was significantly associated with DFS whereas CTS5 ($p = 0.109$) had a non-significant impact (Table S4).

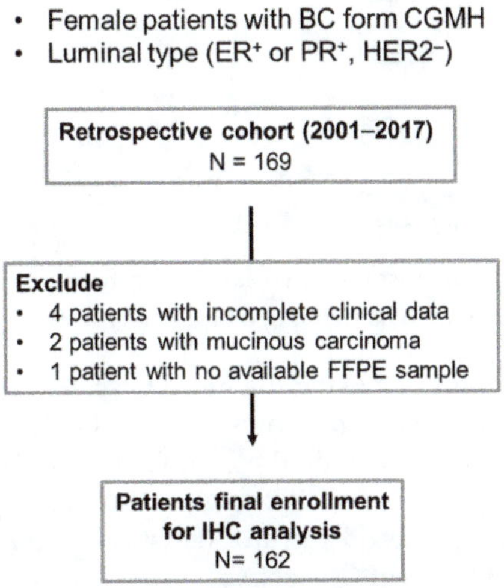

Figure 3. Flow diagram of patient selection in this study. One hundred and sixty-nine $HR^+/HER2^-$ patients who had pathologic reports and no other malignancies diagnosed in 2005–2013 were considered for this retrospective study. Seven were excluded because of incomplete clinical follow-up data ($n = 4$), mucinous carcinoma ($n = 2$), or no available formalin-fixed paraffin-embedded block of the primary tumor ($n = 1$).

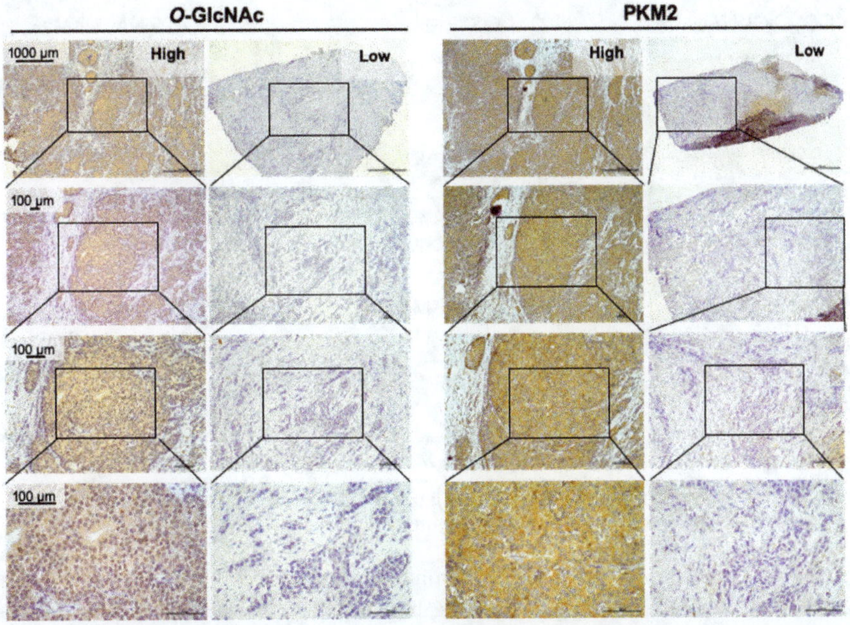

Figure 4. Representative images of IHC profiles. *O*-GlcNAc and PKM2 were immunostained for each of the BC specimens ($n = 162$). Low, Q $\leq$ mean; High, Q > mean. The images are enlarged in series (box, the enlarged portions).

To assess the expression level of *O*-GlcNAc or PKM2 in relation to recurrence risk, patients were stratified into a non-recurrent or a recurrent group. As shown in Figure 5, high expression levels of *O*-GlcNAc ($p = 0.013$) or PKM2 ($p < 0.001$) were positively associated with the risk for cancer recurrence.

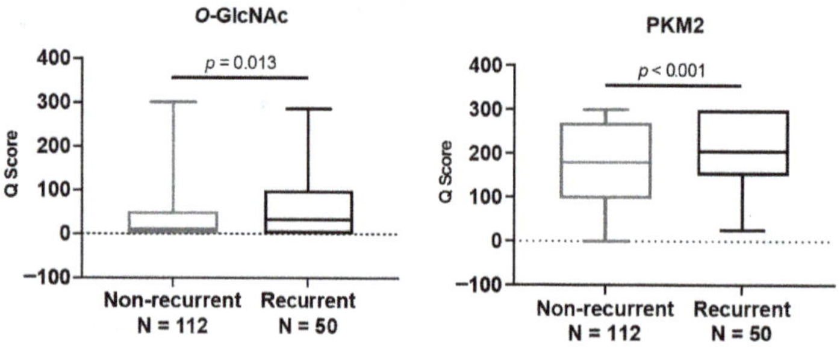

Figure 5. High *O*-GlcNAc or high PKM2 expression is significantly associated with the risk of recurrence. For group comparisons, *p*-values were determined by a two-tailed Student's *t*-test.

Furthermore, samples were stratified into two groups using the mean Q score as a threshold. A Kaplan–Meier survival analysis revealed that high expression of *O*-GlcNAc (*O*-GlcNAcHigh, $p = 0.094$), PKM2 (PKM2High, $p = 0.390$), or the combined double-marker status (*O*-GlcNAcHighPKM2High vs. *O*-GlcNAcLowPKM2Low, $p = 0.083$) were associated with worse overall survival, supporting a trend toward statistical significance (Figure 6A–C). Interestingly, high expression levels of *O*-GlcNAc (*O*-GlcNAcHigh, $p = 0.038$) or PKM2 (PKM2High, $p = 0.032$) were significantly associated with worse DFS (Figure 6D–F). Importantly, the combined double-marker status offered an even greater statistical significance (*O*-GlcNAcHighPKM2High vs. *O*-GlcNAcLowPKM2Low, $p = 0.004$) (Figure 6F). These results suggest that high expression levels of *O*-GlcNAc and PKM2 are associated with a high risk of recurrence and worse DFS.

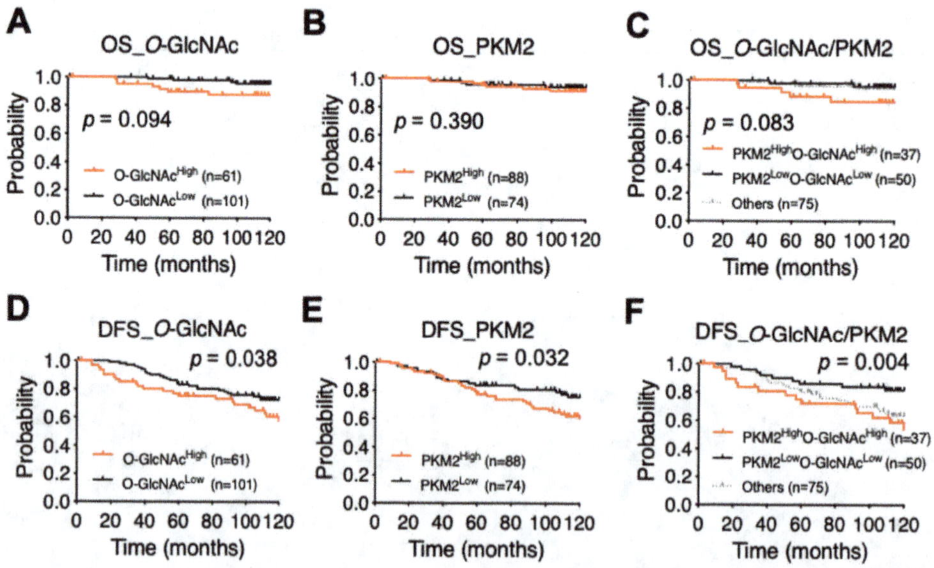

Figure 6. Survival of patients with $ER^+/HER2^-$ luminal BC according to the levels of *O*-GlcNAc and PKM2. (**A–C**) The Kaplan–Meier analysis of overall survival (OS) based on the expression level of *O*-GlcNAc (**A**) or PKM2 (**B**) alone or both (**C**). (**D–F**) Elevated expression of *O*-GlcNAc (**D**) or PKM2 (**E**) alone or both (**F**) is significantly correlated with 10-year DFS. For group comparisons, *p*-values for a single-marker (high vs. low) or double-marker (*O*-GlcNAChighPKM2high vs. *O*-GlcNAClowPKM2low) statuses were determined by log-rank test.

3.3. Logistic Regression and Receiver Operating Characteristic (ROC) Curve Analyses

We next sought to evaluate the impact of PKM2 and *O*-GlcNAc combined with a clinical parameter (invasive tumor size, T stage, or CTS5 that integrates four clinical properties [12]) on the risk of 10-year DFS using multivariate Cox regression analysis. As shown in Table S5, the invasive tumor size-*O*-GlcNAc-PKM2 Cox analysis revealed that invasive tumor size and *O*-GlcNAc served as significant factors, whereas PKM2 was a virtually significant element. Similar results were also found for the T stage-*O*-GlcNAc-PKM2 analysis (Table S6). For the CTS5-*O*-GlcNAc-PKM2 multivariate Cox analysis, *O*-GlcNAc was significantly associated with DFS (Table S7), indicating that *O*-GlcNAc is a good prognostic marker in this multivariate Cox analysis. CTS5 also had a trend to be statistically significant. PKM2 expression nonetheless had no significance. It was likely that there was less information that could be provided by PKM2 in this multivariate analysis, perhaps because of the overlapped signals from *O*-GlcNAcylated PKM2, particularly in the *O*-GlcNAChighPKM2high cases (Figure 4).

Next, we built the logistic regression models using PKM2, *O*-GlcNAc, and/or a clinical parameter (invasive tumor size, T stage, or CTS5) to evaluate the risk of the 10-year DFS outcome. Tables S8–S10 show that each marker (PKM2, *O*-GlcNAc, and an individual clinical parameter (invasive tumor size, T stage, or CTS5)) significantly contributed to the DFS outcome per triple-marker model. Since ROC analysis provides a means to assess the diagnostic ability of a binary classifier system and select possibly optimal models [50], we next conduct ROC analysis to comparing the performance of PKM2 and *O*-GlcNAc in combination with another clinical parameter (invasive tumor size, T stage, or CTS5). Interestingly, the ROC curve analyses revealed that the best performance was seen for the *O*-GlcNAc-PKM2-T stage model (AUC = 0.722), as compared with the *O*-GlcNAc-PKM2-the invasive tumor size model (AUC = 0.699) and the CTS5-*O*-GlcNAc-PKM2 model (AUC = 0.712) (Figure 7). A reduced performance was seen for a single-marker alone (PKM2, *O*-GlcNAc, or CTS5) or the *O*-GlcNAc-PKM2 model (Figure 7). Together, these results suggested that the expression of *O*-GlcNAc and PKM2 provided extra information in addition to the clinical factors. Importantly, T stage, PKM2, and *O*-GlcNAc served as the best prognostic discriminators in the 10-year DFS outcome, offering an improved prognostic indicator for $HR^+/HER2^-$ luminal BC.

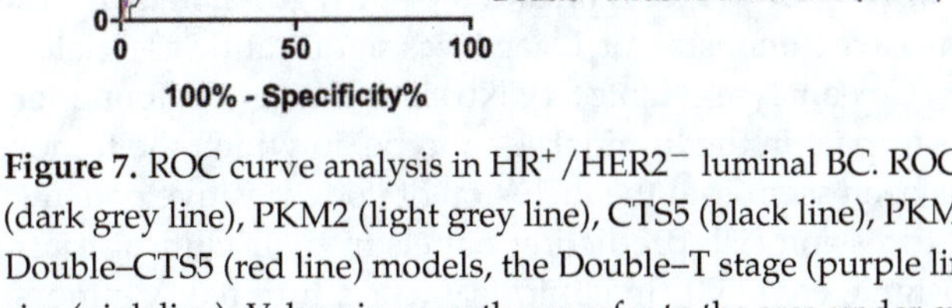

Figure 7. ROC curve analysis in $HR^+/HER2^-$ luminal BC. ROC curve analyses using the *O*-GlcNAc (dark grey line), PKM2 (light grey line), CTS5 (black line), PKM2–*O*-GlcNAc (Double, blue line) the Double–CTS5 (red line) models, the Double–T stage (purple line), and the Double–Invasive tumor size (pink line). Values in parentheses refer to the area under curve (AUC).

4. Discussion

Although the expression profiling of risk genes across BC genomes has provided useful information of high genomic risk for $HR^+/HER2^-$ BC [51], the dysregulated metabolic landscape engaged in BC progression and prognosis remains largely unclear. In this study, analysis of large databases revealed that high expression of PKM2 was significantly associated with worse overall survival in luminal tumors. We thus evaluated the expression of PKM2 (a key Warburg-metabolism protein) and *O*-GlcNAc (a nutrient-status integrator) in a retrospective cohort of luminal $HR^+/HER2^-$ BC. Interestingly, high expression of *O*-GlcNAc ($p = 0.038$) or that of PKM2 ($p = 0.032$) was significantly associated with poor 10-year DFS. Remarkably, the combination of the two markers had an even greater significance ($p = 0.004$). The logistic regression analysis also supported this conclusion. Together, the high clinical relevance of the high expression of PKM2 or *O*-GlcNAc with poor 10-year DFS in this retrospective study agrees well with the findings from survival analysis of the METABRIC dataset, as well as other reports regarding their contribution to more aggressive BC behavior [30,42,43,52]. Importantly, these results suggest that they might serve as potential new prognostic markers in luminal $HR^+/HER2^-$ BC.

Clinicopathological factors, particularly TN, have been commonly used in the decision-making process for selecting adjuvant treatments for $ER^+/HER2^-$ BC [15]. Despite a good prognostic value for those clinical parameters, the overall concordance among different parameters in each patient is often heterogeneous. In a meta-analysis of ER^+ BC patients receiving 5-year endocrine therapy, the risk of late recurrence is found to range from 10% to 41% for up to 20 years, although there is a strong correlation of distant recurrence with the original TN status [8]. Current molecular diagnostics also provides predictive and prognostic values [15–18,20–22]. Despite this, there have been limitations in predicting the risk of recurrence and treatment resistance, particularly low aggressive $ER^+/HER2^-$ tumors [53].

In the present study, we added the expression of PKM2 and *O*-GlcNAc as two potential biomarkers because other groups and we have found their potential relevance in breast cancers [30,31,41–43,46]. We have employed IHC analysis and found that levels of PKM2 and *O*-GlcNAc were highly associated with the disease progression and survival of breast cancer patients. We have repeatedly conducted an immunohistochemical analysis of PKM2 and *O*-GlcNAc levels in breast cancer samples and found our results were consistent and reproducible. We have also conducted multi-levels of experiments in validating our findings, including gel filtration, western blot analysis, and IHC of tissue blocks to confirm our antibody tool is reliable. Compared to molecular diagnostics using mRNA- and DNA-based markers, we consider our markers to have great advantages in clinical practice because of the simple and cost-effective approach using IHC has also been widely used in routine diagnoses, such as HER2 staining, offering a great advantage in routine clinical practice.

Maximum likelihood estimation (MLE) provides a robust approach to determine the optimal cutoff for Cox model analysis. The key property of an MLE is a normal-distribution sampling when (1) the parameter, along with all other parameters in the model, is not at a boundary, and (2) sample size is usually assumed large in order to converge [54]. The two parameters (PKM2 and *O*-GlcNAc) in this cohort study were not normally distributed (the p-value of the normality test: *O*-GlcNAc, $p < 0.001$; PKM2, $p < 0.001$), possibly because of the small sample size. There were several boundaries in the PKM2 data ($Q = 300$, $n = 40$), which limited the subsequent Cox regression and logistic regression analysis. Therefore, no cutoff values were used in performing Cox regression and logistic regression analysis.

Notably, *O*-GlcNAc, PKM2, invasive tumor size, or T stage was significantly associated with the DFS outcome in univariate Cox analyses (Table S4). No significance was found for the N stage. Nodal status has less impact in the luminal A subtype, in which the tumor biology is less aggressive. This has been seen from the inclusion of node-positive patients in commercially available gene expression risk predicting panels in their clinical trials (Oncotype Dx, MammaPrint, Prosigna, etc.) [53]. In clinical practice, luminal A tumors are endocrine-sensitive, and the omission of chemotherapy in node-positive patients is also common. These patients enjoy a substantially better prognosis despite lymph node metastasis. On the other hand, the HR^+ cases were analyzed in this study. If a tumor is ER-negative, it was recruited because PR was positive. The progesterone pathway downstream of ER is still active despite a negative ER expression. However, the major reason for no impact from ER status is the small number of ER-negative cases ($n = 4$) in this study. We were, however, not able to evaluate the impact of Ki-67 in this investigation because of many missing values (n = 83).

Multivariate Cox regression analysis revealed that *O*-GlcNAc and a clinical parameter (invasive tumor size, T stage, or CTS5) had significant impacts on the DFS outcome and that PKM2 was virtually a significant factor in the triple-marker models.

Further logistic regression models and ROC curve analyses, interestingly, revealed that the T stage-*O*-GlcNAc-PKM2 triple model exhibited the best performance (Table S7, AUC = 0.722) when compared with the invasive tumor size-*O*-GlcNAc-PKM2 model (AUC = 0.699) and the CTS5-*O*-GlcNAc-PKM2 model (AUC = 0.712). These results suggested that *O*-GlcNAc, PKM2, and T stage together serve as good prognostic discriminators in ER^+/HER^- patients. It is likely that *O*-GlcNAc and PKM2 provide extra metabolic information in addition to the clinical information provided by the T stage. Given an intrinsically heterogeneous nature in breast tumors, further investigation is needed to substantiate our findings using a large-size cohort.

The complex interplay of prognostic factors and adjuvant treatments might dwindle the pure prognostic value of PKM2 and *O*-GlcNAc, which could have been shown in an untreated population. Despite this, we consider that new biomarkers must be evaluated over contemporary treatment to be clinically useful, which is critical to the rational development of therapeutic treatments. Taken together, the information of the expression of PKM2 and *O*-GlcNAc offers useful complementary information to clinicopathological variables.

Genomic assays providing individual risk estimates have been used to aid in adjuvant treatment decisions, particularly regarding the indication of adjuvant chemotherapy in $ER^+/HER2^-$ BC [15]. These assays comprise proliferation-related genes, which are associated with chemosensitivity, as well as proliferation-independent genes related to immune activity; thus, they are also predictive of chemotherapy benefits in different risk groups [16,19]. Our results demonstrated that the expression of PKM2 and *O*-GlcNAc could provide extra information to clinicopathological features to predict the prognostic outcome of BC patients representing an additional layer of information from metabolism. It is likely that crosstalk exists between metabolism and signaling that affects tumor progression [55,56], microenvironmental change [57], and perhaps endocrine therapy resistance [58,59], which in turn contribute to recurrence. Further investigation is needed to better understand the mechanisms by which *O*-GlcNAcylation and PKM2 contribute to the recurrence of luminal BC.

Our study population was based on a Taiwanese cohort of Chinese Han ethnic background in East Asia, where the frequencies of premenopausal patients and the luminal subtype in young patients are higher than those in the West [60]. It is speculated that there might be a complex interplay among the genetic background and environmental factors under the active ovarian function of young women in this region, which leads to a high premenopausal incidence of BC.

The Asian Breast Cancer Cooperative Group 2019 consensus recommends that the treatment of Asian women with luminal BC, particularly for those at the premenopausal stage, requires special considerations, distinct from international guidelines [61].

The strength of this study is that the clinical outcome data were available for all patients and tissue samples were well-characterized. We followed McGuire's guidelines to explore *O*-GlcNAc and PKM2 statuses as the new prognostic markers [62]. The *O*-GlcNAc and PKM2 statuses were measured in the same laboratory, with all personnel blinded to clinical outcome data. Our study translates a simple metabolism-based IHC analysis in the context of recurrence to clinical applications. The limitation of this study is that we have a selection of 162 $HR^+/HER2^-$ patients with a minimum follow-up of 10 years available from a single medical center in this retrospective analysis. A definitive study of the double marker status, including patients from multi-clinical centers, will be required to provide a solid foundation in a different cohort of patients. The need to further validate the prognostic value of the double-marker status to predict the risks of recurrence in a different cohort study population is important to ascertain this metabolism-based assy.

In summary, *O*-GlcNAc and PKM2 served as potentially independent prognostic markers in $HR^+/HER2^-$ luminal BC in this pilot study. The combination of *O*-GlcNAc-PKM2 with CTS5 provides excellent prognostic accuracy. These results highlight the potential benefits of a metabolism-based risk assay to improve decision-making regarding adjuvant treatment options.

Author Contributions: W.-C.W., W.-L.K., L.-L.T., C.-C.C., M.-L.C., W.-J.L., C.-Y.K. and H.-J.K. designed the study. W.-L.K. provided clinical resources. C.-C.C., H.-H.C., and R.-T.C. initiated IHC staining and analysis. C.-J.C. and Y.-C.H. advised the IHC experiment and scored the clinical subject for further analysis. L.-L.T., M.-J.W., Y.-L.C., H.-Y.T. and W.-P.H. performed all statistical data analysis and compilation. W.-C.W., W.-L.K. and L.-L.T. wrote the manuscript with the comments from all authors. All authors have read and agreed to the published version of the manuscript.

References

1. Matikas, A.; Foukakis, T.; Swain, S.; Bergh, J. Avoiding over- and undertreatment in patients with resected node-positive breast cancer with the use of gene expression signatures: Are we there yet? *Ann. Oncol* **2019**, *30*, 1044–1050. [CrossRef] [PubMed]
2. Inwald, E.C.; Koller, M.; Klinkhammer-Schalke, M.; Zeman, F.; Hofstadter, F.; Gerstenhauer, M.; Brockhoff, G.; Ortmann, O. 4-IHC classification of breast cancer subtypes in a large cohort of a clinical cancer registry: Use in clinical routine for therapeutic decisions and its effect on survival. *Breast Cancer Res. Treat.* **2015**, *153*, 647–658. [CrossRef] [PubMed]
3. Ribelles, N.; Perez-Villa, L.; Jerez, J.M.; Pajares, B.; Vicioso, L.; Jimenez, B.; de Luque, V.; Franco, L.; Gallego, E.; Marquez, A.; et al. Pattern of recurrence of early breast cancer is different according to intrinsic subtype and proliferation index. *Breast Cancer Res.* **2013**, *15*, R98. [CrossRef] [PubMed]
4. Cao, M.D.; Lamichhane, S.; Lundgren, S.; Bofin, A.; Fjosne, H.; Giskeodegard, G.F.; Bathen, T.F. Metabolic characterization of triple negative breast cancer. *BMC Cancer* **2014**, *14*, 941. [CrossRef]
5. Chu, Q.D.; Smith, M.H.; Williams, M.; Panu, L.; Johnson, L.W.; Shi, R.; Li, B.D.; Glass, J. Race/Ethnicity has no effect on outcome for breast cancer patients treated at an academic center with a public hospital. *Cancer Epidemiol. Biomark. Prev.* **2009**, *18*, 2157–2161. [CrossRef] [PubMed]
6. Parker, J.S.; Mullins, M.; Cheang, M.C.; Leung, S.; Voduc, D.; Vickery, T.; Davies, S.; Fauron, C.; He, X.; Hu, Z.; et al. Supervised risk predictor of breast cancer based on intrinsic subtypes. *J. Clin. Oncol.* **2009**, *27*, 1160–1167. [CrossRef]
7. Chin, K.; DeVries, S.; Fridlyand, J.; Spellman, P.T.; Roydasgupta, R.; Kuo, W.L.; Lapuk, A.; Neve, R.M.; Qian, Z.; Ryder, T.; et al. Genomic and transcriptional aberrations linked to breast cancer pathophysiologies. *Cancer Cell* **2006**, *10*, 529–541. [CrossRef]
8. Pan, H.; Gray, R.; Braybrooke, J.; Davies, C.; Taylor, C.; McGale, P.; Peto, R.; Pritchard, K.I.; Bergh, J.; Dowsett, M.; et al. 20-Year Risks of Breast-Cancer Recurrence after Stopping Endocrine Therapy at 5 Years. *N. Engl. J. Med.* **2017**, *377*, 1836–1846. [CrossRef]
9. Galea, M.H.; Blamey, R.W.; Elston, C.E.; Ellis, I.O. The Nottingham Prognostic Index in primary breast cancer. *Breast Cancer Res. Treat.* **1992**, *22*, 207–219. [CrossRef]
10. Lee, A.H.; Ellis, I.O. The Nottingham prognostic index for invasive carcinoma of the breast. *Pathol. Oncol. Res.* **2008**, *14*, 113–115. [CrossRef]
11. Dowsett, M.; Goldhirsch, A.; Hayes, D.F.; Senn, H.J.; Wood, W.; Viale, G. International Web-based consultation on priorities for translational breast cancer research. *Breast Cancer Res.* **2007**, *9*, R81. [CrossRef]
12. Dowsett, M.; Sestak, I.; Regan, M.M.; Dodson, A.; Viale, G.; Thurlimann, B.; Colleoni, M.; Cuzick, J. Integration of Clinical Variables for the Prediction of Late Distant Recurrence in Patients With Estrogen Receptor-Positive Breast Cancer Treated With 5 Years of Endocrine Therapy: CTS5. *J. Clin. Oncol* **2018**, *36*, 1941–1948. [CrossRef] [PubMed]
13. Wang, C.; Chen, C.; Lin, Y.; Zhou, Y.; Mao, F.; Zhu, H.; Zhang, X.; Shen, S.; Huang, X.; Wang, X.; et al. Validation of CTS5 model in large-scale breast cancer population and the impact of menopausal and HER2 status on its prognostic value. *Sci. Rep.* **2020**, *10*, 4660. [CrossRef] [PubMed]
14. Sestak, I.; Crager, M.; Cuzick, J.; Dowsett, M.; Shak, S.; Tang, G.; Gray, R.; Sparano, J.A. Validation of the clinical treatment score post 5 years (CTS5) in women with hormone receptor positive, HER2-negative, node-negative disease from the TAILORx study [abstract]. In *Proceedings of the 2019 San Antonio Breast Cancer Symposium: San Antonio, TX*; AACR: Philadelphia, PA, USA, 2019; p. Abstract nr GS4-03.

15. Sestak, I. Risk stratification in early breast cancer in premenopausal and postmenopausal women: Integrating genomic assays with clinicopathological features. *Curr. Opin. Oncol.* **2019**, *31*, 29–34. [CrossRef] [PubMed]
16. Sparano, J.A.; Gray, R.J.; Makower, D.F.; Pritchard, K.I.; Albain, K.S.; Hayes, D.F.; Geyer, C.E., Jr.; Dees, E.C.; Goetz, M.P.; Olson, J.A., Jr.; et al. Adjuvant Chemotherapy Guided by a 21-Gene Expression Assay in Breast Cancer. *N. Engl. J. Med.* **2018**, *379*, 111–121. [CrossRef] [PubMed]
17. Sparano, J.A.; Gray, R.J.; Ravdin, P.M.; Makower, D.F.; Pritchard, K.I.; Albain, K.S.; Hayes, D.F.; Geyer, C.E., Jr.; Dees, E.C.; Goetz, M.P.; et al. Clinical and Genomic Risk to Guide the Use of Adjuvant Therapy for Breast Cancer. *N. Engl. J. Med.* **2019**, *380*, 2395–2405. [CrossRef]
18. Francis, P.A.; Pagani, O.; Fleming, G.F.; Walley, B.A.; Colleoni, M.; Lang, I.; Gomez, H.L.; Tondini, C.; Ciruelos, E.; Burstein, H.J.; et al. Tailoring Adjuvant Endocrine Therapy for Premenopausal Breast Cancer. *N. Engl. J. Med.* **2018**, *379*, 122–137. [CrossRef]
19. Cardoso, F.; van't Veer, L.J.; Bogaerts, J.; Slaets, L.; Viale, G.; Delaloge, S.; Pierga, J.Y.; Brain, E.; Causeret, S.; DeLorenzi, M.; et al. 70-Gene Signature as an Aid to Treatment Decisions in Early-Stage Breast Cancer. *N. Engl. J. Med.* **2016**, *375*, 717–729. [CrossRef]
20. Sestak, I.; Martin, M.; Dubsky, P.; Kronenwett, R.; Rojo, F.; Cuzick, J.; Filipits, M.; Ruiz, A.; Gradishar, W.; Soliman, H.; et al. Prediction of chemotherapy benefit by EndoPredict in patients with breast cancer who received adjuvant endocrine therapy plus chemotherapy or endocrine therapy alone. *Breast Cancer Res. Treat.* **2019**, *176*, 377–386. [CrossRef]
21. Ohnstad, H.O.; Borgen, E.; Falk, R.S.; Lien, T.G.; Aaserud, M.; Sveli, M.A.T.; Kyte, J.A.; Kristensen, V.N.; Geitvik, G.A.; Schlichting, E.; et al. Prognostic value of PAM50 and risk of recurrence score in patients with early-stage breast cancer with long-term follow-up. *Breast Cancer Res.* **2017**, *19*, 120. [CrossRef]
22. Sgroi, D.C.; Sestak, I.; Cuzick, J.; Zhang, Y.; Schnabel, C.A.; Schroeder, B.; Erlander, M.G.; Dunbier, A.; Sidhu, K.; Lopez-Knowles, E.; et al. Prediction of late distant recurrence in patients with oestrogen-receptor-positive breast can- cer: A prospective comparison of the breast-cancer index (BCI) assay, 21-gene recurrence score, and IHC4 in the TransATAC study population. *Lancet Oncol.* **2013**, *14*, 1067–1076. [CrossRef]
23. Mishra, P.; Ambs, S. Metabolic Signatures of Human Breast Cancer. *Mol. Cell. Oncol.* **2015**, *2*, e992217. [CrossRef]
24. Collin, L.J.; Cronin-Fenton, D.P.; Ahern, T.P.; Christiansen, P.M.; Damkier, P.; Ejlertsen, B.; Hamilton-Dutoit, S.; Kjaersgaard, A.; Silliman, R.A.; Sorensen, H.T.; et al. Cohort Profile: The Predictors of Breast Cancer Recurrence (ProBe CaRE) Premenopausal Breast Cancer Cohort Study in Denmark. *BMJ Open* **2018**, *8*, e021805. [CrossRef]
25. Semenza, G.L. Hypoxia-inducible factors: Coupling glucose metabolism and redox regulation with induction of the breast cancer stem cell phenotype. *EMBO J.* **2017**, *36*, 252–259. [CrossRef]
26. Gandhi, N.; Das, G.M. Metabolic Reprogramming in Breast Cancer and Its Therapeutic Implications. *Cells* **2019**, *8*, 89. [CrossRef] [PubMed]
27. Fardini, Y.; Dehennaut, V.; Lefebvre, T.; Issad, T. O-GlcNAcylation: A New Cancer Hallmark? *Front. Endocrinol. (Lausanne)* **2013**, *4*, 99. [CrossRef] [PubMed]
28. Singh, J.P.; Zhang, K.; Wu, J.; Yang, X. O-GlcNAc signaling in cancer metabolism and epigenetics. *Cancer Lett.* **2015**, *356*, 244–250. [CrossRef] [PubMed]
29. Nagel, A.K.; Ball, L.E. Intracellular protein O-GlcNAc modification integrates nutrient status with transcriptional and metabolic regulation. *Adv. Cancer Res.* **2015**, *126*, 137–166. [CrossRef] [PubMed]
30. Gu, Y.; Mi, W.; Ge, Y.; Liu, H.; Fan, Q.; Han, C.; Yang, J.; Han, F.; Lu, X.; Yu, W. GlcNAcylation plays an essential role in breast cancer metastasis. *Cancer Res.* **2010**, *70*, 6344–6351. [CrossRef] [PubMed]
31. Champattanachai, V.; Netsirisawan, P.; Chaiyawat, P.; Phueaouan, T.; Charoenwattanasatien, R.; Chokchaichamnankit, D.; Punyarit, P.; Srisomsap, C.; Svasti, J. Proteomic analysis and abrogated expression of O-GlcNAcylated proteins associated with primary breast cancer. *Proteomics* **2013**, *13*, 2088–2099. [CrossRef]
32. Krzeslak, A.; Forma, E.; Bernaciak, M.; Romanowicz, H.; Brys, M. Gene expression of O-GlcNAc cycling enzymes in human breast cancers. *Clin. Exp. Med.* **2012**, *12*, 61–65. [CrossRef]
33. Kanwal, S.; Fardini, Y.; Pagesy, P.; N'Tumba-Byn, T.; Pierre-Eugene, C.; Masson, E.; Hampe, C.; Issad, T. O-GlcNAcylation-inducing treatments inhibit estrogen receptor alpha expression and confer resistance to 4-OH-tamoxifen in human breast cancer-derived MCF-7 cells. *PLoS ONE* **2013**, *8*, e69150. [CrossRef]
34. Iqbal, M.A.; Gupta, V.; Gopinath, P.; Mazurek, S.; Bamezai, R.N. Pyruvate kinase M2 and cancer: An updated assessment. *FEBS Lett.* **2014**, *588*, 2685–2692. [CrossRef]
35. Prakasam, G.; Iqbal, M.A.; Bamezai, R.N.K.; Mazurek, S. Posttranslational Modifications of Pyruvate Kinase M2: Tweaks that Benefit Cancer. *Front. Oncol.* **2018**, *8*, 22. [CrossRef] [PubMed]

36. Mazurek, S. Pyruvate kinase type M2: A key regulator of the metabolic budget system in tumor cells. *Int J. Biochem. Cell Biol.* **2011**, *43*, 969–980. [CrossRef]
37. Li, Z.; Yang, P.; Li, Z. The multifaceted regulation and functions of PKM2 in tumor progression. *Biochim. Biophys. Acta* **2014**, *1846*, 285–296. [CrossRef] [PubMed]
38. Gao, X.; Wang, H.; Yang, J.J.; Liu, X.; Liu, Z.R. Pyruvate kinase M2 regulates gene transcription by acting as a protein kinase. *Mol. Cell* **2012**, *45*, 598–609. [CrossRef] [PubMed]
39. Jiang, Y.; Li, X.; Yang, W.; Hawke, D.H.; Zheng, Y.; Xia, Y.; Aldape, K.; Wei, C.; Guo, F.; Chen, Y.; et al. PKM2 regulates chromosome segregation and mitosis progression of tumor cells. *Mol. Cell* **2014**, *53*, 75–87. [CrossRef]
40. Jiang, Y.; Wang, Y.; Wang, T.; Hawke, D.H.; Zheng, Y.; Li, X.; Zhou, Q.; Majumder, S.; Bi, E.; Liu, D.X.; et al. PKM2 phosphorylates MLC2 and regulates cytokinesis of tumour cells. *Nat. Commun.* **2014**, *5*, 5566. [CrossRef]
41. Wang, H.J.; Hsieh, Y.J.; Cheng, W.C.; Lin, C.P.; Lin, Y.S.; Yang, S.F.; Chen, C.C.; Izumiya, Y.; Yu, J.S.; Kung, H.J.; et al. JMJD5 regulates PKM2 nuclear translocation and reprograms HIF-1alpha-mediated glucose metabolism. *Proc. Natl. Acad. Sci. USA* **2014**, *111*, 279–284. [CrossRef]
42. Chen, T.J.; Wang, H.J.; Liu, J.S.; Cheng, H.H.; Hsu, S.C.; Wu, M.C.; Lu, C.H.; Wu, Y.F.; Wu, J.W.; Liu, Y.Y.; et al. Mutations in the PKM2 exon-10 region are associated with reduced allostery and increased nuclear translocation. *Commun. Biol.* **2019**, *2*, 105. [CrossRef] [PubMed]
43. Yang, Y.; Wu, K.; Liu, Y.; Shi, L.; Tao, K.; Wang, G. Prognostic significance of metabolic enzyme pyruvate kinase M2 in breast cancer: A meta-analysis. *Medicine (Baltimore)* **2017**, *96*, e8690. [CrossRef] [PubMed]
44. Wang, Y.; Liu, J.; Jin, X.; Zhang, D.; Li, D.; Hao, F.; Feng, Y.; Gu, S.; Meng, F.; Tian, M.; et al. O-GlcNAcylation destabilizes the active tetrameric PKM2 to promote the Warburg effect. *Proc. Natl. Acad. Sci. USA* **2017**, *114*, 13732–13737. [CrossRef] [PubMed]
45. Dong, T.; Kang, X.; Liu, Z.; Zhao, S.; Ma, W.; Xuan, Q.; Liu, H.; Wang, Z.; Zhang, Q. Altered glycometabolism affects both clinical features and prognosis of triple-negative and neoadjuvant chemotherapy-treated breast cancer. *Tumour Biol.* **2016**, *37*, 8159–8168. [CrossRef] [PubMed]
46. Lin, Y.; Liu, F.; Fan, Y.; Qian, X.; Lang, R.; Gu, F.; Gu, J.; Fu, L. Both high expression of pyruvate kinase M2 and vascular endothelial growth factor-C predicts poorer prognosis in human breast cancer. *Int. J. Clin. Exp. Pathol.* **2015**, *8*, 8028–8037.
47. Curtis, C.; Shah, S.P.; Chin, S.F.; Turashvili, G.; Rueda, O.M.; Dunning, M.J.; Speed, D.; Lynch, A.G.; Samarajiwa, S.; Yuan, Y.; et al. The genomic and transcriptomic architecture of 2,000 breast tumours reveals novel subgroups. *Nature* **2012**, *486*, 346–352. [CrossRef]
48. Sung, W.W.; Wang, Y.C.; Cheng, Y.W.; Lee, M.C.; Yeh, K.T.; Wang, L.; Wang, J.; Chen, C.Y.; Lee, H. A polymorphic -844T/C in FasL promoter predicts survival and relapse in non-small cell lung cancer. *Clin. Cancer Res.* **2011**, *17*, 5991–5999. [CrossRef]
49. Chen, C.J.; Sung, W.W.; Su, T.C.; Chen, M.K.; Wu, P.R.; Yeh, K.T.; Ko, J.L.; Lee, H. High expression of interleukin 10 might predict poor prognosis in early stage oral squamous cell carcinoma patients. *Clin. Chim. Acta* **2013**, *415*, 25–30. [CrossRef]
50. Zou, K.H.; O'Malley, A.J.; Mauri, L. Receiver-operating characteristic analysis for evaluating diagnostic tests and predictive models. *Circulation* **2007**, *115*, 654–657. [CrossRef]
51. Stover, D.G.; Coloff, J.L.; Barry, W.T.; Brugge, J.S.; Winer, E.P.; Selfors, L.M. The Role of Proliferation in Determining Response to Neoadjuvant Chemotherapy in Breast Cancer: A Gene Expression-Based Meta-Analysis. *Clin. Cancer Res.* **2016**, *22*, 6039–6050. [CrossRef]
52. Chaiyawat, P.; Netsirisawan, P.; Svasti, J.; Champattanachai, V. Aberrant O-GlcNAcylated Proteins: New Perspectives in Breast and Colorectal Cancer. *Front. Endocrinol. (Lausanne)* **2014**, *5*, 193. [CrossRef] [PubMed]
53. Laws, A.; Garrido-Castro, A.; Poorvu, P.; Winer, E.; Mittendorf, E.; King, T. Utility of the 21-Gene Recurrence Score in Node- Positive Breast Cancer. *Oncology (Williston Park)* **2021**, *35*, 77–84. [CrossRef]
54. Martin, V.; Hurn, S.; Harris, D. *Econometric Modelling with Time Series: Specification, Estimation and Testing*; Themes in modern econometrics; Cambridge University Press: Cambridge, UK, 2013; p. xxxv.
55. Chen, Y.C.; Li, H.; Wang, J. Mechanisms of metformin inhibiting cancer invasion and migration. *Am. J. Transl. Res.* **2020**, *12*, 4885–4901.
56. He, Y.; Tan, X.; Hu, H.; Wang, Q.; Hu, X.; Cai, X.; Guan, Y.; Chen, B.; Jing, X. Metformin inhibits the migration and invasion of esophageal squamous cell carcinoma cells by downregulating the protein kinase B signaling pathway. *Oncol. Lett.* **2018**, *15*, 2939–2945. [CrossRef]
57. Zhu, J.; Thompson, C.B. Metabolic regulation of cell growth and proliferation. *Nat. Rev. Mol. Cell Biol.* **2019**, *20*, 436–450. [CrossRef]
58. Menendez, J.A.; Mehmi, I.; Papadimitropoulou, A.; Vander Steen, T.; Cuyas, E.; Verdura, S.; Espinoza, I.; Vellon, L.; Atlas, E.; Lupu, R. Fatty Acid Synthase Is a Key Enabler for Endocrine Resistance in Heregulin-Overexpressing Luminal B-Like Breast Cancer. *Int. J. Mol. Sci.* **2020**, *21*, 7661. [CrossRef] [PubMed]

59. de Heer, E.C.; Jalving, M.; Harris, A.L. HIFs, angiogenesis, and metabolism: Elusive enemies in breast cancer. *J. Clin. Investig.* **2020**, *130*, 5074–5087. [CrossRef] [PubMed]
60. Lin, C.H.; Yap, Y.S.; Lee, K.H.; Im, S.A.; Naito, Y.; Yeo, W.; Ueno, T.; Kwong, A.; Li, H.; Huang, S.M.; et al. Contrasting Epidemiology and Clinicopathology of Female Breast Cancer in Asians vs the US Population. *J. Natl. Cancer Inst.* **2019**, *111*, 1298–1306. [CrossRef]
61. Yeo, W.; Ueno, T.; Lin, C.H.; Liu, Q.; Lee, K.H.; Leung, R.; Naito, Y.; Park, Y.H.; Im, S.A.; Li, H.; et al. Treating HR+/HER2- breast cancer in premenopausal Asian women: Asian Breast Cancer Cooperative Group 2019 Consensus and position on ovarian suppression. *Breast Cancer Res. Treat.* **2019**, *177*, 549–559. [CrossRef] [PubMed]
62. McGuire, W.L. Breast cancer prognostic factors: Evaluation guidelines. *J. Natl. Cancer Inst.* **1991**, *83*, 154–155. [CrossRef] [PubMed]

14

Clinical Impact of FDG-PET/CT Compared with CE-CT in Response Monitoring of Metastatic Breast Cancer

Mohammad Naghavi-Behzad [1,2,3,4,*], Hjalte Rasmus Oltmann [1], Tural Asgharzadeh Alamdari [1], Jakob Lykke Bülow [1], Lasse Ljungstrøm [1], Poul-Erik Braad [1,2], Jon Thor Asmussen [5], Marianne Vogsen [1,2,3,4,6], Annette Raskov Kodahl [1,4,6], Oke Gerke [1,2] and Malene Grubbe Hildebrandt [1,2,3,4,7]

[1] Department of Clinical Research, University of Southern Denmark, 5000 Odense, Denmark; Hjalte.rasmus.oltmann@rsyd.dk (H.R.O.); Tural.asgharzadeh.alamdari@rsyd.dk (T.A.A.); Jakob.lykke.bulow2@rsyd.dk (J.L.B.); Lasse.ljungstrom@rsyd.dk (L.L.); Poul-erik.braad@rsyd.dk (P.-E.B.); Marianne.vogsen@rsyd.dk (M.V.); Annette.kodahl@rsyd.dk (A.R.K.); Oke.Gerke@rsyd.dk (O.G.); Malene.Grubbe.Hildebrandt@rsyd.dk (M.G.H.)

[2] Department of Nuclear Medicine, Odense University Hospital, 5000 Odense, Denmark

[3] Open Patient Data Explorative Network (OPEN), Odense University Hospital, 5000 Odense, Denmark

[4] Centre for Personalized Response Monitoring in Oncology, Odense University Hospital, 5000 Odense, Denmark

[5] Department of Radiology, Odense University Hospital, 5000 Odense, Denmark; Jon.asmussen@rsyd.dk

[6] Department of Oncology, Odense University Hospital, 5000 Odense, Denmark

[7] Centre for Innovative Medical Technology, Odense University Hospital, 5000 Odense, Denmark

* Correspondence: Mnb91@rsyd.dk or Dr.naghavii@gmail.com;

Simple Summary: The method of treatment evaluation in patients with chronic breast cancer may affect clinical decision making and treatment protocols. In this study, we compared the two imaging modalities for the evaluation of treatment responses in 65 patients with spread breast cancer. We included 34 patients who underwent contrast-enhanced computed tomography (CE-CT) and 31 patients who underwent positron emission tomography/computed tomography (FDG-PET/CT). Then, we compared the response categories and clinical effects within the two modalities during a follow-up period of an average of 17.3 months. Our results showed that CE-CT modality reported more scans as stable disease, while FDG-PET/CT modality reported regressive metastatic disease more often. This means that FDG-PET/CT responds more precisely with respect to the changes in patients' clinical condition, while CE-CT tends to report stable disease in most of the scans. Therefore, FDG-PET/CT may be a more suitable imaging modality than CE-CT for the evaluation of treatment in patients with metastatic breast cancer.

Abstract: We compared response categories and impacts on treatment decisions for metastatic breast cancer (MBC) patients that are response-monitored with contrast-enhanced computed-tomography (CE-CT) or fluorodeoxyglucose-positron emission tomography/computed tomography (FDG-PET/CT). A comparative diagnostic study was performed on MBC patients undergoing response monitoring by CE-CT (n = 34) or FDG-PET/CT (n = 31) at the Odense University Hospital (Denmark). The responses were assessed visually and allocated into categories of complete response (CR/CMR), partial response (PR/PMR), stable disease (SD/SMD), and progressive disease (PD/PMD). Response categories, clinical impact, and positive predictive values (PPV) were compared for follow-up scans. A total of 286 CE-CT and 189 FDG-PET/CT response monitoring scans were performed. Response categories were distributed into CR (3.8%), PR (8.4%), SD (70.6%), PD (15%), and others (2.1%) by CE-CT and into CMR (22.2%), PMR (23.8%), SMD (31.2%), PMD (18.5%), and others (4.4%) by FDG-PET/CT, revealing a significant difference between the groups ($P < 0.001$). PD and PMD caused changes of treatment in 79.1% and 60%, respectively ($P = 0.083$). PPV for CE-CT and FDG-PET/CT was 0.85 (95% CI: 0.72–0.97) and 0.70 (95% CI: 0.53–0.87), respectively ($P = 0.17$). FDG-PET/CT indicated regression of disease more frequently than CE-CT, while CE-CT indicated stable disease more often. FDG-PET/CT seems to be more sensitive than CE-CT for monitoring response in metastatic breast cancer.

Keywords: FDG-PET/CT; response monitoring; metastatic breast cancer; clinical impact

1. Introduction

Breast cancer is the most common cancer type among women in Europe and the leading cause of female cancer death in most European countries [1,2]. Despite optimized treatment for early-stage breast cancer, these patients still have a substantial risk of relapse. Metastatic breast cancer (MBC) is considered incurable and requires life-long medical treatment along with a reliable modality for the evaluation of treatment effects [3]. Longitudinal response monitoring should assess therapy effects over several treatment intervals with the intention of improving clinical decision making in MBC patients [4,5].

Contrast-enhanced computed tomography (CE-CT) and the corresponding Response Evaluation Criteria in Solid Tumors (RECIST 1.1) have been suggested for response monitoring of solid tumors [6,7]. Although most international guidelines do not provide specific recommendations on the choice of modality for response monitoring of MBC [8], the CE-CT and RECIST tend to be the most widely used methods in clinical practice and experimental trials [8–10].

Up to 70% of MBC patients experience bone involvement during their disease period [11], which is more common in hormone receptor-positive disease [12]. Bone lesions are hardly detected and monitored by CE-CT since active malignant lesions in the bones are difficult to distinguish from osteosclerotic recovering lesions [10,13,14]. This poses a challenge when assessing whether bone metastases are progressing, stable, or have responded to the treatment [15].

^{18F}Fluorodeoxyglucose positron emission tomography with integrated computed tomography (FDG-PET/CT) has proven higher sensitivity compared to conventional imaging procedures such as CE-CT regarding the detection of distant metastasis in MBC patients [14,16]. A meta-analysis compared the sensitivity of FDG-PET/CT and CE-CT for detecting bone metastases and observed FDG-PET/CT as the superior modality with higher sensitivity (89.7% vs. 72.9%) [13]. It has also been shown that FDG-PET/CT is a better predictor of progression-free and disease-specific survival than CE-CT [17]. Hence, FDG-PET/CT has been suggested to be advantageous to CE-CT for response monitoring of MBC patients [17–19], but to our knowledge, no previous studies compared these methods concerning longitudinal response monitoring.

In patients with metastatic breast cancer, we aimed to explore the impact of response monitoring on treatment decisions by comparing CE-CT with FDG-PET/CT. The study objectives were to compare response categories, image-guided treatment decisions, and positive predictive values (PPV) for CE-CT and FDG-PET/CT, respectively.

2. Materials and Methods

This comparative diagnostic study was carried out at the Departments of Nuclear Medicine and Oncology at Odense University Hospital (Odense, Denmark) from September 2017 until June 2019. A longitudinal response assessment was retrospectively compared for MBC patients monitored primarily with CE-CT or FDG-PET/CT over several treatment intervals. The study protocol was approved by the Danish Patients' Safety Authority (approval code: 3-3013-2448/1), and written consent forms were obtained from enrolled patients.

2.1. *Study Design and Subjects*

Women who received treatment for MBC at the Department of Oncology between September 2017 and December 2017 and had undergone CE-CT or FDG-PET/CT for treatment response monitoring were considered eligible for the study.

The inclusion criteria were biopsy-verified MBC (de novo or recurrent); baseline and at least one follow-up scan for response monitoring; use of either FDG-PET/CT or CE-CT as the main response monitoring modality; standard response monitoring protocol with regular imaging intervals (9–12 weeks on average) depending on treatment regime [20]; and regular clinical follow-up. The exclusion criteria were other known disseminated malignancy; monitoring mainly by magnetic resonance imaging (MRI) due to brain metastases; missing clinical data; and response monitoring by both modalities (CE-CT and FDG-PET/CT).

The modality used for response monitoring was generally decided by the oncologist who met the patient at the initial visit. Patients were mainly treated by the same oncologist during follow-up visits and the response monitoring modality was chosen with no internal algorithm to guide the choice of response monitoring modality. Patients were allocated arbitrarily to the treating oncologists with no distinctions due to clinical or performance status. Hence, the choice was mainly at the discretion of the oncologist based on personal preferences to choose either CE-CT or FDG-PET/CT as the response monitoring modality.

The patients were divided into the CE-CT and FDG-PET/CT groups defined by the imaging modality used for response monitoring. One scan performed on the opposite imaging modality was accepted for both groups.

The radiologists and nuclear medicine specialists made qualitative visual assessments in the clinical routine for the CE-CT and FDG-PET/CT scans, respectively. CE-CT assessments were categorized according to scan report into response categories of complete response (CR), partial response (PR), stable disease (SD), progressive disease (PD), mixed response (MR), or equivocal answer (EA). RECIST 1.1 criteria were applied when measurable lesions were present, allowing RECIST evaluation [6]. If the RECIST category differed from the visual response category, the worst prognostic response category was registered to render the response category more in line with the decision made in the clinic.

The corresponding categories were defined for qualitative visual assessments of FDG-PET/CT. The metabolic activity was taken into account as complete metabolic response (CMR), partial metabolic response (PMR), stable metabolic disease (SMD), progressive metabolic disease (PMD), mixed metabolic response (MMR), and equivocal metabolic answer (EMA). The follow-up scans were compared to the baseline and preceding scans, and the decision of multi-disciplinary radiology conference was considered in cases of uncertainty.

Response categories were subsequently dichotomized into groups of progressive and non-progressive diseases. Hence, all scans reporting PD/PMD were categorized as progressive disease, whereas all other categories were defined as non-progressive disease, the latter including MR/MMR and EA/EMA.

Clinical decisions were made by the oncologist based on the scan report, the patient's clinical performance status, the patient's request, and the potential toxicity of ongoing treatment. Treatment decisions were recorded for each interval and were labeled as *progression-induced change of treatment* if the oncologist decided to change the treatment due to the progression observed during imaging and/or signs of clinical progression. Reasons other than clinical progression for change of treatment, including side effects, completion of chemotherapy cycles, patients' request, no available treatment, and complete remission, were not considered as *progression-induced change of treatment*.

2.2. Imaging Techniques

2.2.1. FDG-PET/CT

Patients fasted for six hours before each scan. The tracer 18F-FDG was administered intravenously at a dose of 4 MBq/kg. Patients then rested and rehydrated with 800 mL of water. Scans were performed 60 min ($\pm$15 min) after 18F-FDG injection. A low-dose CT scan was performed from the skull to the proximal femora immediately followed by a PET scan of the same area. FDG-PET/CT scans were performed by using either General Electric Discovery STE, Discovery VCT, or Discovery RX (GE Medical Systems, Milwaukee, USA) with the following settings: CT-scan 140 kVp and 30–110 mA Smart mA; rotation time 0.8 sec.; pitch 1.375:1; Noise Index 25; and detector coverage 40 mm. Transverse images were reconstructed by using filtered back projection with a standard filter, slice thickness of 3.75 mm, and interval of 3.27 mm. PET scans were performed in 3D with a scan time of 2.5 min/frame. Images were reconstructed iteratively by using the GE VUE Point algorithm with 2 iterations, 21 or 28 subsets, and slice thickness of 3.3 mm. PET/CT acquisitions and reconstructions were performed in compliance with EANM guidelines, and the image quality was validated against EARL criteria [21].

2.2.2. CE-CT

The diagnostic CT scans were obtained on either GE VCT, GE VCT XT, GE HD 750HD, Siemens Somatom Definition Flash, or Siemens Somatom Force. The settings for the GE scanners were as follows: 120 kV and 100–750 mA Smart mA; Auto mA; rotation time 0.5 s; pitch 0.984:1; Noise Index from 40 to 47 depending on the scanner type; and either HD 750 or VCT due to the detector specification. The ASiR level was set to 40% and detector coverage to 40 mm. Scans were generally performed over the thorax, abdomen, and pelvis in baseline and all follow-up scans. There were three reconstructions made with Soft, Stnd., and Lung algorithm. Soft was used for 0.625 mm axial slices and 5 mm coronal, and Sagittal. Stnd. and Lung was reconstructed in 5 mm axial slices. The settings for the Siemens Flash scanner were as follows: 120 kV; ref mas 150; rotation time 0.5 s; and pitch 0.9. The detector coverage was 40 mm 0.6 mm × 128, SAFIRE level 3. The settings for the Siemens FORCE scanner were as follows: 120 kV; ref mas 110; rotation time 0.5 s; and pitch 0.6. The detector coverage was 60 mm 0.6 mm × 192, ADMIRE level 2. Reconstructions for the Flash scanner were made with I31f medium Smooth and I50f medium Sharp ASA kernels. I31f was used for 0.625 mm and 5 mm axial, coronal, and sagittal slices. The lung window was reconstructed with I50f medium Sharp ASA in 5 mm axial slices. Reconstructions for the Force scanner are reconstructions made with Br40 and Bl57 kernels. Br40 was used for 0.625 mm and 5 mm axial, coronal, and sagittal slices. The lung window was reconstructed with Bl57 in 5 mm axial slices. The contrast enhancement scheme for diagnostic CT was generally contrast medium Optiray 300 (1 mL/kg on patients' weight) and the scan started 70 s after the injection. Flow rate was usually 3 mL/s, while reduced by radiographer's discretion in the case of a fragile vein. Antecubital vein was preferred, unless the patient already had other peripheral venous access. Iomeron or Omnipaque were administered in similar doses in patients with previous allergic reactions [6].

2.3. *Data Collection and Variables*

Data were extracted from medical records and scan reports. Extracted data included age, performance status [22], and clinical and histopathological data. For patients with more than one primary breast cancer, we used the data for the primary cancer that had most likely resulted in metastasis (i.e., had the same molecular profile as metastasis). In a few patients with de novo metastatic cancer, information from the primary breast biopsy was used since biopsy was not obtained from the metastatic lesion due to local procedure.

2.4. *Outcome Measures and Statistical Analyses*

Study groups were checked for comparability regarding baseline characteristics. Response categories were compared between the study groups. The response monitoring period was defined as the time interval between the first treatment line and the last available scan. A reference standard for true and false progression was assessed using information from subsequent follow-up scans. Hence, true progression could be applied in two situations: (1) when progression (PD/PMD) caused treatment change, and the subsequent scan revealed regression (PR/PMR or CR/CMR); and (2) when progression (PD/PMD) did not results in treatment change, and the subsequent scan revealed further progression (PD/PMD). False progression could be applied when progression (PD/PMD) did not result in treatment change, and the subsequent scan revealed non-progressive disease (SD/SMD, PR/PMR, or CR/CMR). Then, the positive predictive value (PPV) could be compared for the CE-CT and FDG-PET/CT groups, respectively. The PPV was calculated as $\frac{\text{True progression}}{\text{True progression} + \text{False progression}}$. The PPVs for CE-CT and FDG-PET/CT were supplemented by Wilson-score-based 95% confidence intervals (95% CIs). A chi-squared test was used to test for differences in distributions between groups. All data were analyzed by using STATA/IC software (version 15.0, StataCorp, College Station, TX, USA). *P*-values less than 0.05 were considered statistically significant.

3. Results

3.1. Baseline Characteristics

A total of 109 patients were eligible for the study, while 44 patients were subsequently excluded for different reasons, as shown in Figure 1. Of the 65 included patients who were response monitored between 2009 and 2017, 34 were enrolled in the CE-CT group and 31 in the FDG-PET/CT group. Clinical and histopathological characteristics of the primary tumor and metastatic disease are summarized in Tables 1 and 2, respectively. The study groups were comparable regarding most of the baseline characteristics.

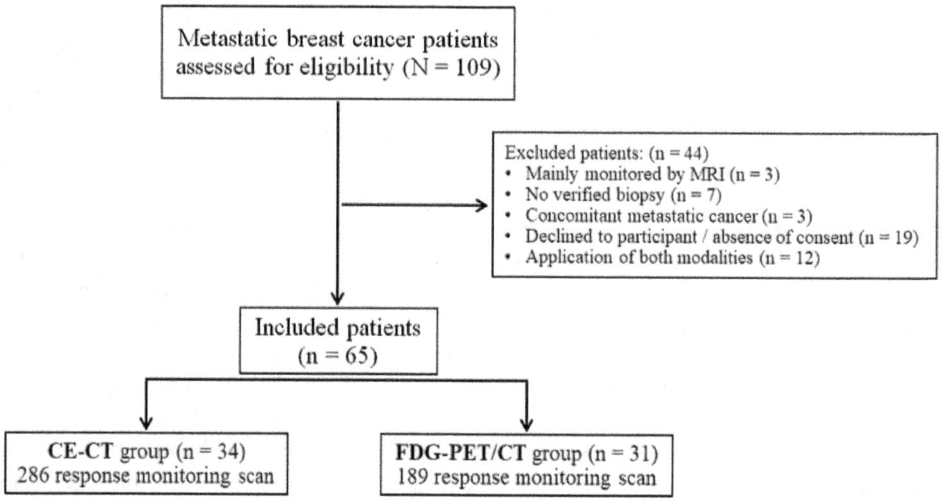

Figure 1. Patient flowchart and distribution of the included patients to study groups (CE-CT: contrast-enhanced computed tomography; FDG-PET/CT: Fluorodeoxyglucose positron emission tomography with integrated computed tomography; MRI: magnetic resonance imaging).

3.2. Treatment Protocol and Metastatic Site

Exposure to different treatment types and metastatic sites reported during the follow-up period are reflected in Table 3. Received treatments were comparable between the study groups without any significant difference. However, CE-CT reported metastatic bone (58% vs. 47.6%; $P = 0.022$) and liver (19.2% vs. 7.9%; $P = 0.001$) metastases significantly more frequently than FDG-PET/CT during response monitoring scans.

3.3. Response Monitoring Scans

A total of 333 CE-CT scans and 230 FDG-PET/CT scans, including baseline and response monitoring scans, were performed in 65 patients with median response monitoring periods of 23 (range: 6–90) and 11 (2–103) months for patients monitored with CE-CT and FDG-PET/CT, respectively ($P = 0.007$). FDG-PET/CT was performed once in 10 out of 34 (29.4%) patients in the CE-CT group, while CE-CT was performed once in 13 out of 31 (41.9%) patients in the FDG-PET/CT group. An illustration of response evaluation intervals with response categories for each patient is shown in Figure 2. The figure illustrates that SD (yellow color) is highly represented in the CE-CT group, while PMR (green color) is highly represented in the FDG-PET/CT group.

Table 1. Clinicopathological characteristics of primary breast cancer.

Characteristics [a]		Study Groups		P-Value
		CE-CT	PET/CT	
Primary tumor size (mm)		18 (3–65)	20 (1–80)	0.85
Bilateral cancer		2 (5.9)	5 (16.1)	0.24
Histopathology	Ductal	26 (76.5)	23 (74.2)	0.59
	Lobular	5 (14.7)	3 (9.7)	
	Adenocarcinoma	3 (8.8)	3 (9.7)	
	Unknown	0 (0)	2 (6.5)	
Primary surgery (lumpectomy/mastectomy)		23 (67.6)	27 (87.1)	0.06
Estrogen receptor status	Positive	31 (91.2)	25 (80.7)	0.43
	Negative	2 (5.9)	3 (9.7)	
	Unknown	1 (2.9)	3 (9.7)	
HER-2 status	Positive	5 (14.7)	6 (19.4)	0.94
	Negative	21 (61.8)	18 (58.1)	
	Unknown	8 (23.5)	7 (22.6)	
Tumor grade	Grade 1	6 (17.7)	6 (19.4)	0.98
	Grade 2	14 (41.2)	11 (35.5)	
	Grade 3	7 (20.6)	8 (25.8)	
	Unknown	7 (20.6)	6 (19.4)	
Ki-67 proliferation (%)		20 (1–80)	50 (10–95)	0.16
Lymph node involvement	None	7 (20.6)	6 (19.4)	0.71
	Micro-metastasis	4 (11.8)	3 (9.7)	
	Macro-metastasis	13 (38.2)	16 (51.6)	
	Unknown	10 (29.4)	6 (19.4)	
Treatment protocol	Neo-adjuvant treatment	2 (5.88)	8 (25.8)	0.09
	Endocrine treatment	23 (67.7)	17 (54.8)	
	No treatment / unknown	9 (26.5)	6 (19.4)	
Radiotherapy (breast/breast + axilla)		20 (58.8)	21 (67.7)	0.31

CE-CT: contrast-enhanced computed tomography; FDG-PET/CT: fluorodeoxyglucose positron emission tomography with integrated computed-tomography; HER-2: human epidermal growth factor receptor-2. [a] Data were shown as median (interquartile range) or frequency (percentage).

3.4. *Response Categories, Clinical Impact, and Positive Predictive Value*

A total of 286 CE-CT and 189 FDG-PET/CT response monitoring scans were performed. RECIST was applied in the response evaluation of 178 out of 286 (62.2%) CE-CT scans and by visual assessment in the remaining scans (37.8%), while response evaluation was performed by visual assessment in all FDG-PET/CT scans. The decision on response categories was different between RECIST and visual assessment in 13 CE-CT scans; however, the difference was balanced regarding the report of worse response category by either of them.

Table 2. Clinicopathological characteristics of metastatic disease [a].

Characteristics		Study Groups		*P*-Value
		CE-CT	PET/CT	
Year of diagnosis		2015 (2010–2017)	2016 (2009–2017)	0.02
Age at diagnosis (year)		67.0 (31.0–84.5)	63.4 (32.9–85.8)	0.69
Performance status	0	12 (35.3)	13 (41.9)	0.36
	1	10 (29.4)	13 (41.9)	
	≥2	3 (8.8)	1 (3.2)	
	Unknown	9 (26.5)	4 (12.9)	
Time until relapse [b] (months)		78.0 (0–271.4)	81.8 (0–307.5)	0.71
Histopathology	Ductal	4 (11.8)	5 (16.1)	0.86
	Lobular	4 (11.8)	2 (6.5)	
	Adenocarcinoma	18 (52.9)	18 (58.1)	
	Unknown	8 (23.5)	6 (19.4)	
De novo metastatic cancer		8 (25.5)	4 (12.9)	0.35
Estrogen receptor status	Positive	30 (88.2)	28 (90.3)	0.50
	Negative	2 (5.9)	3 (9.7)	
	Unknown	2 (5.9)	0 (0)	
HER-2 status	Positive	5 (14.7)	6 (19.4)	0.46
	Negative	22 (64.7)	22 (71.0)	
	Unknown	7 (20.6)	3 (9.7)	
Origin of biopsy	Bone	5 (14.7)	13 (41.9)	0.07
	Liver	6 (17.7)	3 (9.7)	
	Lung/Pleural fluid	8 (23.5)	7 (22.6)	
	Breast/lymph nodes	15 (44.1)	8 (25.7)	
Region of metastases at baseline scan	Bone-only metastasis	4 (11.8)	4 (12.9)	0.89
	Bone	22 (64.7)	21 (67.7)	0.80
	Liver	8 (25.5)	8 (25.8)	0.83
	Lung	10 (29.4)	11 (35.5)	0.60
	Regional lymph nodes	12 (35.3)	9 (29.0)	0.59
	Distant lymph nodes	18 (52.9)	17 (54.8)	0.88
	Pleura/pleural effusion	3 (8.8)	6 (19.4)	0.22
	Breast/local recurrence	7 (20.6)	6 (19.4)	0.90
	Soft tissue	1 (2.9)	4 (12.9)	0.13
	Others [c]	2 (5.9)	3 (9.7)	0.57

CE-CT: contrast-enhanced computed tomography; FDG-PET/CT: fluorodeoxyglucose positron emission tomography with integrated computed-tomography, HER-2: human epidermal growth factor receptor-2. [a] Data shown as median (interquartile range) and frequency (%). [b] Time until relapse for patients with primary disseminated disease was considered zero. [c] Others comprised ascites, adrenal glands, thyroid, uterus, colon, and skin.

Table 3. Treatment regimens and detected metastasis during follow-up.

Characteristics		Study Groups	
		CE-CT (286 scan)	FDG-PET/CT (189 scan)
Received treatments during follow-up [a]	Endocrine therapy	29 (85.3)	25 (80.6)
	Bone-targeted therapies	24 (70.6)	23 (74.2)
	Chemotherapy	22 (64.7)	18 (58.1)
	CDK4/6 inhibitors	19 (55.9)	15 (48.4)
	Anti-HER2 therapy	5 (14.7)	6 (19.4)
	Palliative radiotherapy	5 (14.7)	1 (3.2)
Metastatic sites during follow-up [b]	Bone	166 (58.0)	90 (47.6)
	Liver	55 (19.2)	15 (7.9)
	Lung/plural	110 (38.5)	66 (34.9)
	Regional/distant lymph nodes	112 (39.2)	67 (35.4)
	Others [c]	48 (16.8)	28 (14.8)

CE-CT: contrast-enhanced computed tomography, FDG-PET/CT: fluorodeoxyglucose positron emission tomography with integrated computed-tomography. [a] Data shown as frequency (percentage) out of patients' number. [b] Data shown as frequency (percentage) out of number of scans. [c] Others comprised ascites, adrenal glands, thyroid, uterus, colon, soft tissue, and skin.

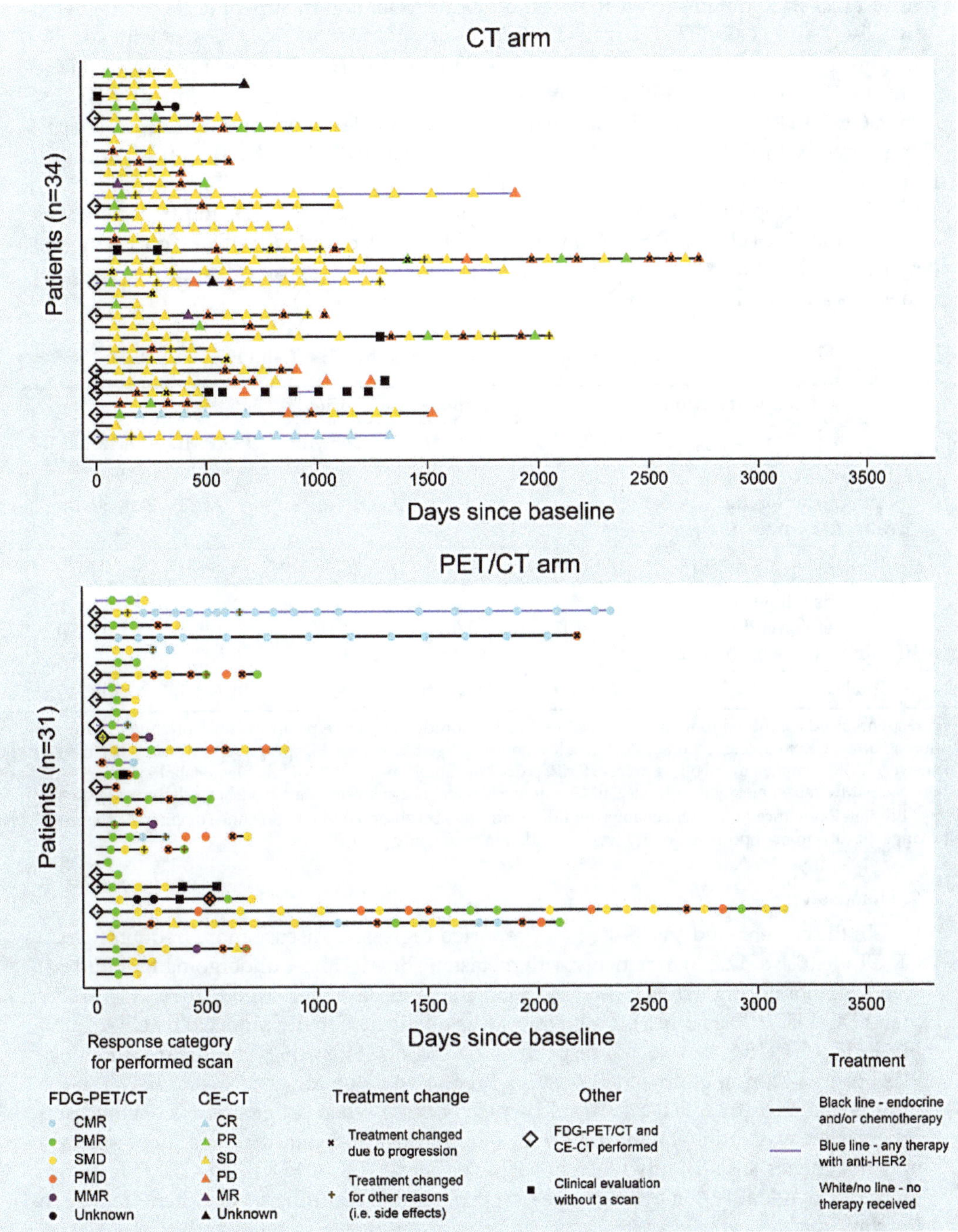

Figure 2. Visualization of response categories and treatment changes for study groups (CE-CT: contrast-enhanced computed tomography; FDG-PET/CT: fluorodeoxyglucose positron emission tomography with integrated computed tomography; CR: complete response; PR: partial response; SD: stable disease; PD: progressive disease; MR: mixed response; CMR: complete metabolic response; PMR: partial metabolic response; SMD: stable metabolic disease; PMD: progressive metabolic disease; MMR: mixed metabolic response).

Within the response monitoring scans, 15.4% (44/286) and 11.6% (22/189) of scans followed by *progression-induced change of treatment* occurred in CE-CT group and FDG-PET/CT group, respectively. Time to the detection of first progression leading *progression-induced treatment change* was 9.3 months shorter in the FDG-PET/CT group (15 patients) with a median of 8.8 (3.5–61.3) months compared to the CE-CT group (20 patients) with a median of 18.1 (2.8–54.9) months ($P = 0.04$). Response categories and treatment decisions followed by CE-CT and FDG-PET/CT scans have been summarized in Table 4. A statistically significant difference in the distribution of response categories was observed between the groups ($P < 0.001$). FDG-PET/CT reported regressive disease more frequently (46.0%) than CE-CT (12.2%) did, while stable disease was reported more often in CE-CT (70.6%) compared with FDG-PET/CT (31.2%). The PPV was 0.85 (95% CI: 0.72–0.97) and 0.70 (95% CI: 0.53–0.87) for CE-CT and FDG-PET/CT, respectively ($P = 0.17$). Additionally, when CE-CT reported PD, treatment was changed in 79.1% (34/43), and treatment was changed in 60% (21/35) ($P = 0.083$) when FDG-PET/CT reported PMD. By observing the patients who had a *progression-induced change of treatment*, progressive disease was reported in 95.5% scans by FDG-PET/CT and 77.3% by CE-CT ($P = 0.08$).

Table 4. Response categories for patients monitored by CE-CT and FDG-PET/CT .

Study Groups	Treatment Actions	Response Categories [a]					
		CR/CMR	PR/PMR	SD/SMD	PD/PMD	MR/MMR	EA/EMA
CE-CT	Scans followed by progression-induced treatment change [b] ($n = 44$)	0 (0)	1 (2.3)	8 (18.2)	34 (77.3)	0 (0)	1 (2.3)
	Total scans [c] ($N = 286$)	11 (3.8)	24 (8.4)	202 (70.6)	43 (15)	2 (0.7)	4 (1.4)
PET/CT	Scans followe by progression-induced treatment change [b] ($n = 22$)	0 (0)	0 (0)	0 (0)	21 (95.5)	1 (4.5)	0 (0)
	Total scans [c] ($N = 189$)	42 (22.2)	45 (23.8)	59 (31.2)	35 (18.5)	4 (2.1)	4 (2.1)

CE-CT: contrast-enhanced computed tomography; FDG-PET/CT: fluorodeoxyglucose positron emission tomography with integrated computed-tomography; CR: complete response; PR: partial response; SD: stable disease; PD: progressive disease; MR: mixed response; EA: equivocal answer; CMR: complete metabolic response; PMR: partial metabolic response; SMD: stable metabolic disease; PMD: progressive metabolic disease; MMR: mixed metabolic response; EMA: equivocal metabolic answer. [a] Data have been shown as frequency (percentage) of each line. [b] Progression-induced treatment change defined as progression observed in imaging and/or clinical progression resulting in treatment change. [c] Scans from opposite modality were excluded in both study groups.

4. Discussion

In the current study, FDG-PET/CT reported regressive disease more frequently than CE-CT (46.0% vs. 12.2%) in patients with metastatic breast cancer undergoing longitudinal response monitoring, while CE-CT deemed stable disease more often (70.6% vs. 31.2%) than FDG-PET/CT (Figure 2). Progression was relatively equally reported by CE-CT and FDG-PET/CT (15% and 18.5%, respectively), and no statistically significant difference was observed for an approached positive predictive value for progression between the groups. Since treatment change would typically occur when progression is deemed and progression was quite equally reported, our findings indicate that treatment strategy may not change significantly when choosing either CE-CT or FDG-PET/CT as response monitoring modality. On average, the first progression resulting in treatment change in the clinic (*progression-induced treatment change*) was detected 9.3 months earlier ($P = 0.04$) in patients response monitored by FDG-PET/CT (15 patients) compared to patients response monitored by CE-CT (20 patients); however, we cannot make firm conclusions due to the lack of sample size and short follow-up time in this sub-group of patients. However, FDG-PET/CT may have the potential to detect progression earlier than CE-CT due to the hypothesis that change in cancer activity would occur before the presentation of morphological changes.

Clinicians were more likely to change treatment when CE-CT deemed progression than when FDG-PET/CT deemed progression (79.1% vs. 60%), while the reporting of progressive disease was more in line with the decision made in the clinic (progression-induced change of treatment) in the FDG-PET/CT group than in the CE-CT group (95.5% vs. 77.3%, $P = 0.08$).

Patients included in this study were biopsy-verified MBC patients in an unselected, unique consecutive cohort monitored with primarily one of the two compared imaging modalities. They were, apparently, by part randomly allocated to monitoring with FDG-PET/CT or CE-CT, and hence the two groups were comparable concerning most characteristics (Tables 1 and 2). However, the patients monitored by CE-CT had a significantly longer follow-up time. This could be explained by the fact that FDG-PET/CT is a more novel option for treatment monitoring than CE-CT, and longer follow-up time for patients monitored by FDG-PET/CT would have been preferable. Clinically relevant data and clinical decision-making data were extracted in order to evaluate the clinical impact of each modality. A considerable large quantity of scans for both modalities was included, and response categories were interpreted by the scan reports representative of routine clinical practice.

The limitations of the study were the single-centre observational design, low sample size, and heterogeneity of the included patients such as a different number of response monitoring series, treatment protocols, time point of diagnosis for metastatic disease (2015 vs. 2016), and follow-up period. Lack of a reference standard for confirmation of true progression/regression was a limitation since we followed the decision made in the clinic with the potential of reporting false positive "true progression". Moreover, we allowed one opposite scan type to be performed in both groups, which may have blurred our findings to some degree. Additionally, the RECIST criteria were applied in 62% of CE-CT scans, and no standardized response evaluation criteria, such as the PET Response Evaluation Criteria in Solid Tumors (PERCIST), were applied for FDG-PET/CT. Furthermore, we have not categorized response evaluations based on different treatments and histopathology profiles, which could impact our results [23].

To our knowledge, this is the first study that compared the impact of response categorization and clinical decision making of using different scan modalities over several treatment intervals in MBC patients. Previously, in a study by Riedl et al., it has been shown that FDG-PET/CT had a higher predictive value than CE-CT for long-term survival when the PERCIST and RECIST were applied [17]. According to their results, CE-CT tended to report SD more often, while FDG-PET/CT reported PMD more often. These patterns are in line with the findings of our study to some degree and could be explained by the inability of CE-CT to distinguish osteoblastic bone lesions from bone healing. They also showed that FDG-PET/CT could be a better predictor for progression-free survival and disease-specific survival compared to CE-CT [17], which was proposed in some other studies as well [24,25]. These results indicate that FDG-PET/CT may be superior to CE-CT in the response assessment of MBC patients [17,24,25].

We observed that clinicians tended to change treatments more often based on progression reported by CE-CT than by FDG-PET/CT. This could be explained by a lack of evidence in this field and the absence of FDG-PET/CT in international and national guidelines as a modality of choice for the response evaluation of MBC patients [26]. Liver metastases were reported more frequently in CE-CT response monitoring scans, which could reflect the lower specificity of CE-CT for the diagnosis of liver metastases compared to FDG-PET/CT [27].

With a major difference in reporting more regressive disease by FDG-PET/CT (23.8% vs. 8.4%) and more stable disease by CE-CT (70.6% vs. 31.2%), it appears that FDG-PET/CT could have the potential to provide an early indication of treatment effect for different treatment options in this group of patients. This may provide the advantage of the knowledge that the treatment has a positive effect on cancer and, thereby, confidence for the clinician and decision-makers of treatment benefit as it may increase the quality of life and treatment motivation for the patients [5,28], and it may have a potential for improving assessment of treatment efficacy in clinical trials.

Since our results were part of the clinical routine, a standardized set of response criteria such as PERCIST was not applied for FDG-PET/CT. However, we showed in previous studies that the clinical application of PERCIST is feasible [29] and has the potential to increase the level of inter-observer agreement and reliability when compared with qualitative visual assessment [30].

Targeted treatment methods, such as anti-HER2 therapy, have been used for a long time in breast cancer resulting in improved survival [31,32]. These treatment lines may require more accurate response monitoring methods to serve as surrogates for survival, to keep patients in the most effective treatment tract over time, and to ensure the cost-effectiveness of modern treatments. Along with the increasing use of molecular directed treatments, we should encourage a move from changes in tumor size towards changes in cancer metabolism when evaluating therapeutic responses [5,33]. Emerging supplemental information is coming from the area of liquid biopsies that could provide more detailed information about active cancer cells and, therefore, be more specific in treatment monitoring [34,35].

The efficacy of using FDG-PET/CT as response monitoring modality may vary for different histopathological profiles of metastases [23]. This restriction refers to the limited performance of FDG-PET/CT due to lower FDG-uptake in patients with invasive lobular carcinoma histotype [36,37].

On the other hand, whole body MRI revealed a comparable diagnostic accuracy to PET/CT regarding the detection of bone metastasis [13,38], and it has been shown that whole body MRI could detect the progression earlier than CE-CT in patients with bone-only MBC [39]. Therefore, whole body MRI could be considered as a potential alternative strategy in the response monitoring of MBC patients, while future prospective studies are needed to compare the clinical impact of all three modalities through comparable groups.

Since optional imaging modalities for response evaluation are suggested by current international guidelines [8], this means that opposing methods might be used in different institutions. Our data suggested that imaging modalities may provide varying information about response to treatment, but it could not show whether any of the modalities detected the progression, resulting in treatment change earlier than the other. The hypothesis that using FDG-PET/CT for monitoring response has an impact on treatment strategy is, therefore, a perspective for future research. Prospective studies with longer follow-up time, applying semi-quantitative response assessments such as the PERCIST criteria to FDG-PET/CT on patients receiving similar treatment types, could potentially result in a better understanding of the clinical impact of FDG-PET/CT in the response monitoring of MBC patients. It would also be valuable to compare the long-term survival and the costs of response monitoring within the modalities along with the clinical impact. The high frequency of bone involvement in these patients is still a strong indicator for further research into the role of FDG-PET/CT in response monitoring of MBC to provide better evidence-based recommendations.

5. Conclusions

In response monitoring of patients with metastatic breast cancer, regressive disease was reported more frequently by FDG-PET/CT, and stable disease was reported more often by CE-CT. Hence, this study indicates that FDG-PET/CT may be more sensitive for confirming treatment effects than the conventional CE-CT. Progressive disease was deemed quite equally, and positive predictive values were quite similar for the two modalities; however, clinicians tended to be more likely to change treatment when CE-CT suggested progression than when FDG-PET/CT suggested progression. Time to detection of treatment failure may impact treatment decisions and should be analyzed for the two modalities in future studies with larger sample size and prospective study design.

Author Contributions: Study concept and design: H.R.O., T.A.A., M.V., and M.G.H.; data collection: H.R.O., T.A.A., J.L.B., L.L., P.-E.B., M.N.-B., and M.V.; statistical analyses: O.G., H.R.O., and M.N.-B.; interpretation of data: H.R.O., T.A.A., M.N.-B., A.R.K., O.G., J.T.A., and M.G.H.; finalization of initial draft: M.N.-B., M.V., O.G., A.R.K., and M.G.H.; critical revision of the manuscript: all of the authors; approval of final draft: all of the authors. All authors have read and agreed to the published version of the manuscript.

References

1. Ferlay, J.; Colombet, M.; Soerjomataram, I.; Dyba, T.; Randi, G.; Bettio, M.; Gavin, A.; Visser, O.; Bray, F. Cancer incidence and mortality patterns in Europe: Estimates for 40 countries and 25 major cancers in 2018. *Eur. J. Cancer* **2018**, *103*, 356–387. [CrossRef]
2. Carioli, G.; Malvezzi, M.; Rodriguez, T.; Bertuccio, P.; Negri, E.; La Vecchia, C. Trends and predictions to 2020 in breast cancer mortality in Europe. *Breast* **2017**, *36*, 89–95. [CrossRef]
3. Harbeck, N.; Gnant, M. Breast cancer. *Lancet* **2017**, *389*, 1134–1150. [CrossRef]
4. Cochet, A.; David, S.; Moodie, K.; Drummond, E.; Dutu, G.; MacManus, M.; Chua, B.; Hicks, R.J. The utility of 18 F-FDG PET/CT for suspected recurrent breast cancer: Impact and prognostic stratification. *Cancer Imaging* **2014**, *14*, 13. [CrossRef]
5. Hildebrandt, M.G.; Lauridsen, J.F.; Vogsen, M.; Holm, J.; Vilstrup, M.H.; Braad, P.-E.; Gerke, O.; Thomassen, M.; Ewertz, M.; Høilund-Carlsen, P.F.; et al. FDG-PET/CT for Response monitoring in metastatic breast cancer: Today, tomorrow, and beyond. *Cancers* **2019**, *11*, 1190. [CrossRef] [PubMed]
6. Eisenhauer, E.A.; Therasse, P.; Bogaerts, J.; Schwartz, L.; Sargent, D.; Ford, R.; Dancey, J.; Arbuck, S.; Gwyther, S.; Mooney, M.; et al. New response evaluation criteria in solid tumours: Revised RECIST guideline (version 1.1). *Eur. J. Cancer* **2009**, *45*, 228–247. [CrossRef] [PubMed]
7. Semiglazov, V. RECIST for Response (Clinical and Imaging) in neoadjuvant clinical trials in operable breast cancer. *J. Natl. Cancer Inst. Monogr.* **2015**, *2015*, 21–23. [CrossRef] [PubMed]
8. Cardoso, F.; Senkus, E.; Costa, A.; Papadopoulos, E.; Aapro, M.; André, F.; Harbeck, N.; Lopez, B.A.; Barrios, C.; Bergh, J.; et al. 4th ESO–ESMO International consensus guidelines for advanced breast cancer (ABC 4). *Ann. Oncol.* **2018**, *29*, 1634–1657. [CrossRef] [PubMed]
9. Schwartz, L.H.; Litière, S.; de Vries, E.; Ford, R.; Gwyther, S.; Mandrekar, S.; Shankar, L.; Bogaerts, J.; Chen, A.; Dancey, J.; et al. RECIST 1.1—Update and clarification: From the RECIST committee. *Eur. J. Cancer* **2016**, *62*, 132–137. [CrossRef]
10. Therasse, P.; Arbuck, S.G.; Eisenhauer, E.A.; Wanders, J.; Kaplan, R.S.; Rubinstein, L.; Verweij, J.; Van Glabbeke, M.; Van Oosterom, A.T.; Christian, M.C.; et al. New guidelines to evaluate the response to treatment in solid tumors. *J. Natl. Cancer Inst.* **2000**, *92*, 205–216. [CrossRef]
11. Van Uden, D.J.P.; van Maaren, M.; Strobbe, L.J.A.; Bult, P.; Van Der Hoeven, J.J.; Siesling, S.; De Wilt, J.H.W.; Blanken-Peeters, C.F.J.M. Metastatic behavior and overall survival according to breast cancer subtypes in stage IV inflammatory breast cancer. *Breast Cancer Res.* **2019**, *21*, 1–9. [CrossRef] [PubMed]
12. Yang, H.; Wang, R.; Zeng, F.; Zhao, J.; Peng, S.; Ma, Y.; Chen, S.; Ding, S.; Zhong, L.; Guo, W.; et al. Impact of molecular subtypes on metastatic behavior and overall survival in patients with metastatic breast cancer: A single-center study combined with a large cohort study based on the Surveillance, Epidemiology and End Results database. *Oncol. Lett.* **2020**, *20*, 1. [CrossRef]
13. Yang, H.-L.; Liu, T.; Wang, X.-M.; Xu, Y.; Deng, S.-M. Diagnosis of bone metastases: A meta-analysis comparing 18FDG PET, CT, MRI and bone scintigraphy. *Eur. Radiol.* **2011**, *21*, 2604–2617. [CrossRef] [PubMed]
14. Hildebrandt, M.G.; Gerke, O.; Baun, C.; Falch, K.; Hansen, J.A.; Farahani, Z.A.; Petersen, H.; Larsen, L.B.; Duvnjak, S.; Buskevica, I.; et al. [18F] fluorodeoxyglucose (FDG)-positron emission tomography (PET)/Computed Tomography (CT) in Suspected Recurrent Breast Cancer: A prospective comparative study of dual-time-point FDG-PET/CT, contrast-enhanced CT, and bone scintigraphy. *J. Clin. Oncol.* **2016**, *34*, 1889–1897. [CrossRef]
15. Bretschi, M.; Fränzle, A.; Merz, M.; Hillengass, J.; Semmler, W.; Bendl, R.; Bäuerle, T. Assessing treatment response of osteolytic lesions by manual volumetry, automatic segmentation, and recist in experimental bone metastases. *Acad. Radiol.* **2014**, *21*, 1177–1184. [CrossRef]
16. Sun, Z.; Yi, Y.L.; Liu, Y.; Xiong, J.P.; He, C.Z. Comparison of whole-body PET/PET-CT and conventional imaging procedures for distant metastasis staging in patients with breast cancer: A meta-analysis. *Eur. J. Gynaecol. Oncol.* **2015**, *36*, 672–676.
17. Riedl, C.C.; Pinker-Domenig, K.; Ulaner, G.A.; Ong, L.T.; Baltzer, P.; Jochelson, M.S.; McArthur, H.L.; Gönen, M.; Dickler, M.; Weber, W.A. Comparison of FDG-PET/CT and contrast-enhanced CT for monitoring therapy response in patients with metastatic breast cancer. *Eur. J. Nucl. Med. Mol. Imaging* **2017**, *44*, 1428–1437. [CrossRef]
18. Joo Hyun, O.; Lodge, M.A.; Wahl, R.L. Practical PERCIST: A simplified guide to pet response criteria in solid tumors 1.0. *Radiology* **2016**, *280*, 576–584. [CrossRef]
19. Paydary, K.; Seraj, S.M.; Zadeh, M.Z.; Emamzadehfard, S.; Shamchi, S.P.; Gholami, S.; Werner, T.J.; Alavi, A. The Evolving Role of FDG-PET/CT in the diagnosis, staging, and treatment of breast cancer. *Mol. Imaging Biol.* **2019**, *21*, 1–10. [CrossRef] [PubMed]
20. Graham, L.J.; Shupe, M.P.; Schneble, E.J.; Flynt, F.L.; Clemenshaw, M.N.; Kirkpatrick, A.D.; Gallagher, C.; Nissan, A.; Henry, L.; Stojadinovic, A.; et al. Current approaches and challenges in monitoring treatment responses in breast cancer. *J. Cancer* **2014**, *5*, 58–68. [CrossRef] [PubMed]
21. Boellaard, R.; Delgado-Bolton, R.; Oyen, W.J.G.; Giammarile, F.; Tatsch, K.; Eschner, W.; Verzijlbergen, F.J.; Barrington, S.F.; Pike, L.C.; Weber, W.A.; et al. FDG PET/CT: EANM

procedure guidelines for tumour imaging: Version 2.0. *Eur. J. Nucl. Med. Mol. Imaging* **2015**, *42*, 328–354. [CrossRef]
22. Sok, M.; Zavrl, M.; Greif, B.; Srpčič, M. Objective assessment of WHO/ECOG performance status. *Support. Care Cancer* **2019**, *27*, 3793–3798. [CrossRef] [PubMed]
23. Groheux, D.; Hindie, E. Breast cancer: Initial workup and staging with FDG PET/CT. *Clin. Transl. Imaging* **2021**, *9*, 221–231. [CrossRef] [PubMed]
24. Mortazavi-Jehanno, N.; Giraudet, A.-L.; Champion, L.; Lerebours, F.; Le Stanc, E.; Edeline, V.; Madar, O.; Bellet, D.; Pecking, A.P.; Alberini, J.-L. Assessment of response to endocrine therapy using FDG PET/CT in metastatic breast cancer: A pilot study. *Eur. J. Nucl. Med. Mol. Imaging* **2012**, *39*, 450–460. [CrossRef]
25. Zhang, F.; Xu, H.; Liu, J.; Xu, Y.; Chen, B.; Yang, Y.; Yan, N.; Song, S.; Lin, Y.; Xu, Y. 18F-FDG PET/CT for the early prediction of the response rate and survival of patients with recurrent or metastatic breast cancer. *Oncol. Lett.* **2018**, *16*, 4151–4158. [CrossRef]
26. Helland, F.; Henriksen, M.H.; Gerke, O.; Vogsen, M.; Høilund-Carlsen, P.F.; Hildebrandt, M.G. FDG-PET/CT Versus contrast- enhanced ct for response evaluation in metastatic breast cancer: A systematic review. *Diagnostics* **2019**, *9*, 106. [CrossRef]
27. Chua, S.C.; Groves, A.M.; Kayani, I.; Menezes, L.; Gacinovic, S.; Du, Y.; Bomanji, J.B.; Ell, P.J. The impact of 18F-FDG PET/CT in patients with liver metastases. *Eur. J. Nucl. Med. Mol. Imaging* **2007**, *34*, 1906–1914. [CrossRef]
28. Avril, S.; Muzic, R.F.; Plecha, D.; Traughber, B.J.; Vinayak, S.; Avril, N. 18F-FDG PET/CT for monitoring of treatment response in breast cancer. *J. Nucl. Med.* **2016**, *57*, 34S–39S. [CrossRef] [PubMed]
29. Vogsen, M.; Bülow, J.; Ljungstrøm, L.; Oltmann, H.; Alamdari, T.; Naghavi-Behzad, M.; Braad, P.-E.; Gerke, O.; Hildebrandt, M. FDG-PET/CT for response monitoring in metastatic breast cancer: The feasibility and benefits of applying percist. *Diagnostics* **2021**, *11*, 723. [CrossRef] [PubMed]
30. Sørensen, J.S.; Vilstrup, M.H.; Holm, J.; Vogsen, M.; Bülow, J.L.; Ljungstrøm, L.; Braad, P.-E.; Gerke, O.; Hildebrandt, M.G. Interrater agreement and reliability of PERCIST and visual assessment when using 18F-FDG-PET/CT for response monitoring of metastatic breast cancer. *Diagnostics* **2020**, *10*, 1001. [CrossRef]
31. Swain, S.M.; Baselga, J.; Kim, S.-B.; Semiglazov, V.; Campone, M.; Ciruelos, E.; Ferrero, J.-M.; Schneeweiss, A.; Heeson, S.; Clark, E. Pertuzumab, Trastuzumab, and Docetaxel in HER2-Positive Metastatic Breast Cancer. *N. Engl. J. Med.* **2015**, *372*, 724–734. [CrossRef] [PubMed]
32. Swain, S.M.; Miles, D.; Kim, S.-B.; Im, Y.-H.; Im, S.-A.; Semiglazov, V.; Ciruelos, E.; Schneeweiss, A.; Loi, S.; Monturus, E.; et al. Pertuzumab, trastuzumab, and docetaxel for HER2-positive metastatic breast cancer (CLEOPATRA): End-of-study results from a double-blind, randomised, placebo-controlled, phase 3 study. *Lancet Oncol.* **2020**, *21*, 519–530. [CrossRef]
33. Ulaner, G.A. PET/CT for Patients With Breast Cancer: Where Is the Clinical Impact? *Am. J. Roentgenol.* **2019**, *213*, 254–265. [CrossRef]
34. Hironaka-Mitsuhashi, A.; Calle, A.S.; Ochiya, T.; Takayama, S.; Suto, A. Towards circulating-tumor DNA-based precision medicine. *J. Clin. Med.* **2019**, *8*, 1365. [CrossRef]
35. Wood-Bouwens, C.M.; Haslem, D.; Moulton, B.; Almeda, A.F.; Lee, H.; Heestand, G.M.; Nadauld, L.D.; Ji, H.P. therapeutic monitoring of circulating dna mutations in metastatic cancer with personalized digital PCR. *J. Mol. Diagn.* **2020**, *22*, 247–261. [CrossRef] [PubMed]
36. Dashevsky, B.Z.; Goldman, D.A.; Parsons, M.; Gonen, M.; Corben, A.D.; Jochelson, M.S.; Hudis, C.A.; Morrow, M.; Ulaner, G.A. Appearance of untreated bone metastases from breast cancer on FDG PET/CT: Importance of histologic subtype. *Eur. J. Nucl. Med. Mol. Imaging* **2015**, *42*, 1666–1673. [CrossRef] [PubMed]
37. Hogan, M.; Goldman, D.A.; Dashevsky, B.; Riedl, C.; Gönen, M.; Osborne, J.; Jochelson, M.; Hudis, C.; Morrow, M.; Ulaner, G.A. Comparison of 18F-FDG PET/CT for Systemic staging of newly diagnosed invasive lobular carcinoma versus invasive ductal carcinoma. *J. Nucl. Med.* **2015**, *56*, 1674–1680. [CrossRef]
38. Jambor, I.; Kuisma, A.; Ramadan, S.; Huovinen, R.; Sandell, M.; Kajander, S.; Kemppainen, J.; Kauppila, E.; Auren, J.; Merisaari, H.; et al. Prospective evaluation of planar bone scintigraphy, SPECT, SPECT/CT, 18F-NaF PET/CT and whole body 1.5T MRI, including DWI, for the detection of bone metastases in high risk breast and prostate cancer patients: SKELETA clinical trial. *Acta Oncol.* **2015**, *55*, 59–67. [CrossRef]
39. Kosmin, M.; Padhani, A.R.; Gogbashian, A.; Woolf, D.; Ah-See, M.-L.; Ostler, P.; Sutherland, S.; Miles, D.; Noble, J.; Koh, D.-M.; et al. Comparison of whole-body MRI, CT, and bone scintigraphy for response evaluation of cancer therapeutics in metastatic breast cancer to bone. *Radiology* **2020**, *297*, 622–629. [CrossRef]

15

Factors Associated with Breast Cancer Screening Adherence among Church-Going African American Women

Pooja Agrawal [1,2], Tzuan A. Chen [1,3], Lorna H. McNeill [4], Chiara Acquati [4,5], Shahnjayla K. Connors [1,6], Vijay Nitturi [1,3], Angelica S. Robinson [7], Isabel Martinez Leal [1,3] and Lorraine R. Reitzel [1,3,*]

1 Department of Psychological, Health and Learning Sciences, University of Houston, Houston, TX 77204, USA; poagrawa@utmb.edu (P.A.); tchen3@central.uh.edu (T.A.C.); connorss@uhd.edu (S.K.C.); vnitturi@central.uh.edu (V.N.); imarti31@central.uh.edu (I.M.L.)
2 School of Medicine, University of Texas Medical Branch, Galveston, TX 77555, USA
3 Health Research Institute, University of Houston, Houston, TX 77204, USA
4 MD Anderson Cancer Center, Department of Health Disparities Research, Houston, TX 77230, USA; lmcneill@mdanderson.org (L.H.M.); cacquati@central.uh.edu (C.A.)
5 Graduate College of Social Work, University of Houston, Houston, TX 77204, USA
6 Department of Social Sciences, University of Houston-Downtown, Houston, TX 77002, USA
7 Department of Radiology, University of Texas Medical Branch, Galveston, TX 77555, USA; an3robin@utmb.edu
* Correspondence: lrreitzel@uh.edu;

Abstract: Relative to White women, African American/Black women are at an increased risk of breast cancer mortality. Early detection of breast cancer through mammography screening can mitigate mortality risks; however, screening rates are not ideal. Consequently, there is a need to better understand factors associated with adherence to breast cancer screening guidelines to inform interventions to increase mammography use, particularly for groups at elevated mortality risk. This study used the Andersen Behavioral Model of Health Services Use to examine factors associated with adherence to National Comprehensive Cancer Network breast cancer screening guidelines amongst 919 African American, church-going women from Houston, Texas. Logistic regression analyses measured associations between breast cancer screening adherence over the preceding 12 months (adherent or non-adherent) and predisposing (i.e., age, education, and partner status), enabling (i.e., health insurance status, annual household income, employment status, patient-provider communication, and social support), and need (i.e., personal diagnosis of cancer, family history of cancer, and risk perception) factors, separately and conjointly. Older age (predisposing: OR = 1.015 (1.007–1.023)), having health insurance and ideal patient–provider communication (enabling: OR = 2.388 (1.597–3.570) and OR = 1.485 (1.080–2.041)), and having a personal diagnosis of cancer (need: OR = 2.244 (1.058–4.758)) were each associated with greater odds of screening adherence. Only having health insurance and ideal patient-provider communication remained significantly associated with screening adherence in a conjoint model; cancer survivorship did not moderate associations between predisposing/enabling factors and screening adherence. Overall, results suggest that interventions which are designed to improve mammography screening rates amongst African American women might focus on broadening health insurance coverage and working to improve patient–provider communication. Implications for multi-level intervention approaches, including the role of churches in their dissemination, are proposed.

Keywords: breast cancer screening; mammogram; cancer health equity; African American women; cancer survivorship; Andersen Behavioral Model; predisposing factors; enabling factors; need factors

1. Introduction

Breast cancer is the most commonly diagnosed cancer among women in the United States, except for skin cancers [1]. The average risk of a woman developing breast cancer in her lifetime is approximately 13% and the American Cancer Society (ACS) estimates that 281,550 new cases of invasive breast cancer and 49,290 cases of ductal carcinoma in situ (DCIS) will be diagnosed in 2021 [1]. Breast cancer is also the second leading cause of cancer death in women after lung cancer [1]. It is estimated that 43,600 women will die from breast cancer in 2021 [1].

African American/Black (hereafter referred to as African American) women have an unequal burden of breast cancer mortality. The overall breast cancer incidence rate in African American women is 126.5 cases per 100,000 compared to 130.1 in White women [2]. Although the incidence rate is lower among African American women, breast cancer mortality is approximately 40% higher compared with White women [2]. African American women are also twice as likely as women of other racial and ethnic backgrounds to be diagnosed with triple-negative breast cancer [2,3] and tend to receive a diagnosis of breast cancer at more advanced stages [4].

Although African American women present with more aggressive cancers as compared to White women, disparities in mortality remain after accounting for tumor stage and characteristics. Thus, the racial disparity may be partially attributed to other factors, such as rates of screening mammograms [5]. Prior to 2015, African American women had lower rates of mammography screening as compared to White women [6]. In more recent years, the rates of mammography screening have increased among African American women, but nevertheless remain below the 81% Healthy People 2020 objective [6,7].

There are several working recommendations for who should be screened for breast cancer, at what age, and at what frequency, and these recommendations may differ based on the associated professional groups espousing them. A relatively clear recommendation is that of the National Comprehensive Cancer Network (NCCN), which recommends annual screening mammography beginning at age 40 years for all women [8]. These recommendations are also consistent with those of the American College of Radiology and the Society of Breast Imaging [9]. Routine breast cancer screening, such as that promoted by the NCCN, can reduce mortality and improve survival outcomes [10].

Given the disproportionally high rate of mortality among African American women with breast cancer, it is important to examine factors that are associated with breast cancer screening adherence in order to better understand factors affecting adherence to recommended screening guidelines in this population. The Andersen Behavioral Model of Health Services Use can be used to examine factors that lead to the use of health services [11–13], including obtaining cancer screenings as recommended [14,15]. According to this model, health service utilization depends on three separate categories: predisposing, enabling, and need factors [11–13]. Predisposing factors are existing conditions/characteristics that influence people to use or not use services (e.g., age, partner status, education, race/ethnicity, religiosity and fatalism) [11–13]. Enabling factors are those that facilitate or impede the use of services, including financial means to access services (e.g., income and insurance status) [11–13]. Need factors are those that laypeople or health care providers recognize as requiring medical treatment and can be divided into perceived and evaluated need (e.g., diagnosis of a medical condition, such as cancer, or family history) [11–13].

The Andersen model is helpful to compare whether one category of factors has a greater effect on breast cancer screening rates over another, an aim that has not been explored previously among African American women. For example, enabling factors may have the largest influence on screening for African American women, who are more likely to encounter various societal and systemic barriers that lead to increased risk for being uninsured and low-income relative to White women [16–18]. Even if breast cancer screenings are available free of charge, low-income individuals may face barriers to receiving them (e.g., no childcare to allow a health provider visit, difficulty with obtaining transportation) [19]. On the other hand, need factors may drive breast cancer screening adherence given the burden of breast cancer mortality experienced by this group, or they may moderate the association between enabling and/or predisposing factors and screening adherence.

Few previous studies have employed a theoretical framework, such as the Andersen model, as a guide to selecting variables that may be associated with breast cancer screening adherence [14]. One notable recent study that used the Andersen model to examine factors associated with breast cancer screening among Indigenous women found that, among predisposing factors, age was a significant predictor of breast cancer screening [14]. Among enabling factors, women with more formal education were more likely to undergo breast cancer screening [19]. Among need factors, participants with family cancer history were more likely to undergo breast cancer screening [19]. The extent to which this would generalize to African American women is not known; however, similar to Indigenous women, some African American women have lower median wages and employment rates than White women. Thus, these factors are also critically important to examine in this racial group [20].

With regard to studies on factors that influence the use of mammography screening among African American women specifically, one important work is Orji and colleagues' literature review on this topic [19]. This literature review identified 24 articles published between 2005 and 2017; however, only 45.9% used a theory to guide variable selection and analysis [19]. Notably, the literature review itself used the Andersen model to synthesize prior work [19]. They reported that among predisposing factors, educational achievement, basic knowledge of breast cancer, and recommended screening frequency were positively associated with mammography screening, with 25% of the studies finding a positive association between education and screening adherence [19]. Medical mistrust was negatively associated with mammography use. Age, breast cancer beliefs (e.g., family teachings, the idea that surgery could cause cancer to spread), religiosity and fear and fatalism had mixed results, indicating a need for further research [19]. Among enabling factors, 10 (42%) of the studies identified health insurance as positively associated with mammography intentions or screening history [19]. Accessibility of care, income, and healthcare utilization (e.g., receiving regular medical checkups or physician visits within the last year) were other enabling factors found to be positively associated with mammography screening. Among need factors, physician recommendation and personal/family history of breast cancer were positively associated with mammography screening, while pain and discomfort caused by mammography and familial responsibilities (e.g., family duties or caretaking demands) were negatively associated with mammography screening [19]. Although Orji's and colleagues' work was a significant step forward in summarizing factors associated with breast cancer screening adherence among African American women across extant studies, it is notable that many of these studies did not comprehensively examine predisposing, enabling, and need factors and most of the included studies (58.4%) had relatively small sample sizes (i.e., less than 300 women) [19].

The current study builds upon the extant literature regarding African American women and factors associated with breast cancer screening using the Andersen framework while adding to the literature by examining additional variables that were not explored previously, such as the role of the patient–provider relationship (i.e., how often the patient felt listened to or respected by the physician), a potential enabling variable of relevance [15]. Specifically, the purpose of the current study was to: (1) Examine associations between predisposing, enabling, and need factor variables and with breast cancer screening adherence; (2) Explore whether predisposing, enabling, and/or need factor categories have the strongest association with breast cancer screening adherence; and (3) Investigate the potential moderating effect of need factors on the associations between predisposing factors and enabling factors, respectively, and breast cancer screening adherence among a large convenience sample of >900 church-going African American women. While religiosity and fatalism have been measured in prior studies among African American women with mixed results, this study is one of only a few studies conducted among a church-based sample [21,22]. This is important because 47% of African Americans in the United States attend religious services at least once a week [23,24]. Furthermore, there may be less variability in constructs previously yielding mixed results, such as religiosity, in homogeneous church-based samples relative to more heterogeneous community-based samples.

Better understanding of the associations between factors and breast cancer screening adherence among a church-based sample of African American women may have several practical applications. For example, it may help inform cancer-reducing interventions delivered within the church or church ministry, which can be tailored to reflect connections with relevant scripture. Moreover, churches may be an important means of dissemination of health information, such as cancer screening guidelines, which can be promoted to groups of women at elevated risk of screening non-adherence. Additionally, the identification of predisposing, enabling, and/or need factors essential to improving breast cancer screening among African American women may also help physicians provide increased support and health education to their patients in order to increase adherence to screening recommendations [14,21,25,26]. Further, the potential findings of this study may help inform policies to remove economic barriers that limit access to screening.

2. Materials and Methods

2.1. Design

Participants comprised a convenience sample from three churches in Southwest Houston, Texas, with predominantly African American membership that agreed to participate in data collection aimed at understanding health and cancer risk among African American adults. Recruitment occurred through printed and televised media in the churches and in-person solicitation. Participants were required to be ≥18 years old, living in the Houston area with a functional telephone number, and an attendee of one of the participating churches. Surveys were completed on-site using a computerized questionnaire format. As compensation, participants received a $30 gift card.

A previous publication details the parent study design and the characteristics of the participating churches and their participants [27]. In short, the underlying parent study, Creating a Higher Understanding of cancer Research and Community Health (Project CHURCH), was a community-based participatory research project with an aim of understanding disparities in cancer risk factors and engaging African Americans as partners in the research process in order to reduce barriers to research participation and improve research outcomes. Project CHURCH used a longitudinal cohort design and started in 2008 with a large Houston mega-church, expanding to add two additional, smaller churches in 2012. Procedures were informed by the church and scientific advisory board. Overall, Project CHURCH enrolled ~1500 adults from the original church, and around 400 adults in each of the smaller churches. About 70% of participants were women, mirroring their proportion amongst church attendees [27]. This study was approved by the IRBs associated with the University of Texas MD Anderson Cancer Center (protocol code 2007-0970, approved 2/28/08; protocol code 2012-0051, approved 2/14/12) and the University of Houston (protocol code 14423-EX, approved 7/10/14).

The number of participants targeted for these data collections varied based on the size of the participating churches and totaled 2254 (N = 1666 women). For the present study, only women 40 years of age or older (N = 1108) and with complete data on all included measures (N = 919) comprised the final analytic sample.

2.2. Measures

2.2.1. Predisposing Factors

Predisposing factors included age (in years), educational achievement (≤high school degree, some college, vs. ≥Bachelor's degree), and partner status (married or living with partner vs. divorced, widowed, separated, and never married). Factors were included in the predisposing category based on precedent from previous research and guidance by the Andersen model [11–13,19].

2.2.2. Enabling Factors

Enabling factors included whether the participant was covered by health insurance over the last year (no vs. yes), annual household income (<\$40,000, \$40–\$79,999, vs. ≥\$80,000) employment status (not employed vs. employed for wages/self-employed), patient–provider communication, and social support.

Patient–provider communication was included as an enabling factor due to a similar categorization in a prior study on prostate cancer screening [15]. Patient–provider communication was measured by four items from the Consumer Assessment of Healthcare Providers and Systems (CAHPS) survey. Participants were asked how often their health care provider or doctor over the prior year: (1) listened carefully to them, (2) explained things in a way they could understand, (3) showed respect for what they had to say, (4) spent enough time with them, with response choices of: never, sometimes, usually, and always. Cronbach's alpha for these four items in this sample was 0.90. Based on convention [28], the measure was scored based on whether each participant selected "always" to each item vs. did not select "always" for each item, essentially capturing ideal versus not always ideal patient–provider communication.

Social support was included as an enabling factor as recommended by an updated version of the Andersen model [13]. Social support was measured through the Interpersonal Support Evaluation List (ISEL)-12, which consists of 12 items and 3 subscales [29]. The three subscales were the tangible support subscale (availability of material aid), the belonging subscale (availability of companions with whom one may engage in activities), and the appraisal subscale (availability of emotional support). Items were rated on a four-point scale (1 = definitely false to 4 = definitely true), with subscale scores ranging from 4 to 16. Higher scores indicated greater social support [30]. Cronbach's alpha for ISEL-12 subscales in this sample were 0.63 (tangible support), 0.70 (belonging support), and 0.70 (appraisal support).

2.2.3. Need Factors

Need factors included a personal diagnosis of cancer (any type; no vs. yes), family history of cancer (any type; yes vs. no), and risk perception. Personal cancer history and family history of cancer were included in need factors based on similar categorization in a previous study, and because need factors include an individual's perceived or evaluated need [14]. Risk perception was measured through three discrete items from the Health Information National Trends Survey (HINTS) [31]. The first item was: "How likely do you think it is that you will develop any type of cancer in the future? Would you say your chance of getting cancer is ... " Answer options ranged from 1 = very low, 2 = somewhat low, 3 = moderate, 4 = somewhat high, to 5 = very high. The second item asked: "Compared to the average person your age, would you say that you are ... " Answer options ranged from 1 = more likely to get cancer, 2 = less likely, to 3 = about as likely. The final item was: "How often do you worry about getting some type of cancer?" Answer options were: 1 = never, 2 = rarely, 3 = sometimes, 4 = often, and 5 = all the time. Each of the risk perception items were respectively included in the analysis.

2.2.4. Breast Cancer Screening Adherence

Receipt of breast cancer screening was measured by asking participants whether they had ever had a mammogram (0 = no; 1 = yes) and, for those endorsing "yes" to the lifetime mammography item, when their most recent mammogram had taken place. Those reporting having received a mammogram 1 year ago or less were considered adherent, whereas those indicating their last mammogram was >1 year ago were considered not adherent, in accordance with NCCN screening recommendations [7].

2.2.5. General Participant Characteristics

Data were also collected about the number of family members under the age of 18 in the household and reasons for obtaining the most recent mammogram for descriptive purposes.

2.3. Data Analysis

The descriptive statistics of participants' characteristics and study variables were assessed. The comparisons between those excluded due to missingness vs. analytic sample on participant characteristics were examined. Participant characteristics relative to breast cancer screening adherence were examined using t-test or chi-square test for continuous and categorical variables, respectively.

For the main analyses (Aim 1), separate logistic regression analyses were conducted to measure associations between breast cancer screening adherence and predisposing factors (i.e., age, education, and partner status), enabling factors (i.e., health insurance status, annual household income, employment status, patient–provider communication, and ISEL social support subscales), and need factors (i.e., personal diagnosis of cancer, family history of cancer, and risk perception). Next (Aim 2), predisposing, enabling, and needs factors were all included in the logistic regression analysis predicting breast cancer screening adherence. Lastly (Aim 3), to examine the moderation effect of need factors, the interaction terms of the significant need factor and predisposing/enabling factor were included in the models. Separate moderation effects were examined. Continuous variables were mean-centered prior to moderation analyses, and church site (1, 2, or 3) was included as a covariate in all logistic regression analyses. All analyses used two-tailed tests of significance with a statistical significance level designated at $p < 0.05$. All analyses were conducted using SAS version 9.4 [32].

3. Results

Of the 1108 total female participants aged 40 and above in the parent study, 919 (82.94%) had full information on all the measures included in this study. Women 40 or older with missing data ($N = 189$) differed statistically from those who had all data ($N = 919$) on ISEL belonging subscale scores, recruitment site, health insurance status, and screening adherence. Specifically, those with missing data reported higher ISEL belonging subscale scores (13.65 vs. 13.22, $p = 0.0304$), were less likely to have health insurance (74.47% vs. 88.36%, $p < 0.0001$), were more likely to be recruited from church site 3 (29.10% vs. 19.15%, $p = 0.0071$) and were less likely to be screening adherent (56.38% vs. 67.03%, $p = 0.0052$) relative to participants who had full data on all the measures.

3.1. Participant Characteristics

Participants ranged from age 40 to 86 (M = 53.12, SD = 8.56). Of the 919 participants, 67.03% ($N = 616$) were screening adherent. Overall, 11.43% of this group ($N = 105$) reported education $\leq$ high school, 40.70% some college ($N = 374$), and 47.88% $\geq$ bachelor's degree ($N = 440$). Additionally, 42.66% ($N = 392$) reported they were married/living with a partner, 88.36% ($N = 812$) reported they were insured, 69.75% ($N = 641$) reported they were employed, 32.21% ($N = 296$) reported ideal patient-provider communication, 5.01% ($N = 46$) had been diagnosed with at least 1 cancer, and 59.74% ($N = 549$) reported a family history of cancer(s). Participant characteristics by breast cancer screening adherence status are shown in Table 1.

Table 1. Participant Characteristics Relative to NCCN Breast Cancer Screening Adherence Status ($N = 919$).

	All	Non-Adherent	Adherent	
	919	303	616	*p*-Value
		Mean (SD)/% [n]		
Age	53.12 (8.56)	51.14 (8.29)	54.09 (8.53)	<0.0001
Education				0.0961
≤High school	11.43 [105]	11.88 [36]	11.20 [69]	
Some college	40.70 [374]	45.21 [137]	38.47 [237]	
≥Bachelor's degree	47.88 [440]	42.90 [130]	50.32 [310]	
Partner Status				0.1461
Not married/living with a partner	57.34 [527]	60.73 [184]	55.68 [343]	
Married/living with a partner	42.66 [392]	39.27 [119]	44.32 [273]	
Number of family members <18 years old in house	0.48 (0.86)	0.54 (0.94)	0.45 (0.82)	0.1270
Church Site				0.0109
Site 1	67.36 [619]	70.30 [213]	65.91 [406]	
Site 2	13.49 [124]	15.84 [48]	12.34 [76]	
Site 3	19.15 [176]	13.86 [42]	21.75 [134]	
Health Insurance Coverage				<0.0001
No	11.64 [107]	20.13 [61]	7.47 [46]	
Yes	88.36 [812]	79.87 [242]	92.53 [570]	
Annual Household Income				0.0853
<$40,000	28.18 [259]	31.68 [96]	26.46 [163]	
$40,000–$79,999	38.19 [351]	39.27 [119]	37.66 [232]	
≥$80,000	33.62 [309]	29.04 [88]	35.88 [221]	
Employment Status				0.3874
Unemployed	30.25 [278]	28.38 [86]	31.17 [192]	
Employed	69.75 [641]	71.62 [217]	68.83 [424]	
Patient-Provider Communication				0.0033
Not always ideal	67.79 [623]	74.26 [225]	64.61 [398]	
Ideal	32.21 [296]	25.74 [78]	35.39 [218]	
Social Support				
ISEL Tangible	13.93 (2.42)	13.67 (2.58)	14.06 (2.32)	0.0276
ISEL Belonging	13.22 (2.60)	13.06 (2.82)	13.30 (2.49)	0.2191
ISEL Appraisal	14.02 (2.55)	13.80 (2.79)	14.12 (2.42)	0.0853
Personal Diagnosis of Cancer				0.0472
No	94.99 [873]	97.03 [294]	93.99 [579]	
Yes	5.01 [46]	2.97 [9]	6.01 [37]	
Family Diagnosis of Cancer				0.6668
No	40.26 [370]	41.25 [125]	39.77 [245]	
Yes	59.74 [549]	58.75 [178]	60.23 [371]	
Chance of Getting Cancer				0.8358
Very low	37.65 [346]	38.61 [117]	37.18 [229]	
Somewhat low	24.59 [226]	25.74 [78]	24.03 [148]	
Moderate	28.84 [265]	26.73 [81]	29.87 [184]	
Somewhat high	7.62 [70]	7.92 [24]	7.47 [46]	
Very high	1.31 [12]	0.99 [3]	1.46 [9]	
Likelihood of getting cancer compared to average person your age				0.8131
More likely to get cancer	7.83 [72]	8.58 [26]	7.47 [46]	
Less likely	57.13 [525]	56.11 [170]	57.63 [355]	
About as likely	35.04 [322]	35.31 [107]	34.90 [215]	
How often worry about getting cancer				0.660
Never	26.22 [241]	29.37 [89]	24.68 [152]	
Rarely	35.04 [322]	33.99 [103]	35.55 [219]	
Sometimes	31.56 [290]	30.03 [91]	32.31 [199]	
Often	5.11 [47]	4.62 [14]	5.36 [33]	
All the time	2.07 [19]	1.98 [6]	2.11 [13]	
Main reason for mammogram [1]				<0.0001
Part of the routine physical exam	84.98 [781]	71.95 [218]	91.4 [563]	
Last mammogram was not normal	4.24 [39]	5.28 [16]	3.73 [23]	
A specific problem	3.81 [35]	3.96 [12]	3.73 [23]	
Something you heard/saw/read	0.33 [3]	0.66 [2]	0.16 [1]	
Family history	1.09 [10]	1.32 [4]	0.97 [6]	
You never had one and thought you should	0.44 [4]	1.32 [4]	0 [0]	

[1] 47 women (5.11% of sample) who were non-adherent with NCCN breast cancer screening guidelines did not provide responses for the main reason for their most recent mammogram. ISEL = Interpersonal Support Evaluation List. SD = Standard deviation.

Compared with participants who were screening non-adherent, participants who were breast cancer adherent were older (54.09 vs. 51.14, $p < 0.0001$) and had higher ISEL tangible support scores (14.06 vs. 13.67, $p = 0.0276$). Chi-square tests revealed significant associations between screening adherence and church site ($p = 0.0109$), health insurance status ($p < 0.0001$), patient–provider communication ($p = 0.0033$), and personal diagnosis of cancer ($p = 0.0472$). Those reporting screening adherence were more likely to have been recruited from church site 3 (21.75% vs. 13.86%), have health insurance (92.53% vs. 79.87%), report ideal patient–provider communication (35.39% vs. 25.74%), and have been a cancer survivor (6.01% vs. 2.97%) relative to participants who were non-adherent with NCCN breast cancer screening recommendations.

3.2. *Aim 1: Predisposing, Enabling, and Need Factors and Breast Cancer Screening Adherence*

Logistic regression analyses revealed that among the predisposing variables, older participants had greater odds of breast cancer screening adherence (OR: 1.015, 95% CI: 1.007–1.023). Among the enabling factors, participants who were insured and who had ideal patient–provider communication had 2.388 (95% CI: 1.597–3.570) and 1.485 (95% CI: 1.080–2.041) times greater odds of breast cancer screening adherence, respectively. Finally, among the need factors, cancer survivors had 2.244 (95% CI: 1.058–4.758) greater odds of breast cancer screening adherence relative to those who had never been diagnosed with cancer(s) (Table 2).

Table 2. Logistic Regression Analyses—Predicting Breast Cancer Screening Adherence ($N = 919$).

Factor	Effect	Estimate	SE	OR	95% CI	*p*-Value
Predisposing Factor	Church site 2	−0.213	0.205	0.808	(0.540, 1.208)	0.299
	Church site 3 (ref: Church site 1)	0.393	0.201	1.481	(0.998, 2.197)	0.051
	Age	0.015	0.004	1.015	(1.007, 1.023)	<0.0001
	Education (≥Bachelor's degree) (ref: ≤High School)	−0.017	0.215	0.983	(0.644, 1.499)	0.936
	Education (Some college) (ref: ≤High School)	−0.317	0.214	0.729	(0.479, 1.108)	0.138
	Partner status (Married/Living with a partner) (ref: Other [1])	0.145	0.144	1.156	(0.873, 1.532)	0.311
Enabling Factor	Church site 2	−0.188	0.214	0.828	(0.545, 1.259)	0.378
	Church site 3 (ref: Church site 1)	0.433	0.202	1.541	(1.038, 2.288)	0.032
	Health insurance coverage (ref: No)	0.870	0.205	2.388	(1.597, 3.570)	<0.0001
	Annual household income ($40,000–$79,999) (ref: <$40,000)	0.064	0.188	1.066	(0.737, 1.542)	0.734
	Annual household income (≥$80,000) (ref: <$40,000)	0.242	0.204	1.274	(0.855, 1.898)	0.235
	Employment status (ref: Unemployed)	−0.256	0.167	0.774	(0.558, 1.075)	0.126
	Patient-provider communication (ref: Not Always Ideal)	0.395	0.162	1.485	(1.080, 2.041)	0.015
	ISEL Tangible support	0.009	0.039	1.009	(0.936, 1.089)	0.807
	ISEL Belonging	−0.032	0.036	0.969	(0.902, 1.040)	0.385
	ISEL Appraisal	0.012	0.037	1.012	(0.941, 1.088)	0.756
Need Factor	Church site 2	−0.074	0.222	0.929	(0.601, 1.435)	0.740
	Church site 3 (ref: Church site 1)	0.656	0.218	1.927	(1.258, 2.953)	0.003
	Personal diagnosis of cancer (ref: No)	0.808	0.384	2.244	(1.058, 4.758)	0.035
	Family members diagnosed with cancer (ref: No)	0.228	0.164	1.256	(0.911, 1.730)	0.164
	Chance of getting cancer (Somewhat low) (ref: Very low)	0.093	0.199	1.097	(0.744, 1.619)	0.641
	Chance of getting cancer (Moderate) (ref: Very low)	−0.083	0.311	0.921	(0.501, 1.693)	0.790

Table 2. *Cont.*

Factor	Effect	Estimate	SE	OR	95% CI	*p*-Value
	Chance of getting cancer (Somewhat high) (ref: Very low)	−0.099	0.189	0.905	(0.625, 1.312)	0.600
	Chance of getting cancer (Very high) (ref: Very low)	0.436	0.732	1.547	(0.369, 6.492)	0.551
	Likelihood of getting cancer compared to average person your age (About as likely) (ref: More likely to get cancer)	0.208	0.209	1.232	(0.817, 1.856)	0.319
	Likelihood of getting cancer compared to average person your age (Less likely) (ref: More likely to get cancer)	0.397	0.171	1.487	(1.064, 2.078)	0.020
	How often worry about getting cancer (All the time) (ref: Never)	0.199	0.552	1.220	(0.413, 3.602)	0.719
	How often worry about getting cancer (Often) (ref: Never)	0.353	0.367	1.423	(0.693, 2.922)	0.337
	How often worry about getting cancer (Rarely) (ref: Never)	0.158	0.180	1.171	(0.822, 1.666)	0.382
	How often worry about getting cancer (Sometimes) (ref: Never)	0.205	0.199	1.228	(0.832, 1.812)	0.301
All	Church site 2	−0.128	0.237	0.880	(0.553, 1.401)	0.590
	Church site 3 (ref: Church site 1)	0.515	0.237	1.673	(1.052, 2.661)	0.030
	Age	0.004	0.008	1.004	(0.989, 1.020)	0.579
	Education (≥Bachelor's degree) (ref: ≤High School)	−0.018	0.266	0.982	(0.583, 1.655)	0.946
	Education (Some college) (ref: ≤High School)	−0.289	0.248	0.749	(0.461, 1.217)	0.243
	Partner status (Married/Living with a partner) (ref: Other [1])	0.102	0.166	1.108	(0.801, 1.533)	0.537
	Health insurance coverage (ref: No)	0.827	0.227	2.286	(1.464, 3.570)	<0.0001
	Annual household income ($40,000–$79,999) (ref: <$40,000)	0.003	0.203	1.003	(0.673, 1.494)	0.989
	Annual household income (≥$80,000) (ref: <$40,000)	0.144	0.243	1.155	(0.717, 1.861)	0.553
	Employment status (ref: Unemployed)	−0.227	0.178	0.797	(0.562, 1.131)	0.204
	Patient-provider communication (ref: Not Always Ideal)	0.424	0.166	1.528	(1.104, 2.115)	0.011
	ISEL Tangible support	0.000	0.041	1.000	(0.922, 1.085)	0.992
	ISEL Belonging	−0.039	0.038	0.962	(0.893, 1.036)	0.303
	ISEL Appraisal	0.005	0.040	1.005	(0.930, 1.086)	0.900
	Personal diagnosis of cancer (ref: No)	0.711	0.392	2.036	(0.944, 4.392)	0.070
	Family members diagnosed with cancer (ref: No)	0.172	0.177	1.187	(0.839, 1.680)	0.334
	Chance of getting cancer (Somewhat low) (ref: Very low)	−0.008	0.211	0.992	(0.655, 1.500)	0.968
	Chance of getting cancer (Moderate) (ref: Very low)	−0.211	0.347	0.810	(0.410, 1.598)	0.543
	Chance of getting cancer (Somewhat high) (ref: Very low)	−0.140	0.198	0.869	(0.589, 1.282)	0.480
	Chance of getting cancer (Very high) (ref: Very low)	0.227	0.794	1.254	(0.264, 5.950)	0.776

Table 2. *Cont.*

Factor	Effect	Estimate	SE	OR	95% CI	p-Value
	Likelihood of getting cancer compared to average person your age (About as likely) (ref: More likely to get cancer)	−0.118	0.319	0.888	(0.475, 1.660)	0.711
	Likelihood of getting cancer compared to average person your age (Less likely) (ref: More likely to get cancer)	0.056	0.332	1.058	(0.552, 2.028)	0.865
	How often worry about getting cancer (All the time) (ref: Never)	0.465	0.585	1.593	(0.506, 5.015)	0.427
	How often worry about getting cancer (Often) (ref: Never)	0.444	0.384	1.559	(0.734, 3.310)	0.248
	How often worry about getting cancer (Rarely) (ref: Never)	0.159	0.191	1.172	(0.807, 1.704)	0.405
	How often worry about getting cancer (Sometimes) (ref: Never)	0.202	0.210	1.224	(0.812, 1.847)	0.335

Note. SE = Standard Error; OR = Odds Ratio; CI = Confidence Interval; [1] Other included divorced, widowed, separated, and never married. ISEL = Interpersonal Support Evaluation List. SE = Standard Error. OR = Odds Ratio. CI = Confidence Interval. Ref = Reference group.

3.3. *Aim 2: Predisposing, Enabling, vs. Need Factors and Breast Cancer Screening Adherence*

When all factors were simultaneously included in the model, logistic regression analysis showed that two enabling factors, health insurance and patient-provider communication, were significantly associated with screening adherence. Specifically, participants who had health insurance (OR: 2.286, 95% CI: 1.464–3.570) and who reported ideal patient–provider communication (OR: 1.528, 95% CI: 1.104–2.115) had greater odds of breast cancer screening adherence (Table 2).

3.4. *Aim 3: Moderation Effects of Personal Cancer Diagnosis (i.e., Survivorship)*

The only significant need factor, personal diagnosis of cancer, was examined as a moderator in the association of the significant predisposing factors and enabling factors, respectively, with breast cancer screening adherence. To examine the moderation effect, the interaction terms of personal diagnosis of cancer and age/health insurance/patient-provider communication were included separately in the models. None of the interaction terms were significant, implying that a personal diagnosis of cancer did not moderate the relationship between age (p = 0.0679), health insurance (p = 0.695), or patient-provider communication (p = 0.425) and breast cancer screening adherence (data not shown).

4. Discussion

Among this sample of church-going African American women, 67% reported receiving a screening mammogram within the last year. This finding was slightly lower but comparable to the 68.1% of African American women in the United States who reported receiving a mammogram within the past 2 years (data from 2018) [33]. However, prevalence rates remain well below the Healthy People 2020 objective of 81%, indicating a considerable need for interventions that increase breast cancer screening [6,7]. Better understanding of factors associated with breast cancer screening adherence amongst African American women, who are at relatively higher risk for breast cancer mortality compared with White women [2], is important to inform intervention development and delivery. The present study, conducted solely among church-going African American women from three churches in Houston, Texas, investigated health care utilization factors that could help inform these future interventions to increase breast cancer screening rates.

Among predisposing factors, increased age was associated with greater odds of receiving a screening mammogram within the last year. Some previous studies have also found that increased age is associated with screening adherence among African American women [34,35]. Decreased adherence to screening among younger women may be due to disputed screening guidelines about the age at which screening should be initiated (e.g., the U.S. Preventive Services Task Force (USPSTF) recommends biennial screening mammography for women aged 50 to 74 years [36].) Previous studies conducted among African American women have also found that older women tend to have a greater number of visits to their physician and often obtain mammograms as a result of physician recommendations [37]. Other studies among African American women, however, have found that older age is associated with a lower motivation to screen and the receipt of fewer mammograms [38,39]. Additional research is needed to understand why these inconsistencies exist and to provide tailored interventions to both older and younger African American women to increase their screening adherence.

Among enabling factors, participants who were insured and who reported ideal levels of patient–provider communication were more likely to be breast cancer screening adherent. Numerous studies have found insurance status to be associated with receipt of breast cancer screening [19]. Orji and colleagues' literature review found that health insurance was the most frequently identified influence on mammography among African American women, with 42% (N = 10) of the included studies finding a significant association between health insurance and mammography intentions or adherence [19]. This is not surprising given that cost has been cited as a barrier to breast cancer screening among African American women [40,41]. Given that at least 8% of African American women in the United States were uninsured in 2019, future interventions designed to increase mammography rates may consider targeting uninsured women for free mammograms through mobile mammography units, community partnerships, or national programs [18,42–44]. Women who had ideal patient–provider communication also had greater odds of screening adherence. This indicates that a strong relationship between the patient and physician may influence a woman's likeliness to obtain a mammogram, a finding seen in a previous study among African American women, but which has never been tested in the context of the Andersen model [45]. Consequently, future interventions to increase screening adherence may include the training of physicians to relay information in a manner that builds trust and respect through patient-centered communication [46,47]. Building trust and respect in the context of a clinical encounter, particularly when patient and provider race/ethnicity is mismatched, may be a time-intensive and ongoing endeavor; healthcare facilities employing physicians should promote ways in which spending this "extra time" can be incentivized (or at least not actively disincentivized). Likewise, women who do not report ideal patient–provider communication might be advised to seek another physician with whom more ideal communication might be possible. Alternatively, women may benefit from coaching regarding how they can be empowered to obtain clearer information from physicians in the context of medical visits in order to become more informed about their options and eligibility for breast cancer screening. This is especially important as most women in this sample reported receiving their last mammogram in the context of a routine physical exam (84.98%). It also bears mentioning that attention to "next steps" in the process is also critical for saving lives, which includes ensuring access to free diagnostic exams and breast biopsies in the event of a screening abnormality.

When need factors were assessed, those reporting a personal diagnosis of cancer were more likely to be screening adherent. Similar results have been reported in previous studies involving African American women, finding that women who reported personal exposure to breast cancer (through own diagnosis or knowing someone with breast cancer) were more likely to have had a mammogram in the past than women without personal exposure [48,49]. Additionally, previous evidence has supported that African American women with a history of chronic illnesses such as cancers were more regularly screened [49]. These findings indicate that personal diagnoses of cancer may contribute to increased knowledge that could potentially elevate the importance of regular screening. It should be noted that our cancer survivorship variable encompassed all cancer types, similar to at least one prior work [14], but in contrast to another contribution where breast cancer survivorship was specifically included [48]. However, having received a prior diagnosis of any cancer is a risk factor for the development of other/recurrent cancers [50], and thus may affect cancer screening adherence in general. Moreover, most survivors in this sample were breast cancer survivors (31/46 = 67.39%); thus, only 1.63% (15/919) of the sample were survivors of other cancers. Future studies with a larger group of survivors might consider an examination of breast cancer survivorship versus other cancer survivorship as relevant need factors.

Overall, the current work is the first study to examine factors associated with breast cancer screening using the Andersen model pursuant to Orji and colleagues' recent literature review [19]. Although each of the above described predisposing, enabling, and need variables contributed unique variance within their overarching grouping to the prediction of breast cancer screening adherence, health insurance and patient-provider communication were the two variables that remained significant in the context of all others. These results suggest two potentially changeable factors that may increase adherence to screening—irrespective of a personal history of cancer—that might be prioritized in intervention design. A multi-level ecological intervention with the ability to: (1) address national and local policies and practices reducing un-insurance rates and/or targeting uninsured women for free cancer screenings; (2) train medical providers on culturally-appropriate and respectful ways to interact with patients; and (3) empower patients to seek and develop ideal health communication with their physicians, may contribute to improving breast cancer screening rates amongst African American women and reduce the gap between the status quo and Healthy People 2020 objectives [9,10].

Given the importance of churches in African American communities, these settings may be useful as a method of dispersing information about mammography screening to women with the goal of increasing screening awareness and adherence [24]. Previous research among this group has found that church-based breast cancer screening education programs positively affected mammography attainment [51]. Darnell and colleagues' study found that African Americans who reported receiving information about mammograms numerous times at their churches were more likely to report mammography use within the prior year than those who encountered such information less frequently [52]. Future interventions may consider taking advantage of the reach and influence of churches to promote mammography screening among African American women, potentially with a particular focus on the development of health literacy and self-advocacy in the context of patient–provider interactions [53].

A limitation of this study is its cross-sectional nature as temporal relations cannot be determined. Other aspects of limitation include the use of self-reported measures for receiving screening mammograms, the timeframe of which may be affected by recollection bias. Additional factors not accounted for or assessed in this study (e.g., psychosocial factors, social network characteristics, mental health symptoms or diagnoses) may have affected the variables in this study, however, we did not examine these factors as they have not been traditionally included in the Andersen model. Statistical analysis was limited to variables collected in all three churches; therefore, some of the variables that have been previously included in the Andersen model could not be analyzed (e.g., health care utilization). Furthermore, this study used convenience sampling to select participants and was limited to church-going African American women in the South, which may affect generalizability to all African American church-going women, or to those who attend churches with lower proportions of African American membership. Moreover, this study did not collect information on which breast cancer screening guidelines were promoted within the respective participant treatment settings and/or followed by participants; thus, it is possible some women were following different screening guidelines than those promoted by the NCCN with which they were indeed adherent. Additionally, this study was largely a replication study, wherein factors examined in other studies were primarily included with the exploration of only a limited number of novel variables (e.g., patient–provider communication). Additional novel constructs may be important to examine in future work, and qualitative feedback from church attendees may be important in ascertaining factors of relevance. Finally, the present work used two-tailed tests based on prior mixed results in other studies, the direct (and novel) application of the Andersen framework in an African American sample, and the addition of limited new constructs; future confirmatory work would benefit from directional hypotheses, the use of one-tailed tests, and considerations for multiple testing.

Limitations are balanced by study strengths, including a large sample of church-going African American women from multiple recruitment sites, the use of a theoretical model guiding variable selection, and inclusion of factors such as patient-provider communication, which have not been extensively examined in the context of breast cancer screening among African American women. Future studies may consider using a longitudinal study design and including these additional variables.

5. Conclusions

In conclusion, this study expands upon existing literature by supporting the association between older age, health insurance coverage, ideal patient–provider communication, and cancer survivorship with adherence to mammography screening in a large sample of church-going African American women. Results have implications for intervention targeting and design. Specifically, (1) educational campaigns to reinforce the importance of establishing yearly mammogram screening behaviors might be best directed toward younger African American church-going women; such efforts might be powerful if congregant cancer survivors are part of educational campaigns; (2) policies and practices that reach and expand preventive (and diagnostic/curative) breast healthcare to uninsured African American women are needed; and (3) methods to enhance patient–provider communication may be important to increasing adherence to mammogram screening guidelines for those reporting less than ideal interactions with healthcare providers. Future interventions aimed at increasing mammogram screening rates among African American women should consider the potential role of the church as an ideal and culturally-relevant setting to provide information and connection to preventative care to their congregants.

Author Contributions: Conceptualization, P.A., C.A., S.K.C. and L.R.R.; Data curation, T.A.C. and L.H.M.; Formal analysis, T.A.C.; Funding acquisition, P.A., L.H.M. and L.R.R.; Investigation, L.H.M.; Methodology, L.H.M. and L.R.R.; Project administration, L.H.M.; Resources, L.H.M. and L.R.R.; Software, T.A.C. and L.H.M.; Supervision, L.H.M. and L.R.R.; Validation, T.A.C. and L.H.M.; Visualization, T.A.C.; Writing—original draft, P.A., T.A.C., V.N. and L.R.R.; Writing—review & editing, P.A., T.A.C., L.H.M., C.A., S.K.C., V.N., A.S.R., I.M.L. and L.R.R. All authors have read and agreed to the published version of the manuscript.

References

1. Siegel, R.L.; Miller, K.D.; Fuchs, H.E.; Jemal, A. Cancer Statistics, 2021. *CA Cancer J. Clin.* **2021**, *71*, 7–33. [CrossRef] [PubMed]
2. American Cancer Society. Cancer Facts & Figures for African Americans 2019–2021. *Am. Cancer Soc.* **2019**, *40*, 3.
3. De Santis, C.E.; Ma, J.; Goding Sauer, A.; Newman, L.A.; Jemal, A. Breast cancer statistics, 2017, racial disparity in mortality by state. *CA Cancer J. Clin.* **2017**, *67*, 439–448. [CrossRef] [PubMed]
4. Daly, B.; Olopade, O.I. A perfect storm: How tumor biology, genomics, and health care delivery patterns collide to create a racial survival disparity in breast cancer and proposed interventions for change. *CA Cancer J. Clin.* **2015**, *65*, 221–238. [CrossRef]
5. Davis, C.; Emerson, J.S.; Husaini, B.A. Breast cancer screening among African American women: Adherence to current recom- mendations. *J. Health Care Poor Underserved* **2005**, *16*, 308–314. [CrossRef] [PubMed]
6. Centers for Disease Control Prevention and National Center for Health Statistics. Table 70 Use of mammography among women aged 40 and over, by selected characteristics: United States, selected years 1987–2015. In *Health, United States, 2016, with Chartbook on Long-Term Trends in Health*; US Department of Health and Human Services, Ed.; U.S. Government Printing Office: Atlanta, GA, USA, 2017; pp. 267–269. ISBN 9780160939778.

7. Office of Disease Prevention and Health Promotion Cancer—Healthy People 2020. Available online: https://www.healthypeople. gov/2020/topics-objectives/topic/cancer/objectives (accessed on 9 July 2021).
8. National Comprehensive Cancer Network. NCCN Guidelines for Breast Cancer Version 5. 2021. Available online: https://www.nccn.org/professionals/physician_gls/pdf/breast.pdf (accessed on 9 July 2021).
9. Monticciolo, D.L.; Newell, M.S.; Hendrick, R.E.; Helvie, M.A.; Moy, L.; Monsees, B.; Kopans, D.B.; Eby, P.R.; Sickles, E.A. Breast Cancer Screening for Average-Risk Women: Recommendations From the ACR Commission on Breast Imaging. *J. Am. Coll. Radiol.* **2017**, *14*, 1137–1143. [CrossRef]
10. Marmot, M.G.; Altman, D.G.; Cameron, D.A.; Dewar, J.A.; Thompson, S.G.; Wilcox, M. The benefits and harms of breast cancer screening: An independent review. *Br. J. Cancer* **2013**, *108*, 2205–2240. [CrossRef]
11. Anderson, J.G. Health services utilization: Framework and review. *Health Serv. Res.* **1973**, *8*, 184–199.
12. Andersen, R.M. Revisiting the behavioral model and access to medical care: Does it matter? *J. Health Soc. Behav.* **1995**, *36*, 1–10. [CrossRef]
13. Andersen, R.M.; Davidson, P.L.; Baumeister, S.E. Improving Access to Care. In *Changing the U.S. Health Care System: Key Issues in Health Services Policy and Management*, 4th ed.; Jossey-Bass: San Francisco, CA, USA, 2013; pp. 33–70. ISBN 9781118128916.
14. Lee, Y.-S.; Roh, S.; Moon, H.; Lee, K.H.; McKinley, C.; LaPlante, K. Andersen's Behavioral Model to Identify Correlates of Breast Cancer Screening Behaviors among Indigenous Women. *J. Evid. Based Soc. Work* **2020**, *17*, 117–135. [CrossRef]
15. Ogunsanya, M.E.; Jiang, S.; Thach, A.V.; Bamgbade, B.A.; Brown, C.M. Predictors of prostate cancer screening using Andersen's Behavioral Model of Health Services Use. *Urol. Oncol.* **2016**, *34*, 529.e9–529.e14. [CrossRef]
16. National Partnership for Women & Families. Black Women Experience Pervasive Disparities in Access to Health Insurance. Available online: https://www.nationalpartnership.org/our-work/resources/health-care/black-womens-health-insurance- coverage.pdf (accessed on 9 July 2021).
17. Semega, J.; Kollar, M.; Emily, A.S.; Creamer, J. Income and Poverty in the United States 2019: Report Number P60270. US Census Bur. 15SEP2020. Available online: https://www.census. gov/library/publications/2020/demo/p60-270.html (accessed on 9 July 2021).
18. Keisler-Starkey, K.; Bunch, L.N. *Health Insurance Coverage in the United States: 2019*; US Census Bur: Washington, DC, USA, 2020.
19. Orji, C.C.; Kanu, C.; Adelodun, A.I.; Brown, C.M. Factors that Influence Mammography Use for Breast Cancer Screening among African American Women. *J. Natl. Med. Assoc.* **2020**, *112*, 578–592. [CrossRef]
20. US Census Bureau PINC-01. Selected Characteristics of People 15 Years and Over, by Total Money Income, Work Experience, Race, Hispanic Origin, and Sex. Available online: https://www.census.gov/data/tables/time-series/demo/income-poverty/ cps-pinc/pinc-01. html#par_textimage_14 (accessed on 9 July 2021).
21. Bowie, J.V.; Wells, A.M.; Juon, H.-S.; Sydnor, K.D.; Rodriguez, E.M. How old are African American women when they receive their first mammogram? Results from a church-based study. *J. Community Health* **2008**, *33*, 183–191. [CrossRef] [PubMed]
22. Husaini, B.A.; Emerson, J.S.; Hull, P.C.; Sherkat, D.E.; Levine, R.S.; Cain, V.A. Rural-urban differences in breast cancer screening among African American women. *J. Health Care Poor Underserved* **2005**, *16*, 1–10. [CrossRef] [PubMed]
23. Pew Research Center Attendance at Religious Services by Race/Ethnicity. Available online: https://www.pewforum.org/ religious-landscape-study/compare/attendance-at-religious-services/by/racial-and-ethnic-composition/ (accessed on 9 July 2021).
24. Nguyen, A.W.; Taylor, R.J.; Chatters, L.M.; Hope, M.O. Church support networks of African Americans: The impact of gender and religious involvement. *J. Community Psychol.* **2019**, *47*, 1043–1063. [CrossRef] [PubMed]
25. Annamalai, A.; Singh, N.; O'Malley, S.S. Smoking Use and Cessation among People with Serious Mental Illness. *Yale J. Biol. Med.* **2015**, *88*, 271–277.
26. Mandelblatt, J.S.; Yabroff, K.R. Effectiveness of interventions designed to increase mammography use: A meta-analysis of provider-targeted strategies. *Cancer Epidemiol. Biomark.* **1999**, *8*, 759–767.
27. McNeill, L.H.; Reitzel, L.R.; Escoto, K.H.; Roberson, C.L.; Nguyen, N.; Vidrine, J.I.; Strong, L.L.; Wetter, D.W. Engaging Black Churches to Address Cancer Health Disparities: Project CHURCH. *Front. Public Health* **2018**, *6*, 191. [CrossRef]
28. US Department of Health and Human Services. *CAHPS 2.0 Survey and Reporting Kit*; US Department of Health and Human Services: Rockville, MD, USA, 1999.

29. Cohen, S.; Hoberman, H.M. Positive events and social supports as buffers of life change stress. *J. Appl. Soc. Psychol.* **1983**, *13*, 99–125. [CrossRef]
30. Cohen, S.; Kamarck, T.; Mermelstein, R. A global measure of perceived stress. *J. Health Soc. Behav.* **1983**, *24*, 385–396. [CrossRef]
31. Nelson, D.; Kreps, G.; Hesse, B.; Croyle, R.; Willis, G.; Arora, N.; Rimer, B.; Vish Viswanath, K.; Weinstein, N.; Alden, S. The health information national trends survey (HINTS): Development, design, and dissemination. *J. Health Commun.* **2004**, *9*, 443–460. [CrossRef]
32. SAS Institute. *SAS Software. Version 9.4. ODS Graphics Procedures Guide*, 3rd ed.; SAS Institute Inc.: Cary, NC, USA, 2014.
33. Table 33 Use of mammography among women aged 40 and over, by selected characteristics: United States, selected years 1987–2018. In *Vital Statistics of the United States 2018: Births, Life Expectancy, Deaths, and Selected Health Data*; Hattis, S.H. (Ed.) Bernan Press: Atlanta, GA, USA, 2018; pp. 286–287. ISBN 9781598889925.
34. Halbert, C.H.; Kessler, L.; Wileyto, E.P.; Weathers, B.; Stopfer, J.; Domchek, S.; Collier, A.; Brewster, K. Breast cancer screening behaviors among African American women with a strong family history of breast cancer. *Prev. Med.* **2006**, *43*, 385–388. [CrossRef] [PubMed]
35. Husaini, B.A.; Sherkat, D.E.; Bragg, R.; Levine, R.; Emerson, J.S.; Mentes, C.M.; Cain, V.A. Predictors of Breast Cancer Screening in a Panel Study of African American Women. *Women Health* **2001**, *34*, 35–51. [CrossRef]
36. Siu, A.L. Screening for Breast Cancer: U.S. Preventive Services Task Force Recommendation Statement. *Ann. Intern. Med.* **2016**, *164*, 279–296. [CrossRef]
37. Danigelis, N.L.; Worden, J.K.; Mickey, R.M. The importance of age as a context for understanding African-American women's mammography screening behavior. *Am. J. Prev. Med.* **1996**, *12*, 358–366. [CrossRef]
38. Chowdhury, R.; David, N.; Bogale, A.; Nandy, S.; Habtemariam, T.; Tameru, B. Assessing the Key Attributes of Low Utilization of Mammography Screening and Breast-self Exam among African-American Women. *J. Cancer* **2016**, *7*, 532–537. [CrossRef] [PubMed]
39. Klassen, A.C.; Smith, K.C.; Shariff-Marco, S.; Juon, H.-S. A healthy mistrust: How worldview relates to attitudes about breast cancer screening in a cross-sectional survey of low-income women. *Int. J. Equity Health* **2008**, *7*, 5. [CrossRef] [PubMed]
40. Mishra, S.I.; DeForge, B.; Barnet, B.; Ntiri, S.; Grant, L. Social determinants of breast cancer screening in urban primary care practices: A community-engaged formative study. *Women's Health Issues* **2012**, *22*, e429–e438. [CrossRef] [PubMed]
41. Patel, K.; Kanu, M.; Liu, J.; Bond, B.; Brown, E.; Williams, E.; Theriot, R.; Bailey, S.; Sanderson, M.; Hargreaves, M. Factors influencing breast cancer screening in low-income African Americans in Tennessee. *J. Community Health* **2014**, *39*, 943–950. [CrossRef]
42. Howard, D.H.; Ekwueme, D.U.; Gardner, J.G.; Tangka, F.K.; Li, C.; Miller, J.W. The impact of a national program to provide free mammograms to low-income, uninsured women on breast cancer mortality rates. *Cancer* **2010**, *116*, 4456–4462. [CrossRef] [PubMed]
43. Wagner, M.; Anderson, K.H.; Broxton, L. Assessment of Barriers to Screening Mammograms for Rural, Poor, Uninsured Women and a Community Plan of Action. *J. Community Health Nurs.* **2016**, *33*, 42–53. [CrossRef]
44. Stanley, E.; Lewis, M.C.; Irshad, A.; Ackerman, S.; Collins, H.; Pavic, D.; Leddy, R.J. Effectiveness of a Mobile Mammography Program. *AJR Am. J. Roentgenol.* **2017**, *209*, 1426–1429. [CrossRef] [PubMed]
45. Lende, D.H.; Lachiondo, A. Embodiment and breast cancer among African American women. *Qual. Health Res.* **2009**, *19*, 216–228. [CrossRef]
46. Fox, S.A.; Heritage, J.; Stockdale, S.E.; Asch, S.M.; Duan, N.; Reise, S.P. Cancer screening adherence: Does physician-patient communication matter? *Patient Educ. Couns.* **2009**, *75*, 178–184. [CrossRef]
47. Meguerditchian, A.-N.; Dauphinee, D.; Girard, N.; Eguale, T.; Riedel, K.; Jacques, A.; Meterissian, S.; Buckeridge, D.L.; Abra- hamowicz, M.; Tamblyn, R. Do physician communication skills influence screening mammography utilization? *BMC Health Serv. Res.* **2012**, *12*, 219. [CrossRef]
48. Sadler, G.R.; Ko, C.M.; Cohn, J.A.; White, M.; Weldon, R.; Wu, P. Breast cancer knowledge, attitudes, and screening behaviors among African American women: The Black cosmetologists promoting health program. *BMC Public Health* **2007**, *7*, 57. [CrossRef] [PubMed]
49. Greene, A.L.; Torio, C.M.; Klassen, A.C. Measuring sustained mammography use by urban African-American women. *J. Community Health* **2005**, *30*, 235–251. [CrossRef]
50. Curtis, R.E.; Hoover, R.N.; Kleinerman, R.A.; Harvey, E.B. Second cancer following cancer of the female genital system in Connecticut, 1935–1982. *Natl. Cancer Inst. Monogr.* **1985**, *68*, 113–137. [PubMed]

51. Powell, M.E.; Carter, V.; Bonsi, E.; Johnson, G.; Williams, L.; Taylor-Smith, L.; Hayes, Q.; Hull, P.C.; Cain, V.A.; Husaini, B.A. Increasing mammography screening among African American women in rural areas. *J. Health Care Poor Underserved* **2005**, *16*, 11–21. [CrossRef] [PubMed]
52. Darnell, J.S.; Chang, C.-H.; Calhoun, E.A. Knowledge about breast cancer and participation in a faith-based breast cancer program and other predictors of mammography screening among African American women and Latinas. *Health Promot. Pract.* **2006**, *7*, 201S–212S. [CrossRef]
53. Wynia, M.K.; Osborn, C.Y. Health literacy and communication quality in health care organizations. *J. Health Commun.* **2010**, *15* (Suppl. 2), 102–115. [CrossRef] [PubMed]

Permissions

All chapters in this book were first published by MDPI; hereby published with permission under the Creative Commons Attribution License or equivalent. Every chapter published in this book has been scrutinized by our experts. Their significance has been extensively debated. The topics covered herein carry significant findings which will fuel the growth of the discipline. They may even be implemented as practical applications or may be referred to as a beginning point for another development.

The contributors of this book come from diverse backgrounds, making this book a truly international effort. This book will bring forth new frontiers with its revolutionizing research information and detailed analysis of the nascent developments around the world.

We would like to thank all the contributing authors for lending their expertise to make the book truly unique.

They have played a crucial role in the development of this book. Without their invaluable contributions this book wouldn't have been possible. They have made vital efforts to compile up to date information on the varied aspects of this subject to make this book a valuable addition to the collection of many professionals and students.

This book was conceptualized with the vision of imparting up-to-date information and advanced data in this field. To ensure the same, a matchless editorial board was set up. Every individual on the board went through rigorous rounds of assessment to prove their worth. After which they invested a large part of their time researching and compiling the most relevant data for our readers.

The editorial board has been involved in producing this book since its inception. They have spent rigorous hours researching and exploring the diverse topics which have resulted in the successful publishing of this book. They have passed on their knowledge of decades through this book. To expedite this challenging task, the publisher supported the team at every step. A small team of assistant editors was also appointed to further simplify the editing procedure and attain best results for the readers.

Apart from the editorial board, the designing team has also invested a significant amount of their time in understanding the subject and creating the most relevant covers. They scrutinized every image to scout for the most suitable representation of the subject and create an appropriate cover for the book.

The publishing team has been an ardent support to the editorial, designing and production team. Their endless efforts to recruit the best for this project, has resulted in the accomplishment of this book. They are a veteran in the field of academics and their pool of knowledge is as vast as their experience in printing. Their expertise and guidance has proved useful at every step. Their uncompromising quality standards have made this book an exceptional effort. Their encouragement from time to time has been an inspiration for everyone.

The publisher and the editorial board hope that this book will prove to be a valuable piece of knowledge for researchers, students, practitioners and scholars across the globe.

List of Contributors

Brendah K. Masisi, Rokaya El Ansari, Lutfi Alfarsi, Madeleine L. Craze, Natasha Jewa, Andrew Oldfield, Hayley Cheung, Michael Toss and Andrew R. Green
Nottingham Breast Cancer Research Centre, Academic Unit for Translational Medical Sciences, School of Medicine, University of Nottingham Biodiscovery Institute, University Park, Nottingham NG7 2RD, UK

Emad A. Rakha
Nottingham Breast Cancer Research Centre, Academic Unit for Translational Medical Sciences, School of Medicine, University of Nottingham Biodiscovery Institute, University Park, Nottingham NG7 2RD, UK
Cellular Pathology, Nottingham University Hospitals NHS Trust, Hucknall Road, Nottingham NG5 1PB, UK

Soong June Bae, Sung Gwe Ahn, Jung Hwan Ji, Chihhao Chu and Joon Jeong
Department of Surgery, Gangnam Severance Hospital, Yonsei University College of Medicine
Institute for Breast Cancer Precision Medicine, Yonsei University College of Medicine, 237 Dogok-ro, Gangnam-gu, Seoul 06230, Korea

Dooreh Kim
Department of Surgery, Seoul St. Mary's Hospital, College of Medicine, The Catholic University of Seoul

Janghee Lee
Department of Surgery, Sacred Heart Hospital, Hallym University, Hwaseong 18450, Korea

Yoon Jin Cha
Institute for Breast Cancer Precision Medicine, Yonsei University College of Medicine, 237 Dogok-ro, Gangnam-gu, Seoul 06230, Korea
Department of Pathology, Gangnam Severance Hospital, Yonsei University College of Medicine, 211 Eonju-ro, Gangnam-gu, Seoul 06273, Korea

Hava Gil-Henn and Jonathan Solomon
Cell Migration and Invasion Laboratory, The Azrieli Faculty of Medicine, Bar-Ilan University, Safed 1311502, Israel

Abraham O. Samson
Drug Discovery Laboratory, The Azrieli Faculty of Medicine, Bar-Ilan University, Safed 1311502, Israel

Trishna Saha
Cell Migration and Invasion Laboratory, The Azrieli Faculty of Medicine, Bar-Ilan University, Safed 1311502, Israel
Drug Discovery Laboratory, The Azrieli Faculty of Medicine, Bar-Ilan University, Safed 1311502, Israel

Ivica Ratosa and Gaber Plavc
Department of Radiation Oncology, Institute of Oncology Ljubljana, 1000 Ljubljana, Slovenia
Faculty of Medicine, University of Ljubljana, 1000 Ljubljana, Slovenia

Nina Pislar
Department of Surgery, Institute of Oncology Ljubljana, 1000 Ljubljana, Slovenia

Tina Zagar
Department of Epidemiology and Cancer Registry, Institute of Oncology Ljubljana, 1000 Ljubljana, Slovenia

Andraz Perhavec
Faculty of Medicine, University of Ljubljana, 1000 Ljubljana, Slovenia
Department of Surgery, Institute of Oncology Ljubljana, 1000 Ljubljana, Slovenia

Pierfrancesco Franco
Department of Translational Medicine, University of Eastern Piedmont, 28100 Novara, Italy
Radiation Oncology Unit, AOU "Maggiore della Carità", 28100 Novara, Italy

Antoine Goisnard, Pierre Daumar, Emmanuelle Mounetou and Mahchid Bamdad
Institut Universitaire de Technologie, Université Clermont Auvergne, UMR INSERM-UCA, U1240, Imagerie Moléculaire et Stratégies Théranostiques, 63000 Clermont Ferrand, France

Manon Roux and Marie Depresle
BIOMARQUEURS Company, 5 Avenue Blaise Pascal, 63178 Aubière, France

Clémence Dubois
Institut Universitaire de Technologie, Université Clermont Auvergne, UMR INSERM-UCA, U1240, Imagerie Moléculaire et Stratégies Théranostiques, 63000 Clermont Ferrand, France
BIOMARQUEURS Company, 5 Avenue Blaise Pascal, 63178 Aubière, France

Corinne Aubel
Faculté de Médecine, Université Clermont Auvergne, UMR INSERM-UCA, U1240, Imagerie Moléculaire et Stratégies Théranostiques, 63000 Clermont Ferrand, France

Jean Gauthier and Bernard Vidalinc
BIOMARQUEURS Company, 5 Avenue Blaise Pascal, 63178 Aubière, France
BIOPASS Company, 5 Avenue Blaise Pascal, 63178 Aubière, France

Frédérique Penault-Llorca
Centre de Lutte Contre le Cancer Jean Perrin, Université Clermont Auvergne, UMR INSERM-UCA, U1240, Imagerie Moléculaire et Stratégies Théranostiques, 63000 Clermont Ferrand, France

Sarra Bouaouiche, Silvia Ghione, Randa Sghaier, Cindy Racoeur, Ali Bettaieb and Stéphanie Plenchette
Laboratoire d'Immunologie et Immunothérapie des Cancers (LIIC), EPHE, PSL Research University, 75000 Paris, France
Laboratoire d'Immunologie et Immunothérapie des Cancers (LIIC), EA7269, Université de Bourgogne Franche-Comté, 21000 Dijon, France

Olivier Burgy
INSERM U1231, UFR Sciences de Santé, Université de Bourgogne-Franche Comté, 21000 Dijon, France

Valentin Derangère
Plateforme de Transfert en Biologie du Cancer, Centre Georges-François Leclerc, 21000 Dijon, France

Michaël Pérès and Caroline Imbert
Centre de Recherches en Cancérologie de Toulouse, INSERM UMR1037, CNRS UMR5071, 2 Avenue Hubert Curien, CEDEX 1, 31047 Toulouse, France

Stéphanie Delmas and Maud Chusseau
SeleXel, 1 Place Pierre Potier, BP 50624, CEDEX 1, 31106 Toulouse, France

Elie Marcheteau and Florence Cabon
Centre de Recherches en Cancérologie de Toulouse, INSERM UMR1037, CNRS UMR5071, 2 Avenue Hubert Curien, CEDEX 1, 31047 Toulouse, France
SeleXel, 1 Place Pierre Potier, BP 50624, CEDEX 1, 31106 Toulouse, France
Université Toulouse III—Paul Sabatier, 118 Rte de Narbonne, 31062 Toulouse, France

Thomas Farge, Guillaume Labrousse, Julie Tenet, Justine Noujarède, Céline Colacios and Hervé Prats
Centre de Recherches en Cancérologie de Toulouse, INSERM UMR1037, CNRS UMR5071, 2 Avenue Hubert Curien, CEDEX 1, 31047 Toulouse, France
Université Toulouse III—Paul Sabatier, 118 Rte de Narbonne, 31062 Toulouse, France

Raphaëlle Duprez-Paumier, Camille Franchet and Florence Dalenc
Institut Claudius Regaud, Institut Universitaire du Cancer de Toulouse-Oncopole, 1 Av. Irène Joliot-Curie, 31100 Toulouse, France

Bruno Ségui
Centre de Recherches en Cancérologie de Toulouse, INSERM UMR1037, CNRS UMR5071, 2 Avenue Hubert Curien, CEDEX 1, 31047 Toulouse, France
Université Toulouse III—Paul Sabatier, 118 Rte de Narbonne, 31062 Toulouse, France
Equipe Labellisée par la Fondation ARC—Association Pour la Recherche sur le Cancer, 94803 Villejuif, France

Ana Salomé Correia
OncoPharma Research Group, Center for Health Technology and Services Research (CINTESIS), Rua Dr. Plácido da Costa, 4200-450 Porto, Portugal
Department of Molecular Pathology and Immunology, Institute of Biomedical Sciences Abel Salazar (ICBAS), University of Porto, Rua de Jorge Viterbo Ferreira 228, 4050-313 Porto, Portugal

Rita Matos and Irina Amorim
Department of Molecular Pathology and Immunology, Institute of Biomedical Sciences Abel Salazar (ICBAS), University of Porto, Rua de Jorge Viterbo Ferreira 228, 4050-313 Porto, Portugal
Institute of Molecular Pathology and Immunology of the University of Porto (IPATIMUP), Rua Júlio Amaral de Carvalho 45, 4200-135 Porto, Portugal
i3S, Instituto de Investigação e Inovação em Saúde da Universidade do Porto, Rua Alfredo Allen 208, 4200-135 Porto, Portugal

Nuno Vale
OncoPharma Research Group, Center for Health Technology and Services Research (CINTESIS), Rua Dr. Plácido da Costa, 4200-450 Porto, Portugal
Department of Community Medicine, Health Information and Decision (MEDCIDS), Faculty of Medicine, University of Porto, Al. Prof. Hernâni Monteiro, 4200-319 Porto, Portugal

Beata Smolarz and Hanna Romanowicz
Laboratory of Cancer Genetics, Department of Pathology, Polish Mother's Memorial Hospital Research Institute, Rzgowska 281/289, 93-338 Lodz, Poland

Anna Zadro˙zna-Nowak
Department of Chemotherapy, Copernicus Memorial Hospital, Medical University of Lodz, 93-513 Lodz, Poland

Gabriela Silva, Carolina Matos, Khrystyna Kucheryava and Ana Barbas
iBET, Instituto de Biologia Experimental e Tecnológica, Apartado 12, 2781-901 Oeiras, Portugal

Joana Sales-Dias, Giacomo Domenici, Ana R. Lemos, Maria Raquel Moita, Catarina Brito, Pedro M. F. Sousa and Tiago M. Bandeiras
Instituto de Tecnologia Química e Biológica António Xavier, Universidade Nova de Lisboa, Av. da República, 2780-157 Oeiras, Portugal

Diogo Casal
Departamento de Anatomia, NOVA Medical School (NMS), Universidade NOVA de Lisboa, 1150-082 Lisbon, Portugal
iNOVA4Health, CEDOC, NOVA Medical School (NMS), Universidade NOVA de Lisboa, 1150-082 Lisbon, Portugal

Sara Alves
Departamento de Anatomia, NOVA Medical School (NMS), Universidade NOVA de Lisboa, 1150-082 Lisbon, Portugal
Serviço de Anatomia Patológica, Centro Hospitalar de Lisboa Central-Hospital de São José, 1150-199 Lisbon, Portugal

Clara Barreto
iBET, Instituto de Biologia Experimental e Tecnológica, Apartado 12, 2781-901 Oeiras, Portugal
Unidade de Mama, Instituto CUF de Oncologia, 1998-018 Lisbon, Portugal

Ana T. Matias, Andreia Ferreira, M. Guadalupe Cabral, Cristina Casalou and Duarte C. Barral
iNOVA4Health, CEDOC, NOVA Medical School (NMS), Universidade NOVA de Lisboa, 1150-082 Lisbon, Portugal

Sofia Braga
iNOVA4Health, CEDOC, NOVA Medical School (NMS), Universidade NOVA de Lisboa, 1150-082 Lisbon, Portugal
Unidade de Mama, Instituto CUF de Oncologia, 1998-018 Lisbon, Portugal

Paula A. Videira
UCIBIO, Departamento Ciências da Vida, Faculdade de Ciências e Tecnologia, Universidade NOVA de Lisboa, 2829-516 Caparica, Portugal

Chi-Chang Yu and Shin-Cheh Chen
Department of General Surgery, Chang Gung Memorial Hospital at Linkou, Chang Gung University, Taoyuan 333, Taiwan

Yun-Chung Cheung
Department of Diagnostic Radiology, Chang Gung Memorial Hospital at Linkou, Chang Gung University, Taoyuan 333, Taiwan

Chuen Hsueh
Department of Pathology, Chang Gung Memorial Hospital at Linkou, Chang Gung University, Taoyuan 333, Taiwan

Kamil Grubczak, Anna Kretowska-Grunwald, Dawid Groth, Andrzej Eljaszewicz, Aleksandra Starosz and Jordan M. Holl
Department of Regenerative Medicine and Immune Regulation, Medical University of Bialystok, Jerzego Waszyngtona 13, 15-269 Bialystok, Poland

Izabela Poplawska
Department of Medical Pathomorphology, Medical University of Bialystok, Jerzego Waszyngtona 13, 15-269 Bialystok, Poland

Lukasz Bolkun
Department of Haematology, Medical University of Bialystok, M. Sklodowskiej-Curie 24A, 15-276 Bialystok, Poland

Marta Mysliwiec, Joanna Kruszewska and Marek Z. Wojtukiewicz
Department of Oncology, Medical University of Bialystok, Ogrodowa 12, 15-027 Bialystok, Poland

Marcin Moniuszko
Department of Regenerative Medicine and Immune Regulation, Medical University of Bialystok, Jerzego Waszyngtona 13, 15-269 Bialystok, Poland
Department of Allergology and Internal Medicine, Medical University of Bialystok, M. Sklodowskiej-Curie 24A, 15-276 Bialystok, Poland

Wen-Ling Kuo
Division of Breast Surgery, General Surgery, Department of Surgery, Chang Gung Memorial Hospital Linkou Medical Center, Taoyuan City 33305, Taiwan

Lin-Lu Tseng, Hsin-Hung Cheng, Meng-Jen Wu, Yu-Lun Chen and Wen-Ching Wang
Institute of Molecular and Cellular Biology and Department of Life Sciences, National Tsing-Hua University, Hsinchu City 30013, Taiwan

Che-Chang Chang and Ruei-Ting Chang
The Ph.D. Program for Translational Medicine, College of Medical Science and Technology, Taipei Medical University, Taipei City 11031, Taiwan

Chih-Jung Chen and Yong-Chen Hsu
Department of Pathology and Laboratory Medicine, Taichung Veterans General Hospital, Taichung City 40705, Taiwan
School of Medicine, Chung Shan Medical University, Taichung City 40201, Taiwan

Mei-Ling Cheng
Department of Biomedical Sciences, College of Medicine, Chang Gung University, Taoyuan City 33302, Taiwan
Metabolomics Core Laboratory, Healthy Aging Research Center, Chang Gung University, Taoyuan City 33302, Taiwan

Hsiang-Yu Tang
Metabolomics Core Laboratory, Healthy Aging Research Center, Chang Gung University, Taoyuan City 33302, Taiwan

Wen-Jye Lin and Cheng-Yuan Kao
Immunology Research Center, National Health Research Institutes, Miaoli County 35053, Taiwan

Wen-Ping Hsieh
Institute of Statistics, National Tsing Hua University, Hsinchu City 30013, Taiwan

Hsing-Jien Kung
Graduate Institute of Cancer Biology and Drug Discovery, Taipei Medical University, Taipei City 11031, Taiwan
Department of Biochemistry and Molecular Medicine, University of California Davis School of Medicine, University of California Davis Cancer Centre, Sacramento, CA 95817, USA

Hjalte Rasmus Oltmann, Tural Asgharzadeh Alamdari, Jakob Lykke Bülow and Lasse Ljungstrøm
Department of Clinical Research, University of Southern Denmark, 5000 Odense, Denmark

Poul-Erik Braad and Oke Gerke
Department of Clinical Research, University of Southern Denmark, 5000 Odense, Denmark
Department of Nuclear Medicine, Odense University Hospital, 5000 Odense, Denmark

Mohammad Naghavi-Behzad
Department of Clinical Research, University of Southern Denmark, 5000 Odense, Denmark
Department of Nuclear Medicine, Odense University Hospital, 5000 Odense, Denmark
Open Patient Data Explorative Network (OPEN), Odense University Hospital, 5000 Odense, Denmark
Centre for Personalized Response Monitoring in Oncology, Odense University Hospital, 5000 Odense, Denmark

Jon Thor Asmussen
Department of Radiology, Odense University Hospital, 5000 Odense, Denmark

Marianne Vogsen
Department of Clinical Research, University of Southern Denmark, 5000 Odense, Denmark
Department of Nuclear Medicine, Odense University Hospital, 5000 Odense, Denmark
Open Patient Data Explorative Network (OPEN), Odense University Hospital, 5000 Odense, Denmark
Centre for Personalized Response Monitoring in Oncology, Odense University Hospital, 5000 Odense, Denmark
Department of Oncology, Odense University Hospital, 5000 Odense, Denmark

Annette Raskov Kodahl
Department of Clinical Research, University of Southern Denmark, 5000 Odense, Denmark
Centre for Personalized Response Monitoring in Oncology, Odense University Hospital, 5000 Odense, Denmark
Department of Oncology, Odense University Hospital, 5000 Odense, Denmark

Malene Grubbe Hildebrandt
Department of Clinical Research, University of Southern Denmark, 5000 Odense, Denmark
Department of Nuclear Medicine, Odense University Hospital, 5000 Odense, Denmark
Open Patient Data Explorative Network (OPEN), Odense University Hospital, 5000 Odense, Denmark
Centre for Personalized Response Monitoring in Oncology, Odense University Hospital, 5000 Odense, Denmark
Centre for Innovative Medical Technology, Odense University Hospital, 5000 Odense, Denmark

Pooja Agrawal
Department of Psychological, Health and Learning Sciences, University of Houston, Houston, TX 77204, USA
School of Medicine, University of Texas Medical Branch, Galveston, TX 77555, USA

Tzuan A. Chen
Department of Psychological, Health and Learning Sciences, University of Houston, Houston, TX 77204, USA
Health Research Institute, University of Houston, Houston, TX 77204, USA

Lorna H. McNeill
MD Anderson Cancer Center, Department of Health Disparities Research, Houston, TX 77230, USA

Chiara Acquati
MD Anderson Cancer Center, Department of Health Disparities Research, Houston, TX 77230, USA
Graduate College of Social Work, University of Houston, Houston, TX 77204, USA

Shahnjayla K. Connors
Department of Psychological, Health and Learning Sciences, University of Houston, Houston, TX 77204, USA
Department of Social Sciences, University of Houston-Downtown, Houston, TX 77002, USA

Vijay Nitturi, Isabel Martinez Leal and Lorraine R. Reitzel
Department of Psychological, Health and Learning Sciences, University of Houston, Houston, TX 77204, USA
Health Research Institute, University of Houston, Houston, TX 77204, USA

Angelica S. Robinson
Department of Radiology, University of Texas Medical Branch, Galveston, TX 77555, USA

Index